Torsten Engelt
Dr. Claus Köhn
Dr. Samantha B
Dr. Stefano Sco

VIRUS MANIA

**Corona/COVID-19, Measles,
Swine Flu, Avian Flu, Cervical
Cancer, SARS, BSE, Hepatitis C,
AIDS, Polio, Spanish Flu**

How the Medical Industry Continually
Invents Epidemics, Making Billion-
Dollar Profits at Our Expense

3rd English Edition, 2021

Original German Title: Virus-Wahn
Published by Books on Demand

First published in 2007 by Trafford Publishing

© Torsten Engelbrecht, Claus Köhnlein, Samantha Bailey
Translation: Samantha Bailey, Carina Hahn, Megan Chapelas, Danielle Egan
Editing: Torsten Engelbrecht, Samantha Bailey, Carina Hahn, Danielle Egan, David Crowe
Printing, production and layout: BoD – Books on Demand, Norderstedt, Germany
Cover: Heike Müller, Robin Hahn
Photos (cover): Gürsoy Dogtas

ISBN: 978-3-7526-2978-1

For Mark, Weston and Augie
(Samantha Bailey)

For Alexa, Gabriel and Tasha
(Stefano Scoglio)

For Christiane, Theresa, Johanna, Catharina and Julius
(Claus Köhnlein)

For Anela, Liam, Maria, Karen, Eckart and Labolina—
and for all those who are committed to an
equitable and loving coexistence on this planet
(Torsten Engelbrecht)

„Ultimate Scepticism. — But what after all are man's truths?
—They are his *irrefutable* errors."

Friedrich Nietzsche
„The Joyous Science," aphorism 265

Contents

Chapter 12 Total Corona Mania: Worthless PCR Tests, Lethal Drugs—and Mortality Data that Makes a Viral Cause Impossible 367

Epilog Rock Hudson Gave „AIDS" a Face—and His Fallacious Story the Virus Hunters Godlike Status 449

Literature 459

About the Book

If one follows public pronouncements, the world is repeatedly afflicted with new terrible virus diseases. As the latest horror variant, the so-called coronavirus SARS-CoV-2 dominated the headlines. The population is also terrified by reports of measles, swine flu, SARS, BSE, AIDS or polio. However, this virus mayhem ignores very basic scientific facts: the existence, the pathogenicity and the deadly effects of these agents have never been proven. The medical establishment and its loyal media acolytes claim that this evidence has been produced. But these claims are highly suspect because modern medicine has pushed direct virus proof methods aside and uses dubious indirect tools to "prove" the existence of viruses such as antibody tests and the polymerase chain reaction (PCR).

The authors of *Virus Mania*, journalist Torsten Engelbrecht and doctor of internal medicine Claus Köhnlein, MD, the general practitioner and research physician Samantha Bailey, MD, and the expert in microbiology Stefano Scoglio, BSc PhD, show that these alleged contagious viruses may be, in fact, alternatively be seen as particles produced by the cells themselves as a consequence of certain stress factors such as drugs and toxins. These particles are then identified by antibody and PCR tests and (wrongly) interpreted as epidemic-causing viruses by doctors who have been indoctrinated for over 100 years by the theory that microbes are deadly and only modern medications and vaccines will protect us from virus pandemics.

The central aim of this book is to steer the discussion back to a real scientific debate and put medicine back on the path of an impartial analysis of the facts. It will put medical experiments, clinical trials, statistics and government policies under the microscope, revealing that the people charged with protecting our health and safety have deviated from this path.

Along the way, Engelbrecht, Köhnlein, Bailey and Scoglio will analyze all possible causes of illness such as pharmaceuticals, lifestyle drugs, pesticides, heavy metals, pollution, stress and processed (and sometimes genetically modified) foods. All of these can heavily damage the body of humans and animals and even kill them. And these factors are precisely the ones that typically prevail where the victims of alleged viruses live and work. To substantiate these claims, the authors cite dozens of highly

11

renowned scientists, among them the Nobel laureates Kary Mullis, Barbara McClintock, Walter Gilbert, Sir Frank Macfarlane Burnet and microbiologist and Pulitzer Prize winner René Dubos. The book presents approximately 1,100 pertinent scientific references, the majority of which have been published recently.

The topic of this book is of pivotal significance. The pharmaceutical companies and top scientists rake in enormous sums of money by attacking germs and the media boosts its audience ratings and circulations with sensationalized reporting (the coverage of the *New York Times* and *Der Spiegel* are specifically analyzed). Individuals pay the highest price of all, without getting what they deserve and need most to maintain health: enlightenment about the real causes and true necessities for prevention and cure of their illnesses. "The first step is to give up the illusion that the primary purpose of modern medical research is to improve people's health most effectively and efficiently," advises John Abramson of Harvard Medical School. "The primary purpose of commercially-funded clinical research is to maximize financial return on investment, not health."

Virus Mania will inform you on how such an environment took root—and how to empower yourself for a healthy life.

About the Authors

Torsten Engelbrecht works as investigative journalist in Hamburg. In 2009, he received the Alternative Media Award for his article "The Amalgam Controversy." He was trained at the renowned magazine for professional journalists *Message* and was a permanent editor at the *Financial Times Deutschland*, among others. He has written for publications such as *Off-Guardian*, *Süddeutsche Zeitung*, *Neue Zürcher Zeitung*, *Rubikon*, *Greenpeace Magazin* and *The Ecologist*. In 2010 his book "Die Zukunft der Krebsmedizin" (The Future of Cancer Medicine) has been published, with 3 doctors as co-authors. See www.torstenengelbrecht.com.

Dr. Claus Köhnlein, MD, is a medical specialist of internal diseases. He completed his residency in the Oncology Department at the University of Kiel. Since 1993, he has worked in his own medical practice, treating also Hepatitis C and AIDS patients who are skeptical of antiviral medications. Köhnlein is one of the world's most experienced experts when it comes to alleged viral epidemics. In April 2020, he was mentioned in the *OffGuardian* article "8 MORE Experts Questionig the Coronavirus Panic." A *Russia Today* interview with him, published on Youtube in September 2020, on the topic "fatal COVID-19 overtherapy" achieved almost 1.4 million views within a short time.

Dr. Samantha Bailey, MD, is a research physician in New Zealand. She completed her Bachelor of Medicine and Bachelor of Surgery degree at Otago University in 2005. She has worked in general practice, telehealth and in clinical trials for over 12 years with a particular interest in novel tests and treatments for medical diseases. She has the largest YouTube health channel in New Zealand, and creates educational health videos based on questions from her audience. Bailey has also been a co-presenter for a nationwide television health show in New Zealand that debunks common health misconceptions, called *The Checkup.*

Dr. Stefano Scoglio, BSc Phd, is an expert in microbiology and naturopathy. Since 2004, he has been working as a scientific researcher, publishing many articles in international scientific journals and coordinating scientific and clinical research on Klamath algae extracts, and on microalgae-based probiotics, in cooperation with the Italian National Research Center and various Universities. He is the inventor of 7 medical patents. For his important scientific publications, in 2018, Scoglio was nominated for the Nobel Prize in Medicine.

Foreword I
by Prof. Dr. Etienne de Harven, MD

This Book Has To Be Read, Quickly and Worldwide

The book *Virus Mania* by Torsten Engelbrecht and Claus Köhnlein presents a tragic message that will, hopefully, contribute to the re-insertion of ethical values in the conduct of virus research, public health policies, media communications, and activities of the pharmaceutical companies. Obviously, elementary ethical rules have been, to a very dangerous extent, neglected in many of these fields for an alarming number of years.

When American journalist Celia Farber courageously published, in *Harper's Magazine* (March 2006) the article "Out of control—AIDS and the corruption of medical science," some readers probably attempted to reassure themselves that this "corruption" was an isolated case. This is very far from the truth as documented so well in this book by Engelbrecht and Köhnlein. It is only the tip of the iceberg. Corruption of research is a widespread phenomenon currently found in many major, supposedly contagious health problems, ranging from AIDS to Hepatitis C, Bovine spongiform encephalopathy (BSE or "mad cow disease"), SARS, Avian flu and current vaccination practices (human papillomavirus or HPV vaccination).

In research on all of these six distinct public health concerns scientific research on viruses (or prions in the case of BSE) slipped onto the wrong track following basically the same systematic pathway. This pathway always includes several key steps: inventing the risk of a disastrous epidemic, incriminating an elusive pathogen, ignoring alternative toxic causes, manipulating epidemiology with non-verifiable numbers to maximize the false perception of an imminent catastrophe, and promising salvation with vaccines. This guarantees large financial returns. But how is it possible to achieve all of this? Simply by relying on the most powerful activator of human decision making process, i.e. FEAR!

We are not witnessing viral epidemics; we are witnessing epidemics of fear. And both the media and the pharmaceutical industry carry most of the responsibility for amplifying fears, fears that happen, incidentally, to always ignite fantastically profitable business.

14

Research hypotheses covering these areas of virus research are practically never scientifically verified with appropriate controls. Instead, they are established by "consensus." This is then rapidly reshaped into a dogma, efficiently perpetuated in a quasi-religious manner by the media, including ensuring that research funding is restricted to projects supporting the dogma, excluding research into alternative hypotheses. An important tool to keep dissenting voices out of the debate is censorship at various levels ranging from the popular media to scientific publications.

We haven't learnt well from past experiences. There are still many unanswered questions on the causes of the 1918 Spanish flu epidemic, and on the role of viruses in post-WWII polio (DDT neurotoxicity?). These modern epidemics should have opened our minds to more critical analyses. Pasteur and Koch had solidly constructed an understanding of infection applicable to many bacterial, contagious diseases. But this was before the first viruses were actually discovered. Transposing the principles of bacterial infections to viruses was, of course, very tempting but should not have been done without giving parallel attention to the innumerable risk factors in our toxic environment; to the toxicity of many drugs, and to some nutritional deficiencies.

Cancer research had similar problems. The hypothesis that cancer might be caused by viruses was formulated in 1903, more than one century ago. Even today it has never been convincingly demonstrated. Most of the experimental laboratory studies by virus-hunters have been based on the use of inbred mice, inbred implying a totally unnatural genetic background. Were these mice appropriate models for the study of human cancer? (we are far from being inbred!) True, these mice made possible the isolation and purification of "RNA tumor viruses," later renamed "retroviruses" and well characterized by electron microscopy. But are these viral particles simply associated with the murine tumors, or are they truly the culprit of malignant transformation? Are these particles real exogenous infective particles, or endogenous defective viruses hidden in our chromosomes? The question is still debatable. What is certain is that viral particles similar to those readily recognized in cancerous and leukemic mice have never been seen nor isolated in human cancers. Of mice and men.

However, by the time this became clear, in the late 1960s, viral oncology had achieved a dogmatic, quasi-religious status. If viral particles cannot be seen by electron microscopy in human cancers, the problem was with electron microscopy, not with the dogma of viral oncology! This was the time molecular biology was taking a totally dominant posture in viral research. "Molecular markers" for retroviruses were therefore invented (reverse transcriptase for example) and substituted most conveniently for the absent viral particles, hopefully salvaging the central dogma of viral oncology. This permitted the viral hypothesis to survive for another ten years, until the late 1970s, with the help of increasingly generous support from funding agencies and from pharmaceutical companies. However by 1980 the failure of this line of research was becoming embarrassingly evident, and the closing of some viral oncology laboratories would have been inevitable, except that ...

Except what? Virus cancer research would have crashed to a halt except that, in 1981, five cases of severe immune deficiencies were described by a Los Angeles physician, all among homosexual men who were also all sniffing amyl nitrite, were all abusing other drugs, abusing antibiotics, and probably suffering from malnutrition and STDs (sexually transmitted diseases). It would have been logical to hypothesize that these severe cases of immune deficiency had multiple toxic origins. This would have amounted to incrimination of these patients' life-style.

Unfortunately, such discrimination was, politically, totally unacceptable. Therefore, another hypothesis had to be found—these patients were suffering from a contagious disease caused by a new ... retrovirus! Scientific data in support of this hypothesis was and, amazingly enough, still is totally missing. That did not matter, and instantaneous and passionate interest of cancer virus researchers and institutions erupted immediately. This was salvation for the viral laboratories where AIDS now became, almost overnight, the main focus of research. It generated huge financial support from Big Pharma, more budget for the CDC and NIH, and nobody had to worry about the life style of the patients who became at once the innocent victims of this horrible virus, soon labeled as HIV.

Twenty-five years later, the HIV/AIDS hypothesis has totally failed to achieve three major goals in spite of the huge research funding exclusively directed to projects based on it. No AIDS cure has ever been found; no verifiable epidemiological predictions have ever been made; and no HIV vaccine has ever been successfully prepared. Instead, highly toxic (but not curative) drugs have been most irresponsibly used, with frequent, lethal side effects. Yet not a single HIV particle has ever been observed by electron microscopy in the blood of patients supposedly having a high viral load! So what? All the most important newspapers and magazine have displayed attractive computerized, colorful images of

HIV that all originate from laboratory cell cultures, but never from even a single AIDS patient. Despite this stunning omission the HIV/AIDS dogma is still solidly entrenched. Tens of thousands of researchers, and hundreds of major pharmaceutical companies continue to make huge profits based on the HIV hypothesis. And not one single AIDS patient has ever been cured ...

Yes, HIV/AIDS is emblematic of the corruption of virus research that is remarkably and tragically documented in this book. Research programs on Hepatitis C, BSE, SARS, Avian flu and current vaccination policies all developed along the same logic, that of maximizing financial profits. Whenever we try to understand how some highly questionable therapeutic policies have been recommended at the highest levels of public health authorities (WHO, CDC, RKI etc.), we frequently discover either embarrassing conflicts of interests, or the lack of essential control experiments, and always the strict rejection of any open debate with authoritative scientists presenting dissident views of the pathological processes. Manipulations of statistics, falsifications of clinical trials, dodging of drug toxicity tests have all been repeatedly documented. All have been swiftly covered up, and none have been able to, so far, disturb the cynical logic of today's virus research business.

Virus mania is a social disease of our highly developed society. To cure it will require conquering fear, fear being the most deadly contagious virus, most efficiently transmitted by the media.

Errare humanum est sed diabolicum preservare ... (to err is human, but to preserve an error is diabolic).

Prof. Dr. Etienne de Harven, MD, was a pioneer in virology. He was as professor of pathology at the University of Toronto and member of the Sloan Kettering Institute for Cancer Research, New York. He was member of Thabo Mbeki's AIDS Advisory Panel of South Africa and president of Rethinking AIDS (www.rethinkaids.net). Etienne de Harven died in 2019 at the age of 82.

Foreword II
by Dr. Joachim Mutter, MD

This Book Will Instigate an Upheaval of Dogmas

The book *Virus Mania* shows in a simple comprehensible way the diversity of scientific data that proves most of the epidemics presented in the media as horror stories (flu, avian flu, AIDS, BSE, Hepatitis C, etc.) do not actually exist or are harmless. In contrast: Through this scaremongering and through the toxic materials contained in vaccines a vast number of diseases can emerge; diseases that have recently been increasing on a massive scale: allergies, cancer, autism, attention deficit disorder (ADD), attention deficit hyperactivity disorder (ADHD), autoimmune diseases and disorders of the nervous system. The authors, the journalist Torsten Engelbrecht and doctor of internal medicine Claus Köhnlein, succeed in tracking down the real culprits, including the profiteers in this game. They also identify solutions that everybody can easily implement in their daily lives. This work is one of the most important and enlightening books of our times which will instigate an upheaval of the dogmas and delusions that have held for more than 150 years.

Dr. Joachim Mutter, MD, is a specialist in hygiene and environmental medicine with his own practice in Southern Germany (Constance). From 2001 to 2008 he worked as a physician at the University Center for Naturopathy in Freiburg under the direction the pioneer in environmental medicine Prof. Dr. Franz Daschner, MD. From 2004 to 2006 he was an expert at the Robert Koch-Institute.

Introduction

Society under the Spell of a One-Dimensional Microbe Theory

*"We had accepted some half-truths and had stopped searching for the whole
truths. The principal half-truths were that medical research had stamped out
the great killers of the past—tuberculosis, diphtheria, pneumonia, puerperal
sepsis, etc.—and that medical research and our superior system of medical
care were major factors in extending life expectancy. The data on deaths
from tuberculosis show that the mortality rate from this disease has been
declining steadily since the middle of the 19th century and has continued to
decline in almost linear fashion during the past 100 years [till 1970]. There
were increases in rates of tuberculosis during wars and under specified
adverse local conditions. The poor and the crowded always came off worst of
all in war and in peace, but the overall decline in deaths from tuberculosis
was not altered measurably by the discovery of the tuberculosis bacillus,
the advent of the tuberculin test, the appearance of BCG vaccination, the
widespread use of mass screening, the intensive anti-tuberculosis campaigns,
or the discovery of streptomycin. It is important that this point be understood
in its completeness. The point was made years ago by Wade Hamptom Frost,
and more recently by René Dubos, and has been repeatedly stressed through
the years by many observers of the public health. Similar trends in mortality
have been reported with respect to diphtheria, scarlet fever, rheumatic fever,
pertussis, measles, and many others."*[1] [2]
Edward H. Kass, Harvard physician and founding member and
first president of the Infectious Disease Society of America

The founding of The Royal Society in 1660 caused a tectonic shift in Western medicine.
A group of British scientists decided that what counts is "the experimental proof" not
speculative fantasy, superstition and blind faith.[3] [4] The Royal Society called this basic research principle "nullius in verba,"[5] which essentially means "Don't just trust what someone says." In that era, it was still common to accuse women of witchcraft "in the name

19

of God" and burn them at the stake, or to subjugate entire peoples such as the Aztecs or Mayans to Western ideologies. Setting a standard of scientific proof marked the end of the dark ages and had enormous long-term consequences.

Today, considering ourselves enlightened and in the safe hands of our high-tech scientific culture, we look back with misgivings and great discomfort at the abuses of power that occurred in such draconian times. Indeed, the dream that science promises with its principle of proof—namely to free people from ignorance, superstition, tyranny, and not least from physical and psychological suffering—has, in many cases, particularly in wealthy countries, become a reality.[6] Airplanes, tractors, computers, bionic limbs—all these achievements are the product of scientific research. Like our modern legal system, bound by the principle of evidence, science recognizes only one guiding principle: provable fact.

Our enthusiasm for scientific achievements has risen immeasurably. We have granted a godlike status to researchers and doctors, who still had the status of slaves in ancient Rome and even until the early 20th century were mostly poor and powerless.[7] Because of this status, we continue to perceive them as selfless truth-seekers.[8] The English biologist Thomas Huxley, a powerful supporter of Charles Darwin and grandfather of the author Aldous Huxley (*Brave New World*, 1932), described this phenomenon as early as the late 19th century, when he compared science's growing authority to the Church's position of power. For this, he coined the term "Church Scientific."[9] [10]

Today's enlightened civilized individual believes so firmly in the omnipotence of scientists that they no longer question the evidence for certain hypotheses or even whether they make sense. Instead, citizens rely on the latest sensationalized media coverage churned out in daily newspapers and TV newscasts about world-threatening viral epidemics (Corona/COVID-19, swine flu, avian flu, SARS, HIV/AIDS, etc.). For many decades, the media (and scientific reporters above all) have intently cultivated friendly relationships with researchers in the drive to scoop their competitors for provocative headlines. "We scientific reporters all too often serve as living applause for our subject," *New York Times* reporter Natalie Angier says critically about her profession. "Sometimes we write manuscripts that sound like unedited press releases."[11]

Journalists usually assume that scientists engage in rigorous studies and disseminate only provable facts—and that rare instances of fraud will quickly be driven out of the hallowed halls of research. It's an ideal picture, but one that has nothing to do with reality.[12] [13] [14] [15] [16] [17] Uncountable billions of dollars are transformed into "scientific" hypotheses, which are ultimately packaged and hawked by pharmaceutical companies, researchers, health advocates and journalists alike as the ultimate conclusions of truth. In actuality, these theories are often mere speculation, proven false and years later, finally discarded.

"The more willing the people are, the more promises must be made," warned Erwin Chargaff as early as 1978. "A quick route to long life, freedom from all diseases, a cure for cancer—soon, perhaps the elimination of death—and what then?" asked the co-founder of biochemical research and gene-technology, and a repeatedly decorated professor at Columbia University's Biochemical Institute in New York. "But no singer would ever have to promise to make me a better person if I would just listen to her trills."[18]

Since the end of the 1970s, this situation has dramatically worsened.[19] Just as in politics and economics, we in research are also "bombarded, saturated, harried by fraud," writes renowned science historian Horace Judson,[20] whose analyses are corroborated by a number of relevant studies.[21] [22] [23] [24] [25] [26] [27] [2829] [30] [31] "There is widespread and organized crime in the drug industry," states Peter C. Gøtzsche, professor of medicine, longtime director of the world-renowned Nordic Cochrance Center and author of the book "Deadly Medicine and Organised Crime."[32]

"From a global viewpoint, there is corruption at all levels of the public health service, from health ministries to patients—and there are almost no limits to criminal imagination," maintains Transparency International, an institution for protection against corruption, in its annual "Global Corruption Report 2006" (focus on health services).[33]

A close look at this data reveals that our scientific culture is ruled by secretiveness, privilege-granting and lack of accountability, and suffers from a blatant lack of monitoring, often motivated by the prospects that these companies and researchers will make exorbitant profits. All of these questionable factors contribute to the potential for researcher bias and fraud, jeopardizing the scientific proof principle introduced in the 17th century.[34] "Judson paints a dark picture of [biomedical] science today, but we may see far darker days ahead as proof and profit become inextricably mixed," warns the medical publication *Lancet*.[35]

Even when one theoretically assumes ideal researchers and ideal studies, it must be emphasized that medicine remains (is still) a "science of uncertainties,"[36] expressed William Osler (1849-1919), regarded as the father of modern medicine.[37] Nothing has changed.

Donald Miller, Professor of Surgery at the University of Washington, warns that with today's medical research, "scientific standards of proof are not uniform and well defined, in contrast to legal standards. Standards of measurement, ways of reporting and evaluating results, and particular types of experimental practices vary. Science prizes objective certainty. But science does not uniformly adhere to this standard. Subjective opinions and consensus among scientists often supersede the stricture of irrefutability."[38]

Table 1   Examples for Methods for Pharmaceutical Companies to Get the Results from Clinical Trials They Want

Conduct a trial of your drug against a treatment known to be inferior.	Use multiple endpoints (survival time, reduction of blood pressure, etc.) in the trial and select for publication those that give favorable results.
Trial your drugs against too low a dose of a competitor drug.	
Conduct a scientific trial of your drug against too high a dose of a competitor drug (making your drug seem less toxic or deadly).	Conduct trials that are too small to show differences from competitor drugs.
	Do multicenter trials and select for publication results from centers that are favorable.

Source: Smith, Richard, Medical Journals Are an Extension of the Marketing Arm of Pharmaceutical Companies, Plos Medicine, May 2005, p. e138

To effectively combat this systemic problem, much would be gained if it were compulsory to have certain studies replicated, thus reviewing them for their soundness.[39] But, according to Judson, "replication, once an important element in science, is no longer an effective deterrent to fraud because the modern biomedical research system is structured to prevent replication—not to ensure it." Such verification is unattractive, because it doesn't promise gigantic profits, but might only produce similar results to the original research, which is unlikely to be published by a medical journal.[40] But from time to time, these reviews are carried out, with stunning results.

At the beginning of 2005, an investigation disclosed a severely flawed study leading to the approval of viramune, a globally-touted AIDS treatment.[41] The follow-up investigation found that records of severe side effects including deaths were simply swept under the carpet.

At the same time, chief investigator Jonathan Fishbein was greatly hindered, from the highest levels of the National Institutes of Health, in his bid for clarification. The medical system, according to Fishbein, is shaped more by politics of interest, partisanship and intrigue than by sound science. Fishbein called the government's AIDS research agency "a troubled organization," referring to an internal review that found its managers had engaged in unnecessary feuding, sexually explicit language and other inappropriate conduct.[42] [43]

How far this can go becomes apparent when research produced by individual scientists is placed under the microscope. The South Korean veterinarian Hwang Woo Suk, for example, published a paper in the journal *Science* in May 2005 in which he described how he had extracted human stem cells from cloned embryos for the first time. The work was celebrated as a "global sensation" and Hwang as a "cloning pioneer." But at the end of 2005, it was discovered that Hwang had completely forged his experiments.[44] [45]

The medical field is ultimately about illness, dying and death. Naturally, these experiences involve a complex and nuanced range of emotions for individuals, their loved ones and doctors. The process makes us extremely receptive to a belief in salvation through miracle treatments. In this, researchers and physicians take over the roles of priests; the white smock has merely replaced the black robes and black wigs physicians used to wear.[46]

These white knights proclaim their healing messages, and of course require "victims" to carry out their research with billions of dollars of government, i.e. taxpayer funded dollars. "Indeed, so profound is our belief in the cures of science" that it has become "the new secular theology of the 20th century,"[47] according to American media scientist Michael Tracey. "This belief is so inherent within us that we construct any problem, grievance, pain, or fear in conceptual terms that not only allow us to seek the cure, but demand that we do so."[48]

At the heart of this web of feelings and wishes are the fantasies of almightiness that further prop up the medical-industrial complex. This ever more powerful part of the global economy consists of pharmaceutical companies worth billions, their lobby-ists and spin doctors, and an immense army of highly-paid researchers and doctors. In the process, we've turned our bodies into vehicles of consumerism, internalizing a highly-questionable promise inherent to this industry: Science can conquer terrible and puzzling diseases — just like we conquered the moon — if it is just given enough money.[49]

To avoid any misunderstandings: medicine has made tremendous achievements. This applies first and foremost to reparative medicine such as accident surgery, organ trans-plants and laser eye surgery. But, the various perils of modern medicine are all-too evident in the ever-expanding field of so-called preventive and curative treatments, particularly the growing arsenal of pharmaceutical drugs — in other words, medicine that purports to be able to heal.[50]

Take cancer, for example. In 1971, US President Richard Nixon at the behest of pub-lic health officials (and above all, virologists), declared a "War on Cancer." The med-ical establishment vowed there would be a cure at hand by 1975.[51] But we are still waiting. And there is "no evidence of the way cancer comes into being," according to German Cancer Research Center (Deutsches Krebsforschungszentrum).[52] Mainstream cancer theories also show blatant contradictions.[53] Despite this, hundreds of billions of dollars have already flowed into a completely one-sided cancer research focused on wonder-drug production. Above all, this set-up generates gigantic profits for pharma-ceutical companies, researchers and doctors.

In contrast, plausible alternative theories (which may be less profitable, because they focus on lifestyle and environmental factors and not only on fatefully appear-ing genes and viruses as causes) remain almost completely disregarded.[54] [55] For in-stance, although official cancer theories assume that a third of cancer cases could be prevented through a change of diet (above all more fruit and vegetables and less meat),[56] cancer expert Samuel Epstein points out that the American National Cancer Institute spent "just $1 million — that is 0.02 percent of its $4.7 billion budget in 2005 — on education, press work and public relations to encourage eating fruit and vegetables to prevent cancer."[57]

At the same time, the number of people who die from "non-smoking" cancers has noticeably increased since Nixon's 1971 call to battle (even, it is worth noting, when one takes
into consideration that people on average have become older).[58] In Germany more than
200,000 people still die from this terrible disease annually; in the USA there are around
600,000 cancer deaths per year.[59]

The situation doesn't look any better for other widespread illnesses such as diabetes,
heart disease, high blood pressure, or rheumatism. In spite of exorbitant research budgets, the development of a cure is unforeseeable. Cortisone, for instance, does help to
alleviate acute rheumatic or allergic discomfort—but only during the cortisone therapy. If
treatment is discontinued, suffering returns. At the same time, cortisone, which also finds
plenty of use in the treatment of viruses, is, like most reputed miracle cures (aka "magic
bullets"), connected with severe side effects.[60]

Vera Sharav of the New York City-based Alliance for Human Research Protection (AHRP),
an organization that fights for independent and ethically responsible medical science,
warns that "often enough, the medications are so toxic that they produce precisely the
diseases against which, as the pharmaceutical manufacturers' advertising messages aim
to convince us, they are supposed to be so active. And then, new preparation after new
preparation is given."[61]

As relevant studies reveal, drug toxicities are so severe that the American "health" industry's pill craze is responsible for about 800,000 deaths each year, more than any illness
(including cancer and heart attack). And in Germany, tens of thousands of people are
estimated to die each year due to improper treatment and prescription of incorrect medications (there are no exact figures because certain interest groups have successfully
resisted the collection of the relevant information).[62] As Peter C. Gøtzsche, professor of
medicine, points out: "Our prescription drugs are the third leading cause of death after
heart disease and cancer in the United States and Europe."[63]

The fact that a society calling itself enlightened is nevertheless dominated by the belief
that there is a healing pill for every little ache and pain or serious complaint is substantially due to the persuasive craftiness of Big Pharma. Pharmaceutical companies operating in the US spend approximately a third of their expenses on marketing, which means
that dozens of billions US dollars per year are invested in advertising their preparations

as miracle cures to doctors, journalists, consumers and politicians.[64] With this, they have extended their sphere of influence in a most alarming way to include institutions like the World Health Organization (WHO), the Food and Drug Administration (FDA), as well as the US National Institutes of Health (NIH), the independence and integrity of which is particularly important.[65] [66] [67] [68]

A study published in the *Journal of the American Medical Association* (*JAMA*) in April 2006, showed that "conflicts of interest at the FDA are widespread." It was shown that in 73 percent of meetings, at least one member of the consulting team in question had conflicts of interest: being remunerated by Big Pharma, for instance, through consultation fees, research contracts or grants, or stock ownership or options. In nearly a quarter of contracts and grants sums of more than $100,000 changed hands. The study found that these conflicts of interest influenced voting behavior: When panel members with conflicts of interest were excluded from voting, the judgment of the product in question was much less favorable. And even though these conflicts of interest were so extensive, panel members with relevant conflicts of interest were disqualified in only 1 percent of cases.[69] [70]

"Big Pharma money and advertising not only influence the perception of illness, the demand for drugs, and the practice of medicine, but government budgets, including health service and oversight agencies have become dependent on Big Pharma money," says Vera Sharav of the AHRP. "An out of the box analysis opened our eyes to a fundamental conflict of interest that has never been discussed. Public health policies are not merely influenced by Big Pharma; they are formulated so as to increase industry's profits because government budgets are tied to this industry's profits." In this context, a decisive event occurred in 1992 when the US Congress waved through the "Prescription Users Fees Act" (PDUFA), which established the "fast track drug approval service." According to Sharav, "the FDA has received $825 million in industry 'user fees'," and "other government agencies have similarly become financially dependent on Big Pharma."[71]

The issue stirred up so much controversy that the British Parliament also opened an extensive investigation. Their conclusions: the pharmaceutical industry's corrupt practices and its massive influence upon parliaments, authorities, universities, health professionals and the media were sharply criticized.[72]

In fact, "if prescription medicines are so good, why do they need to be pushed so hard?" asks Marcia Angell, former Editor in Chief of the well-known *New England Journal of Medicine (NEJM)*. "Good drugs don't have to be promoted."[73] Her opinions are as simple as they are revealing, but unfortunately they don't register in the consciousness of the modern believer in science. Our society that considers itself particularly enlightened has become senselessly "overmedicated."[74]

This pill-mania exists because we have a distorted comprehension of what causes diseases—a comprehension that has been able to lodge itself firmly in our thought processes over a period of more than 100 years.[75] To understand this, one must look back to the middle of the 19th century, when a true paradigm shift in the way we see disease occurred. There was an about-turn, away from a complex, holistic view concerning how diseases originate, to a monocausal and "one-dimensional" mindset, to use a term from philosopher Herbert Marcuse. Through this, a false awareness arose "which is immune to its falseness" because the dimensions of self-criticism and the ability to look in various alternative directions is missing.[76]

This paradigm shift is largely due to the fact that from approximately the 16th century, in the course of the Enlightenment, the natural sciences began to develop rapidly, and put the population under their spell with descriptions of very specific phenomena. One need only remember the tremendous achievements of the English physicist Isaac Newton, who described gravitation; or the invention of the steam locomotive or even the printing press.

But in the euphoric exuberance of progress, particularly from the middle of the 19th century, this thought pattern of specificity—that very particular chemical or physical phenomena have very specific causes—was simply transferred to the medical sciences. Many researchers and interest groups didn't even consider if this actually made sense.[77]

The dogma of a single cause for diseases was decisively shaped by microbiology, which became predominant at the end of the 19th century, declaring specific microorganisms (viruses, bacteria, fungi) to be the causes of very definite diseases; including mass epidemics such as cholera and tuberculosis.[78] The founders of microbe theory, researchers Louis Pasteur and Robert Koch, ascended in their lifetimes to the heights of medicine's Mount Olympus.

With the microbe theory, the "cornerstone was laid for modern biomedicine's basic formula with its monocausal-microbial starting-point and its search for magic bullets: one disease, one cause, one cure," writes American sociology professor, Steven Epstein.[79]

From the end of the 19th century, the hunt for microbes increasingly provided the thrill, and the same admiration that physicists and chemists had earlier garnered (as in Paris in 1783, when the brothers Montgolfier performed the "miracle" of launching a hot air balloon into the sky).[80]

But as fascinating as this conception of a single cause is, it has very little to do with the complex workings of the human body. A significant majority of diseases have far more than just one cause, so the search for *the single* cause of disease, and by extension for the one miracle-pill, will remain for them a hopeless undertaking.[81] This is particularly true in microbiology, a "scientific No Man's Land,"[82] as the American magazine *The New Yorker* fittingly described it. The field is becoming ever more complex and incomprehensible, as further research penetrates the seemingly infinite microcosmic mini-worlds of cellular components, molecules and microbes.

Bacteria, fungi and viruses are omnipresent—in the air, in our food, in our mucous membranes—but we aren't permanently sick.[83] When a disease generally held to be contagious "breaks out," only some individuals become sick. This is clear evidence that microbes, whatever potential they may have to make you sick, cannot be the lone cause of disease.

Pasteur himself admitted on his deathbed: "The microbe is nothing, the terrain is everything."[84] And indeed, even for mainstream medicine, it is becoming increasingly clear that the biological terrain of our intestines—the intestinal flora, teeming with bacteria—is accorded a decisive role, because it is by far the body's biggest and most important immune system.[85] A whole range of factors (in particular nutrition, stress, lack of activity, drug use, etc.) influence intestinal flora, so it has a decisive influence on all sorts of severe as well as less serious illnesses.[86] [87] [88] [89]

But it is not just this large oversimplification that calls for opposition to the microbe theory.[90] Under closer examination, fundamental assumptions of microbe theory also emerge as pure myth. Edward Kass, professor of medicine at Harvard University, made this the subject of his opening address at a conference of the American Society for Infectious Diseases in 1970. US citizens were becoming increasingly critical of the Vietnam War and many people in the USA began to rebel against the establishment. Maybe this *zeitgeist* spurred Kass to address these issues openly, although they may have stood in glaring opposition to the views of most of his listeners.

Diagram 1   Pertussis: Death Rates of Children Younger than 15
               (England and Wales)

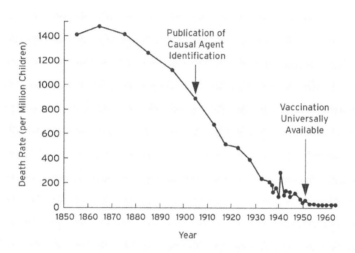

Source: McKeown, Thomas, *Die Bedeutung der Medizin, Suhrkamp, 1979, p. 149*

Kass argued that medical scientists and microbe hunters were not the ones to be praised for stemming the flow of mass diseases like tuberculosis, diphtheria, measles, whooping cough or pulmonary infections. The data unquestionably shows that death rates for these so-called infectious diseases had noticeably decreased from the middle of the 19th century; long before microbe hunters and the medical establishment became active (see diagram 1). The monumental accomplishment of pushing back diseases and raising life expectancy is primarily due to an improvement in general standards of living (improved nutrition, construction of water purification plants, etc.), which gained momentum in in-dustrialized countries precisely in the mid-19th century.[91]

This also explains why deaths from so-called infectious diseases have become a rar-ity in affluent societies (in wealthy countries, they make up less than 1 percent of all mortalities).[92] Yet, in poor third-world regions like Africa, where every third person is malnourished,[93] these same diseases (tuberculosis, leprosy, etc.) that wealthy countries fought during times of recession run rampant.[94] The excessive panic-like fear, which so easily consumes members of affluent societies when the media stokes the flames of the viral-epidemic panic, can in this context, only be described as irrational.

And although the horror scenarios that were painted on the wall by the mainstream media "at the behest" of the virologists in connection with SARS (2002/2003), bird flu (2004/2005) or swine flu (2009/2010) have never become a reality, in 2020 total panic was nonetheless spread again with Corona/COVID-19. In addition, civil rights and freedoms were massively restricted with totalitarian measures.These shocking media reports totally overlook the fact that the existence and pathogenic effects of all these allegedly contagious and even fatal viruses—H5N1 ("avian flu"), H1N1 ("swine flu"), HIV etc.—have never been proven. In fact, very few people actually die from these purported large new epidemics. Strictly speaking, these epidemics are not epidemics whatsoever.

No scientists have even seen the avian flu virus H5N1 in full (with its complete genetic material and virus shell); we don't even know if it could be dangerous to humans, or if it could trigger the already widely reported global pandemic; something that mainstream researchers also admit.[95] And despite this lack of proof, Reinhard Kurth, director of Ger-many's Robert Koch-Institute, which is responsible for microbe epidemics, does not shy from warning that H5N1 "potentially threatens all of humanity."[96] There is also a signif-icant discrepancy between speculation and existing facts in the BSE "epidemic." To date, we are yet to see a single human case of the disease in Germany, only animals that have tested „positive" for the "prion."[97]

With regard to hepatitis C, we are still waiting for the predicted epidemic of liver cirrhosis (serious liver damage).[98] Meanwhile, according to official statistics, since the 1980s nor more than a few hundred people die in Germany each year from so-called AIDS. And what about the horrifying figures of x-million "infected with HIV" in Africa and other developing countries? This is primarily due to the redefinition of patients who suffer from conventional diseases like tuberculosis or leprosy as AIDS patients.[99] The threat of SARS is similarly over hyped: In the first nine months (November 2002-July 2003) after the alleged discovery of the SARS virus at the end of 2002, the World Health Organization found only 800 "probable SARS deaths."[100]

"Years from now, people looking back at us will find our acceptance of the HIV theory of AIDS as silly as we find the leaders who excommunicated Galileo, just because he insisted that the earth was not the center of the universe," predicted Kary Mullis, one of the most significant Nobel laureates of the 20th century who died in 2019. "It has been disappointing that so many scientists have absolutely refused to examine the available evidence in a neutral, dispassionate way, regarding whether HIV causes AIDS."[101]

This deviation from the fundamental principles of scientific research has also happened in other new alleged epidemics like Corona/COVID-19, hepatitis C, SARS, swine flu, avian flu, cervical cancer, Ebola, and BSE.

Mullis' words come from his article titled, "The Medical Establishment vs. the Truth." In it, he discusses how the entire virus-busting industry plies its dogmas, declaring them to be eternal truths, without the support of factual evidence. Of course, this helps to secure the gigantic research budgets and profits of pharmaceutical groups and top scientists.

Federal Funding for HIV has increased significantly over time, rising in the United States from a few hundred thousand in 1982 to more than US$34.8 billion in 2019. Between 1981 and 2006, i.e. in the first 25 years, US taxpayers shelled out $190 billion for AIDS research focused almost exclusively on the deadly virus hypothesis and the development of treatment drugs.[102] The same amount of taxpayer money went to AIDS research in America in the five years between 2014 and 2019.

Yet the growing list of medications haven't demonstrably extended the life of a single patient, and a "cure" is nowhere in sight.[103] The same strategy has been employed with Tamiflu flu medication, which has serious side effects, yet, thanks to skillful public relations work, support of the WHO and the media's avian flu fear mongering, this drug mutated in a short time from shelf warmer to cash cow.[104]

While pharmaceutical groups and top researchers cash in and the media drive their circulation ratings sky high with sensationalized headlines, citizens must foot a gigantic bill without getting what is necessary: enlightenment over the true causes and true solutions. "So what are dedicated clinicians to do?" asks John Abramson of Harvard Medical School. "The first step is to give up the illusion that the primary purpose of modern medical research is to improve Americans' health most effectively and efficiently. In our opinion, the primary purpose of commercially-funded clinical research is to maximize financial return on investment, not health."[105]

This book's central focus is to steer this discussion back to where a scientific debate belongs: on the path to prejudice-free analysis of facts. To clarify one more time, the point is not to show that diseases like cervical cancer, SARS, AIDS or hepatitis C do not exist. No serious critic of reigning virus theories has any doubt that people or animals are or could become sick (although many are not really sick at all, but are only defined as sick, and then are made sick or killed). Instead, the central question is: What really causes these diseases known as cervical cancer, avian flu, SARS, AIDS and hepatitis C? Is it a virus? Is it a virus in combination with other causes? Or is it not a virus at all, but rather something very different?

We will embark on a detailed examination of the scientific hypotheses of science, politics and the media elite, looking at all of the available evidence. At the same time, alternative explanations or causes of ill-health will be described: substances like drugs, medicines, pesticides, heavy metals or inadequate nutrition. All these factors can severely damage or even completely destroy the immune system—and their devastating effects can be encountered in the victims hastily branded with a diagnosis of COVID-19, cervical cancer, avian flu, SARS, AIDS or hepatitis C. Ultimately they are victims of complex, broad socio-economic and political forces and are further marginalized and degraded by a profession that pledges to "do no harm."

Chapter 1 explains what microbes (bacteria, fungi, viruses) actually are, and what role they play in the complete cycle of life and the ways in which the medical establishment and the media have turned these microbes into our worst enemies. In Chapter 2, we'll travel from the middle of the 19th century until modern times, in order to separate myth from reality in microbe theory. Louis Pasteur and Robert Koch rose to become medicine's shining lights, but we cannot leave them out of this analysis since they were certainly not immune from lying and deception. Nor will we shy away from the question of whether polio is a viral disease or if poisons like pesticides have not made at least some contribution to the destruction of the spinal nerves that is so typical of this disease.

With this background knowledge, we dive into the time of modern virus research. Chapter 3 thus begins with the history of HIV/AIDS, which arrived in the early 1980s, triggering an almost unprecedented mass panic that continues to this day. And now the whole world also seems to accept that Hepatitis C, BSE, SARS, avian flu, cervical cancer and COVID-19 are each triggered by a single causative agent (pathogen). In Chapters 4 through 12, we will see that these statements do not hold up and that other explanations make much more sense.

Chapter 1

Medicine Presents a Distorted Picture of Microbes

> *"The gods are innocent of man's suffering. Our diseases and physical pains*
> *are the products of excess!"*
> Pythagoras (570-510 B.C.)

> *"Béchamp was right, the microbe is nothing, the terrain is everything!"*[106]
> Louis Pasteur (1822-1895)

> *"Where there is life, there are germs."*[107]
> Robinson Verner

> *"Diet clearly has a major influence on many diseases and modulates the*
> *complex internal community of microorganisms. These microorganisms,*
> *weighing up to 1 kg in a normal adult human, may total 100 Trillion cells."*[108]
> Jeremy Nicholson
> Professor of Biochemistry

Microbes: Branded as Scapegoats

People are very susceptible to the idea that certain microbes act like predators, stalking our communities for victims and causing the most serious illnesses like COVID-19 (pulmonary infection) or hepatitis C (liver damage). Such an idea is thoroughly simple, perhaps too simple. As psychology and social science have discovered, humans have a propensity for simplistic solutions, particularly in a world that seems to be growing increasingly complicated.[109] It also allows for a concept of the "enemy at the gates" allowing individuals to shift responsibility for their illnesses to a fungus, a bacteria or a virus. "Man prefers to perish rather than change his habits!" the author Leo Tolstoy once said.

This type of scapegoat thinking has often led humanity astray, be it in personal life, in science or in politics. Fishermen and politicians both earnestly assert that seals and dolphins contribute to the depletion of ocean fish stocks. So, each year in Canada, one hundred thousand seals—often just a few days old—are battered to death,[110] while every autumn in Japan, thousands of dolphins are hacked apart while still alive.[111]

But in their blind hatred for the animals, the slaughterers completely overlook the fact that it is their own species – Homo sapiens – who have plundered the world's fish stocks through massive overexploitation using high-technology catch-methods. A German-Canadian study that appeared in *Nature* in 2003, found that industrialized fishing has dramatically reduced the stocks of predators like tuna and swordfishes, marlins, cod, halibut, ray and flounder in the world's oceans since the beginning of commercial fishing in the 1950s—by no less than 90 percent.[112]

Similarly, our modern misconception of the "deadly predatory microbe" ignores the bigger picture. Some microorganisms can be harmful; but it is negligent to ignore the role that individual behaviors play, particularly nutrition, drug consumption, etc. "Whether the method of treatment affects the animal predators in the wilderness or the bacteria in the gut, it is always risky to tamper with the natural balance of forces in nature," wrote microbiologist and Pulitzer Prize winner René Dubos.[113]

Medical and biological realities, like social ones, are just not that simple. Renowned immunology and biology professor Edward Golub's rule of thumb is that, "if you can fit the solution to a complex problem on a bumper sticker, it is wrong! I tried to condense my book *The Limits of Medicine: How Science Shapes Our Hope for the Cure* to fit onto a bumper sticker and couldn't."[114]

The complexities of the world—and above all, the living world—might seem too difficult for any one individual to grasp with even approximate comprehension. Informing ourselves on economics, culture, politics and medical science seems incredibly daunting. Man "is not an Aristotelian god that encompasses all existence; he is a creature with a development who can only comprehend a fraction of reality," wrote social psychologist Elisabeth Noelle-Neumann.[115]

Supposed experts are no exception. Most doctors themselves, for instance, have hardly more than a lay understanding of the concepts that loom on the horizons of molecular biology, including research into microbes and their role in the onset of diseases.

Correspondingly, if you asked most doctors to define the unmistakable characteristics of retroviruses (HIV, for example, is claimed to be one), they'd most likely shrug their shoulders or throw out a bewildering cryptic response. Another challenge for many doctors would be a description of how the polymerase chain reaction (PCR) functions, even though it developed into a key technology in molecular biology in the 1990s, and is brought up again and again in connection with the alleged discovery of the so-called avian flu virus H5N1 (on PCR, see chapter 3, about the "miracle weapons" of the epidemic inventors, as well as chapter 12 about corona/COVID-19).

Ignorance and the desire for oversimplification are root problems in medical science. As early as 1916, the philosopher Ludwig Wittgenstein remarked in his diary: "Humanity has always searched for a science that follows the motto *simplex sigillum veri*," essentially meaning that "there is a strong desire for simplification," as Chargaff commented on Wittgenstein's words.[116] And microbial theory fits exactly into this scheme: one disease, one agent as cause—and ultimately, one miracle pill or vaccine as a solution.[117]

But this oversimplification belies the goings-on in the "invisible" micro-world of cells and molecules. The living world—on both a small and large scale—is just much more complicated than medical science and the media lets on. For this reason, as biochemist Erwin Chargaff points out, "The attempt to find symmetry and simplicity in the world's living tissue has often led to false conclusions."[118] There are even a few people who believe that what is now called 'molecular biology' encompasses all life sciences. But that is not the case, except on a superficial level: everything we can see in our world is somehow made up of molecules. But is that all? Can we describe music by saying that all instruments are made of wood, brass, and so on, and that because of that they produce their sounds?"[119]

Biology—the science of life—isn't even capable of defining its own object of research: life. "We do not have a scientific definition of life," as Erwin Chargaff states. And "indeed, the most precise tests are carried out on dead cells and tissues."[120] This phenomenon is particularly prevalent in bacterial and viral research (and in the whole pharmaceutical development of medicines altogether) where laboratory experiments on tissue samples which are tormented with a variety of often highly reactive chemicals allow few conclusions about reality. And yet, conclusions are constantly drawn—and then passed straight on to the production of medications and vaccines.

Fungi: As in the Forest, So in the Human Body

It's ultimately impossible to find out exactly everything that microbes get up to on a cellular and molecular level in living people or animals. To do this, you would have to chase every single microbe around with mini-cameras. And even if it were possible, you'd merely have little pieces of a puzzle, not an intricate blueprint of the body in its entirety. By focusing on microbes and accusing them of being the primary and lone triggers of disease, we overlook how various factors are linked together, causing illness, such as environmental toxins, the side effects of medications, psychological issues like depression and anxiety and poor nutrition.

If over a longer period of time, for instance, you eat far too little fresh fruits and vegetables, and instead consume far too much fast food, sweets, coffee, soft drinks, or alcohol (and along with them, all sorts of toxins such as pesticides or preservatives), and maybe smoke a lot or even take drugs like cocaine or heroin, your health will eventually be ruined. Drug-addicted and malnourished junkies aren't the only members of society who make this point clear to us. It was also tangibly presented in the 2004 film *Super Size Me*, in which American Morgan Spurlock—the film's director and guinea pig rolled into one—consumed only fast food from McDonald's for 30 days. The result: Spurlock gained 12 kg, his liver fat values were equivalent to those of an alcoholic, his cholesterol increased, he became depressed, suffered from severe headaches and erectile dysfunction.

Despite its drastic effects, people still become addicted to this protein and fat-containing and simultaneously nutrient-deficient foodstuff. Certainly, it may have something to do with the fact that fast-food corporations have billion-dollar annual advertising budgets, that purposefully and successfully target the most vulnerable consumers. Meanwhile, the US government has had an advertising budget of merely $2 million for their campaign "Fruit and Vegetables—five times a day").[121] As laboratory studies on rats and mice show, the contents of hamburgers and French fries can cause reactions in the body that are similar to that of heroin addiction,[122] which has been proven to have a destructive effect upon the immune system.[123]

According to researchers, processed ingredients are significant components in the onset of addiction. "A diet containing salt, sugar and fats caused the animals to become addicted to these foodstuffs," says Ann Kelley, a neurologist at the Wisconsin Medical School who observed alterations in brain chemistry in long-term test series that were similar to long-term use of morphine or heroin.

Sugar "is in a position to be a 'gateway' to other drugs, legal or illegal," according to Thomas Kroiss, president of the Austrian Society for holistic medicine. Sugar robs vitamins from the body, which influences mood as well. Although it is popular in Western cultures it doesn't exist at all in nature, and causes an imbalance when regularly consumed.[124] This prompted the journal *New Scientist* to write that fast foods, like cigarettes, should carry a health advisory warning.[125] But instead of providing more information and carrying out more research (not least into the influence of animal proteins on health not just those found in burgers)[126] [127] [128] on the many dangers of fast foods, McDonald's continues luring children with "Happy Meals" and even promotes the brand by sponsoring large sporting events.

One such event is the Football Champions League, which was supposed to be all about sport—and by extension health. In order to associate the McDonald's brand as being a promoter of health, in 1987 the fast food giant has founded a children's aid program, "McDonald's Kinderhilfe"—for sick children who, according to the fast food giant, "need one thing above all: love and security." Super-celebrities such as athletes Michael Ballack, Henry Maske, Jérôme Boateng and Katarina Witt, as well as supermodel Heidi Klum and the world-famous vocal trio Destiny's Child functioned as brand influencers.[129] [130]

Corporate groups also receive political support. In late 2005, the EU commission announced that they wanted to relax TV advertising regulations, which would mean that advertising could be more specifically targeted to the audience, such as using direct product placement during programs.[131] If these measures had been carried out, European cultures would undoubtedly have found themselves closer to US standards—and the consumer would be even more heavily bombarded with advertising messages from the food, pharmaceutical and other multi-national industries. Such partisan politics certainly has nothing to do with targeted health precautions, although that kind of public service is so urgently needed.

Preventive health care is generally neglected by the very government-sponsored groups charged with protecting the health of citizens. A good and symbolically appropriate example of this is that these bloated bureaucracies pay little attention to intestinal function and health. Even organizations like the generally esteemed Stiftung Warentest, a German consumer protection organization still earnestly clinged to the message that "poor nutrition or a lifestyle that leads to constipation generally has nothing to do with intestinal bacteria." And in general, "shifts in the composition of the intestine's microbes are merely symptoms [that is, consequences] of infections, inflammations or antibiotic treatments, but not their causes. Under normal patterns of life, the intestinal flora regulates itself on its own as soon as the cause of the disturbance has been eliminated," the researchers say.[132] [133]

Stiftung Warentest cannot, however, furnish studies that prove this. And there is also no reason to assume that their statements are well founded. Of course, there are many factors to consider beyond allegedly sole causes of a shift in the intestinal flora from infections or inflammations. A large proportion of the population suffers from intestinal problems like constipation or abnormally high candida infection, so, it's absurd to assume that toxins and antibiotics should pass by the intestinal flora's composition without leaving a trace.

We don't even know precisely what "normal intestinal flora" is. We've yet to become acquainted with all the microbes in the intestinal ecosystem, and it has also been observed that different people have very different intestinal flora.[134] How, then, could we possibly know what "normal" intestinal flora looks like? Or how it constantly regulates itself toward a "normal" level? Individual microbes might remain very stable, as studies suggest,[135] but "stable" doesn't automatically mean "normal" or even "healthy."

It is certain that "artificial sugar, for example, constitutes a terrain for the wrong fungi and bacteria," says physician Thomas Kroiss.[136] Additionally, studies have shown that diets with little to no fresh (raw) food create an unsuitable environment o maintain a fully functioning intestinal flora.[137] Individual behavior (nutrition, activity, stress, etc.) also influences intestinal flora, and can make candida fungi grow.

In this context, it would also be interesting to discover what kind of effect an overly acidic diet has on the intestinal flora and on an individual's health. Previously, studies on factory farm animals show that the acids ingested with food, which are said to speed up growth in pigs or poultry, negatively affect intestinal flora.[138] But, how does it affect the human body?

The human body is like a forest with a buffer system of lungs, kidneys and sweat glands, so that superfluous acids can be released. The German Nutrition Society (DGE, Deutsche Gesellschaft für Ernährung) claimed that an "excessively basic diet brings no provable advantages to your health. Too much acid in the body is nothing to fear in a healthy individual, since buffer systems keep the acid-base level in blood and tissue constant."[139] Still, the DGE cannot deliver any evidence. It is difficult to imagine that a "normal" diet, that only consists of acid-generating foods like meat, fish, eggs, cheese, butter, refined sugar and pills, with few to no base-producing foods like fruit and vegetables will leave no trace in the body.

Even if the buffer systems in a so-called healthy person (whatever that means!) keeps the acid-base level in the blood constant, it cannot be ruled out that tissue may be stressed or even damaged. Many experts, such as the American nutritionist Gary Tunsky are of the opinion that "the fight for health is decided by the pH values."[140] It is worth noting that cancer tissue, for instance, is extremely acidic,[141] and it would be easy to investigate how various basic or acidic diets affect the course of the cancer—but unfortunately this doesn't happen.[142] Meanwhile, the influence on nutrition on the skeletal system has been well investigated.[143] [144] Even osteoporosis tablet manufacturers expressly indicate that one should try to avoid "phosphate and foods containing oxalic acids, in other words [calcium robbers like] meat, sausages, soft drinks, cocoa or chocolate."[145]

"The intestinal flora is among the numerous factors that could take part in the onset and triggering of an illness," states Wolfgang Kruis, intestinal expert and professor of medicine in Cologne.[146] And his colleague Francisco Guarner adds that "the intestinal flora is very significant to an individual's health, something that has been well documented."[147] It is essential in providing nutrients for the development of epithelial cells.[148] And if the intestine is disturbed, this can affect the absorption and processing of important nutrients and vital substances, which in turn can trigger a chain reaction of problems, such as the contamination of body tissue, which then helps certain fungi and bacteria to move in.[149]

An article in the German *Ärzte Zeitung* (*Doctor's Newspaper*) described how a healthy intestinal flora improves overall health by reporting that "four out of five patients had normal and pain free bowel movements again." According to the article, this resounding success could be traced back to giving patients a preparation containing Escherichia coli or E. coli bacteria. In contrast to classic laxatives, bothersome flatulence, intestinal rumbling, abdominal cramps and nausea seldom appeared after the 8-week-long bacterial cure.[150] After all, there are evermore studies to indicate that probiotics (tablets containing live bacterial cultures) and prebiotics (nutrients which are supposed to stimulate certain "good" bacteria already found in the intestines) are of some use to health.[151]

The primary objective should be to study exactly how certain foodstuffs, specific diets, drug consumption, toxins (pesticides, automobile exhaust, etc.), and stress effect the composition of the intestinal flora—and how this in turn influences human health. Researchers are practically unanimous in that the intestinal flora influences health, but they continue to puzzle over *how* this happens.[152] But, evidently, this research work is neglected. Neither the EU[153] (which financially facilitates studies of intestinal flora),[154] nor the German Institute of Human Nutrition[155] (Institut für Ernährungsforschung) in Potsdam were willing to indicate to what extent they are active in this area. Instead the impression is given that the development of marketable products like "functional food ingredients," "specifically designed bacterial strains," or "probiotics and prebiotics" are the primary research targets.[156]

This shows, once again, that the medical industry has little interest in real preventive research.[157] The sale and application of antifungal preparations (just like antibiotics, antiviral medicines, vaccines, probiotics, etc.) makes a lot of money; the advice to eliminate, avoid, or reducerefined sugar or lifestyle drugs, on the other hand, does not make any money at all.[158] And who really wants (or is able) to give up beloved habits? Many people would rather hope for a magic potion that makes all the aches and pains go away fast. Regretfully, this has led to the formation of a medical structure which ultimately only supports concepts that pass through the market's needle eye, and lets company profits and experts' salaries swell.[159] The various hazards of this paradigm are shut out of the public conversation, and, so, we drift further and further from the possibilities of truly effective preventive health.

We must not ignore the fact that people are experiencing higher rates of fungal infections. It's certainly not because fungi have become more aggressive, since they have hardly changed in millions of years. But what has changed is our behavior and with it our physical environment as well. We only have to glance at other areas of nature, where fungi can't tell the difference between a human body and, for example, a forest. Everywhere, balance is at play: Excess substances are continuously generated, and must somehow be diminished again. If this were not the case, the earth would suffocate in the chaos of these excessively produced substances.[160] This is where over 100,000 species of fungi come in and form their own kingdom next to animals and plants,[161] acting like garbage collectors, eating up leaves, dead twigs, branches, tree stumps or pinecones in the forest, and bringing the nutrients back into the life cycle of the plants as re-utilizable humus.

Everything in nature—cells, our bodies, the land—occurs in a balance,[162] which is why "fungal illnesses in compact, healthy plants do not have a chance," as stated in a botany textbook. Yet if "a plant is infested by a fungus, then something must be wrong with the plant's living conditions."[163] This would be the case, for instance, if the plant's soil were overly acidic, something which causes fungi to thrive.

Bacteria: At the Beginning of All Life

For billions of years, nature has functioned as a whole with unsurpassed precision. Microbes, just like humans, are a part of this cosmological and ecological system. If humanity wants to live in harmony with technology and nature, we are bound to understand the supporting evolutionary principles ever better and to apply them properly to our own lives. Whenever we don't do this, we create ostensibly insolvable environmental and health problems.

These are thoughts which Rudolf Virchow (1821-1902), a well-known doctor from Berlin, had when he required in 1875 that "the doctor should never forget to interpret the patient as a whole being."[164] The doctor will hardly understand the patient, then, if he or she does not see that person in the context of a larger environment.

Without the appearance of bacteria, human life would be inconceivable, as bacteria were right at the beginning of the development towards human life:[165]

Progenotes (precursors to bacteria; ca. 3.5 billion years ago) →
Prokaryotes →
Anaerobic bacteria (anaerobe) →
Anaerobic photosynthetic bacteria →
Photosynthetic cyano-bacteria →
Oxygen-rich atmosphere →
Aerobic breathing →
Aerobic prokaryotes →
Eukaryotes (1.6–2.1 billion years ago) →
Many-celled plants and animals →
Mammals →
Humans

With the term progenotes, bacteriologists denote a "pre-preliminary stage," a life form from which prokaryotes (cells without nuclei) arise. Bacteria are known not to have cell nuclei, but they do have deoxyribonucleic acid (DNA) and ribonucleic acid (RNA), the carriers of genetic material. Anaerobic bacteria, as the word "anaerobic" indicates, can get by without oxygen. Only after the earth was supplied with oxygen could aerobic bacteria live; bacteria that formed the foundation for the lives of plants, animals, and humans.[166]

Through this it becomes obvious that bacteria could very well exist without humans; humans, however, could not live without bacteria! It also becomes unimaginable that these mini-creatures, whose life-purpose and task for almost infinite time has been to build up life, are supposed to be the great primary or singular causes of disease and death. Yet, the prevailing allopathic medical philosophy has convinced us of this since the late 19th century, when Louis Pasteur and Robert Koch became heroes. Just a few hours after birth, all of a newborn baby's mucous membrane has already been colonized by bacteria, which perform important protective functions.[167] Without these colonies of billions of germs, the infant, just like the adult, could not survive. And, only a small part of our body's bacteria have even been discovered.[168]

"The majority of cells in the human body are anything but human: foreign bacteria have long had the upper hand," reported a research team from Imperial College in London under the leadership of Jeremy Nicholson in the journal Nature Biotechnology in 2004. In the human digestive tract alone, researchers came upon around 100 trillion microorganisms, which together have a weight of up to one kilogram. "This means that the 1,000-plus known species of symbionts probably contain more than 100 times as many genes as exist in the host," as Nicholson states. It makes you wonder how much of the human body is "human" and how much is "foreign"?

Nicholson calls us "human super-organisms"—as our own ecosystems are ruled by microorganisms. "It is widely accepted," writes the Professor of Biochemistry, "that most major disease classes have significant environmental and genetic components and that the incidence of disease in a population or individual is a complex product of the conditional probabilities of certain gene components interacting with a diverse range of environmental triggers." Above all, nutrition has a significant influence on many diseases, in that it modulates complex communication between the 100 trillion microorganisms in the intestines![169] "The microbes are part of our extended symbiotic genome and as such are in many ways just as important as our genes," says Nicholson.[170]

How easily this bacterial balance can be decisively influenced can be seen with babies: if they are nursed with mother's milk, their intestinal flora almost exclusively contains a certain bacterium (Lactobacillus bifidus), which is very different from the bacterium most prevalent when they are fed a diet including cow's milk. "The bacterium lactobacillus bifidus lends the breast-fed child a much stronger resistance to intestinal infections, for instance," writes microbiologist Dubos.[171]

This is just one of countless examples of the positive interaction between bacteria and humans. "But unfortunately, the knowledge that microorganisms can also do a lot of good for humans never enjoyed much popularity," Dubos points out. "Humanity has made it a rule to take better care of the dangers that threaten life than to take interest in the biological powers upon which human existence is so decisively dependent. The history of war has always fascinated people more than descriptions of peaceful coexistence. And so it comes that no one has ever created a successful story out of the useful role that bacteria play in stomach and intestines. Alone the production of a large part of the food that lands on our plates is dependent on bacterial activity."[172]

However, haven't antibiotics helped or saved the lives of many people? Without a doubt. But, we must note that it was only as recent as 12 February 1941, that the first patient was treated with an antibiotic, specifically penicillin. Therefore, antibiotics have nothing to do with the increase in life expectancy, which really took hold in the middle of the 19th century (in industrialized countries), almost a century before the development of antibiotics.[173]

And, plenty of substances, including innumerable bacteria essential to life are destroyed through the administration of antibiotics, which directly translated from the Greek, means, "against life."[174]

In the USA alone, millions of antibiotics are now unnecessarily administered, as American talk radio host Gary Null outlined in his article "Death by Medicine" (his book later appeared under the same title).[175] [176] [177] This has profound consequences, in fact antibiotics are held responsible for nearly one fifth of the more than 100,000 annual deaths that are traced back to medication side effects in the United States alone.[178] [179]

The over-use of antibiotics is also causing more bacteria to become resistant. Today, 70 percent of microbes held responsible for lung illnesses no longer respond to medications.[180] The increase in resistance prompts the pharmaceutical sector to conduct more intensive research for new antibiotics. But the discovery of such molecules is a long, difficult and costly process (about $600 million per molecule).[181] For many years, no important new antibiotic has come onto the market. At the same time, increasingly stronger preparations are being introduced, which only leads to the bacteria becoming even more resistant and excreting even more toxins.

A key question, such as the causes of pulmonary or middle-ear infection, cannot be answered by simply branding the microbes as lethal enemies and wiping them out. And yet people stick to vilifying the microbes because they are caught in their concept of the enemy and their tunnel vision is directed only at germs.

This is a perception that actually began with Louis Pasteur, who as an acclaimed researcher spread the opinion that bacteria lingered everywhere in the air. And so the idea was born that bacteria (like fungi and viruses subsequently) would fatefully descend upon humans and animals like swarms of locusts.

For about ten years, doctors even speculated that even heart attacks were an infectious disease, triggered by the Chlamydia pneumoniae bacterium. Because of this some patients were treated with antibiotics—but a study published in the *New England Journal of Medicine* stated quite plainly that there is no benefit from this.[182]

Another issue when considering reports that E. coli bacteria have been detected in drinking water, is the false notion that somehow on their forays these germs discovered a stream and then contaminated it. In fact, E. coli gets into drinking water through human or animal excrement, which serves as food for the bacteria.

Bacteria do not live isolated in an open atmosphere. Rather, they always exist together with cells and tissue parts.[183] Just like a fungal culture, a bacterial culture does not simply consist of bacteria or fungi; rather, a terrain always exists as well. And depending on the (toxicity of a) terrain, there are different (toxic) germs. Let's recall a well-known phrase from Claude Bernard (1813-1878), one of the best-known representatives of a holistic approach to health: "The microbe is nothing, the terrain is everything."

If we ask bacteriologists which comes first: the terrain or the bacteria, the answer is always that it is the environment (the terrain) that allows the microbes to thrive. The germs, then, do not directly produce the disease. So, it is evident that the crisis produced by the body causes the bacteria to multiply by creating the proper conditions for actually harmless bacteria to become into poisonous pus-producing microorganisms.

"Under close observation of disease progression, particularly in infective processes, damage to the organism occurs at the beginning of the disease—and only afterwards the bacterial activity begins," says general practitioner Johann Loibner. "Everyone can observe this in himself. If we put dirt into a fresh wound, other bacteria appear as well. After the penetration of a foreign body, very specific germs appear which, after removal or release, go away on their own and do not continue to populate us. If we damage our respiratory mucous membrane through hypothermia, then those bacteria accordingly appear which, depending on the hypothermia's acuteness and length, and the affected individual's condition, can break down the affected cells and lead to expulsion, catarrh."

This explains why the dominant medical thought pattern can't comprehend: that so many different microorganisms can co-exist in our bodies (among them such "highly dangerous" ones as the tuberculosis bacillus, the Streptococcus or the Staphylococcus bacterium) without bringing about any recognizable damage.[184] They only become harmful when they have enough of the right kind of food. Depending on the type of bacterium this food could be toxins, metabolic end products, improperly digested food and much more.

Even surgery makes use of this principle, using little sacks of maggots to clean wounds that are particularly difficult to sanitize. The maggots eat only the dead or "broken" material. They do not touch healthy, living flesh. No surgeon in the world can cleanse such a wound so precisely and safely as these maggots. And when everything is clean, the feast is over; the maggots don't eat you up, because the healthy tissue isn't suitable for them to eat.[185]

Pasteur finally became aware of all of this, quoting Bernard's dictum—"the microbe is nothing, the terrain is everything"—on his deathbed.[186] But Paul Ehrlich (1854-1915), known as the father of chemotherapy, adhered to the interpretation that Robert Koch (just like Pasteur in his "best days") preached: that microbes were the actual causes of disease. For this reason, Ehrlich, whom his competitors called "Dr. Fantasy,"[187] dreamed of "chemically aiming" at bacteria, and decisively contributed to helping the "magic bullets" doctrine become accepted, by treating very specific illnesses successfully with very specific chemo-pharmaceutical preparations.[188] This doctrine was a gold rush for the rising pharmaceutical industry with their wonder-pill production.[189] "But the promise of the magic bullet has never been fulfilled," writes Allan Brandt, a medical historian at Harvard Medical School.[190]

Viruses: Lethal Mini-Monsters?

This distorted understanding of bacteria and fungi and their functions in abnormal processes shaped attitudes toward viruses. At the end of the 19th century, as microbe theory rose to become the definitive medical teaching, no one could actually detect viruses. Viruses measure only 20-450 nanometers (billionths of a meter) across and are thus very much smaller than bacteria or fungi—so tiny, that one can only see them under an electron microscope. And the first electron microscope was not built until 1931. Bacteria and fungi, in contrast, can be observed through a simple light microscope. The first of these was constructed as early as the 17th century by Dutch researcher Antoni van Leeuwenhoek (1632-1723).

"Pasteurians" were already using the expression "virus" in the 19th century, but this is ascribed to the Latin term "virus" (which just means poison) to describe organic structures that could not be classified as bacteria.[191] It was a perfect fit with the concept of the enemy: if no bacteria can be found, then some other single cause must be responsible for the disease. In this case, a quote by Goethe's Mephistopheles comes to mind: "For just where no ideas are, the proper word is never far."[192]

The number of inconsistencies that arise from the theory of death-bringing viruses is illustrated by the smallpox epidemic, which even today people like to draw upon to stir up epidemic panic.[193] But was smallpox really a viral epidemic that was successfully overpowered by vaccines? "Medical historians doubt this," writes journalist Neil Miller in his book "Vaccines: Are They Really Safe & Effective?" "Not only were there no vaccines for scarlet fever or the Black Plague, and these diseases disappeared all the same."[194]

For example, in England, prior to the introduction of mandatory vaccinations in 1953, there were two smallpox deaths per 10,000 inhabitants per year. But at the beginning of the 1870s, nearly 20 years after the introduction of mandatory vaccinations, which had led to a 98 percent vaccination rate,[195] England suffered 10 smallpox deaths per 10,000 inhabitants annually; five times as many as before. "The smallpox epidemic reached its peak after vaccinations had been introduced," summarizes William Farr, who was responsible for compiling statistics in London.[196]

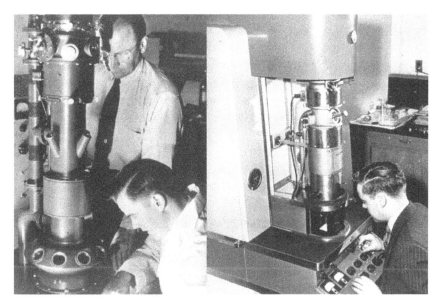

The photo on the left shows the first commercial electron microscope (the EM) from Radio Corporation of America (RCA), in 1940, operated by James Hillier with Alexander Zworykin, RCA's research chief and instigator of the EM project, looking on. This was followed in 1943 by the RCA "universal" EM, the EMU (right), which was capable of both imaging and diffraction. The EM, invented in 1931, first made it theoretically possible to see viruses for the first time. Viruses are not visible with a normal light microscope, but the EM uses fast electrons, which have a much smaller wavelength than visible light, to depict a sample's surface. And since a microscope's resolution is limited by the wavelength, a much higher resolution can be achieved with an EM (currently approximately 0.1 Nanometer = billionth of a meter) than with a light microscope (approximately 0.2 micrometers = millionth of a meter). Source: James Hillier 1915 - 2006: Contributions to Electron Microscopy, *www.microscopy.org*

From an orthodox view, the picture on the Philippines was no less contradictory: the islands experienced their worst smallpox epidemic at the beginning of the 20th century, even though the vaccination rate was at almost 100 percent.[197] And in 1928, a paper was finally published in the *British Medical Journal* that disclosed that the risk of dying from smallpox was five times higher for those who had been vaccinated than for those who had not.[198]

In Germany statistics of smallpox mortalities have been collected since 1816. There were around 6,000 smallpox deaths per year until the end of the 1860s. In the years 1870-1871, the number of victims suddenly jumped 14-fold to nearly 85,000 deaths. What had happened? The Franco-Prussian War was raging, and French prisoners of war were held in German camp under the most miserable conditions with extremely bad nutrition. As a result, the number of smallpox cases in the camps increased exponentially, even though all French and German soldiers had been vaccinated against smallpox. Germans (themselves suffering from the war) were likewise affected by the smallpox, although some of them had also been vaccinated.

When the camps were dissolved directly after the war, the number of smallpox deaths also markedly declined. Three years later, in 1874, there were only 3,345 smallpox deaths in Germany per year. Prevailing medicine says that this reduction was due to the *Reichsimpfgesetz*, a law that among other things stipulated that a child had to be vaccinated "before the end of the calendar year following his year of birth." But in fact, this law first came into effect in 1875, when the smallpox scare was long past. " At that time there must have been Improvements in hygiene, technology, and civilization, which led to the decline in diseases and deaths," says physician Gerhard Buchwald.[199]

Irrespective of this, mainstream viral research and medicine exclusively assumes that viruses are "infectious" pathogenic germs, which actively spread out in the cells in a parasitic way (with the assistance of enzymes and other cellular components) and multiply—ultimately attacking and sometimes killing cells. Or as a well-known German daily newspaper puts it, in the typical sensationalized manner: "Viruses are the earth's wiliest infectious agents: they attack animals and humans to enslave their cells."[200]

As thrilling as this may sound, no scientific backing is provided for this statement. To accept the theory, the existence of these so-called "killer viruses" must first be proven. And this is where the trouble begins because consequential, scientifically-sound evidence has never been provided. It should be as easy as taking a sample of blood from a patient and isolating one of these viruses, in a purified form with its complete genetic material (genome) and virus shell, and then imaging it with an electron microscope. But these critical initial steps have never been done with H5N1 (avian flu),[201] the so-called hepatitis C virus,[202] HIV,[203] [204] and numerous other particles that are officially called viruses and depicted as attack-crazy beasts.

At this point, we encourage our readers to verify dominant virus theories independent-ly — as many people have done, among them Nobel laureates, top microbiologists and researchers from other fields, serious journalists and lay people alike. We've asked for evidence from important institutions like the World Health Organization (WHO), the American Centers for Disease Control (CDC), and its German counterpart, the Robert Koch-Institute (RKI) in Berlin. In the summer of 2005, for example, we contacted the RKI and requested the following information:[205]

1. Please name the studies that indisputably show that the SARS, hepatitis C, Ebola, smallpox and polio viruses and the BSE causative agent have been proven to exist (complete purification, isolation and definition of biochemical properties plus electron micrographs).

2. Please name studies that indisputably show that the viruses named above cause disease (and also that other factors like malnutrition, toxins, etc. do not at least co-determine the course of disease).

3. Please name at least two studies that indisputably show that vaccinations are effective and active.

Unfortunately, to date we have not (despite repeated questioning) yet had a single study named to us.

Readers may wonder how it can be continually claimed that this or that virus exists and has potential to trigger diseases through contagion. An important aspect in this context is that some time ago, mainstream virus-science left the road of direct observation of nature, and decided instead to go with so-called indirect "proof" with procedures such as antibody and PCR tests.

Chapter 1

In this book, we will often stray from the well-traveled road, but at this point we must point out that these methods lead to results which have little to no meaning. Antibody tests just prove the existence of antibodies—and not the virus or particle itself to which the antibody tests react. That means: as long as the virus or cell particle (antigen) has not been precisely defined, no one can say what these antibody tests are reacting to; they are thus "nonspecific" in medical lingo.[206]

It is no different with PCR (polymerase chain reaction), which is used to track down genetic sequences, little genetic snippets, and then replicate them a million-fold. As with antibody tests, PCR probably has significance because it detects a sort of immune reaction (as it is called in technical terms) in the body; or, to put it more neutrally, some sort of disturbance or activity on a cellular level. But a virus with indeterminate characteristics cannot be proven by PCR any more than it can be determined by a little antibody test.[207] Again, this is because the exact virus determination has not been carried out. Even Robert Gallo conceded this in court in 2007.[208]

In terms of genetics, these short DNA or RNA pieces that are found using the PCR do not even satisfy the definition of a gene (of which humans are said to have 20,000 to 50,000, depending on criteria).[209] But even if scientists assume that the genetic sequences discovered in the laboratory belong to the viruses mentioned, this is a long way from proving that the viruses are the causes of the diseases in question, particularly when the patients or animals that have been tested are not even sick, which, often enough is the case.

Another important question must be raised: even when a supposed virus does kill cells in the test-tube (*in vitro*), or results in embryos in a chicken egg culture dying, can we safely conclude that these findings can be carried over to a complete living organism (*in vivo*)? Many issues contradict this theory, such as that the particles termed viruses stem from cell cultures (*in vitro*) whose particles could be genetically degenerate because they have been bombarded with chemical additives like growth factors or strongly oxidizing substances.[210] These effects were demonstrated with antibiotic use in a 2017 study.[211]

In 1995, the German news magazine *Der Spiegel* delved into this problem (something that is worth noting, when one considers that this news magazine usually runs only orthodox virus coverage), quoting researcher Martin Markowitz from the Aaron Diamond

AIDS Research Center in New York: "The scientist [Markovitz] mauls his virus-infected cell cultures with these poisons in all conceivable combinations to test which of them kill the virus off most effectively. 'Of course, we don't know how far these cross-checks in a test-tube will bring us,' says Markowitz. 'What ultimately counts is the patient.' His clinical experience has taught him the difference between test-tube and sick bed. He is more aware than most AIDS researchers of how little the behavior of cultured virus stems in incubator cells has to do with those that grow naturally in a network of hormones, antibodies, scavenger and T cells of the immune system of a living person."[212]

The chemist Andreas Meyerhans, when he was still working at the Institut Pasteur in Paris, used the phrase "To culture is to disturb," which basically means that the results obtained *in vitro* can lead to confusion.[213] [214]

"Unfortunately, the decade is characterized by climbing death rates, caused by lung cancer, heart disease, traffic accidents and the indirect consequences of alcoholism and drug addiction," wrote Sir Frank Macfarlane Burnet, recipient of the Nobel Prize for Medicine, in his 1971 book *Genes Dreams, and Realities*: "The real challenge of the present day is to find remedies for these diseases of civilization. But nothing that comes out of the labs seems to be significant in this context; laboratory research's contribution has practically come to an end. For someone who is well on the way to a career as a lab researcher in infectious disease and immunology, these are not comforting words."

To biomedical scientists and the readers of their papers, Burnet continued, it may be exciting to hold forth on "the detail of a chemical structure from a phage's [viruses from simple organisms; see below] RNA, or the production of antibody tests, which are typical of today's biological research. But modern fundamental research in medicine hardly has a direct significance to the prevention of disease or the improvement of medical precautions."[215]

But mainstream medicine avoids this wisdom like the devil does holy water. Instead, it has tried to demonstrate the pathogenicity (ability to cause disease) of these particles through experiments that could hardly be more arcane. For instance, test substrates were injected directly into the brains of lab animals. This was the procedure used for BSE and polio, for example; and even the famous Louis Pasteur had applied this method in his rabies experiments, in which he injected diseased brain tissue into the heads of dogs (Pasteur became famous through these experiments, and only years after his death were these studies found to be fraudulent).[216] [217] At least the industry now says that "direct injections into the brain" are unrealistic, and thus ultimately provide no evidence of pathogenic effects.[218]

Why not suppose that a virus, or what we term a virus, is a symptom—i.e. a result—of a disease? Medical teaching is entrenched in Pasteur and Koch's picture of the enemy, and has neglected to pursue the thought that the body's cells could produce a virus on its own accord, for instance as a reaction to stress factors. The experts discovered this a long time ago, and speak of "endogenous viruses"—particles that form inside the body's cells themselves.

In this context, the research work of geneticist Barbara McClintock is a milestone. In her Nobel Prize paper from 1983, she reports that the genetic material of living beings can constantly alter, by being hit by "shocks." These shocks can be toxins, but can also be from other materials that produced stress in the test-tube.[219] This in turn can lead to the formation of new genetic sequences, which were unverifiable (*in vivo* and *in vitro*) before.

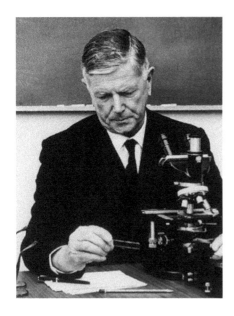

Sir Frank Macfarlane Burnet received the Nobel Prize for medicine in 1960; the photograph shows him in his laboratory in the microbiology department of the University of Melbourne (1965). © *Burnet, F. M. Collection, University of Melbourne Archives 89/34*

Long ago, scientists observed that toxins in the body could produce these physiological reactions, yet current medicine sees this only from the perspective of exogenous viruses. In 1954, the scientist Ralph Scobey reported in the journal *Archives of Pediatrics,* that herpes simplex had developed after the injection of vaccines, the drinking of milk or the ingestion of certain foodstuffs; while herpes zoster (shingles) arose after ingestion or injection of heavy metals like arsenic and bismuth or alcohol.[220]

It is also conceivable that toxic drugs like poppers, recreational drugs commonly used by homosexuals, or immunosuppressive medications like antibiotics and antivirals could trigger what is called oxidative stress. This means that the blood's ability to transport oxygen, so important for the life and survival of cells, is compromised. Simultaneously, nitric oxides are produced, which can severely damage cells. As a result, antibody production is "stirred up," which in turn causes the antibody tests to come out "positive." Also, new genetic sequences are expressed through this process, which are then picked up by the PCR tests[221] [222] — all this, mind you, without a pathogenic virus that attacks from outside.

But prevailing medicine condemns such thoughts as heresy. Just as the orthodoxy fought against McClintock's concept of "jumping genes" for decades, because they did not want a challenge of their model of a completely stable genetic framework. Here, they had not merely ignored McClintock, but even became downright "hostile," according to McClintock.[223] "Looking back, it is painful to see how extremely fixated many scientists are on the dominant assumptions, on which they have tacitly agreed," McClintock wrote in 1973, shortly after the medical establishment admitted, finally, that she had been right. "One simply has to wait for the right time for a change in conception."[224]

However, McClintock had no time to brace herself against the prevailing HIV = AIDS dogma. She did voice criticism that it has never been proven AIDS is triggered by a contagious virus.[225] But the Nobel Prize winner died in 1992, shortly after increased numbers of critics of the HIV = AIDS dogma had come into the game.

Whether Nobel laureate or layperson, ask yourself this simple question: how is it actually imaginable that killer viruses stalk the world bumping off one human cell after another? Viruses — as opposed to bacteria and fungi — do not even have their own metabolic apparatus. By definition, a virus' metabolisms is dependent on the "host" cell. They are composed of only one nucleic acid strand (DNA or RNA genes) and one protein capsule, so are missing the decisive attributes of living beings.

Strictly speaking, they do not count among "microbes," which comes from the Greek: "micro" = small, "bios"=life. How can viruses, like bacteria, be in a position to become active and aggressive of their own accord? Remember, it is said that viruses may have existed for three billion years.[226]

Exactly like bacteria and fungi, viruses are also said to be ubiquitous from the deep sea to the polar ice caps. A 2006 study published in the *Proceedings of the National Academy of Sciences*[227] found that there are more than 20,000 species of bacteria in a liter of seawater—the researchers had expected to find only 1,000 to 3,000 species.

"Just as scientists have discovered through ever more powerful telescopes that stars number in the billions, we are learning that the number of marine organisms invisible to the eye exceeds all expectations and their diversity is much greater than we could have imagined," says lead author Mitchell Sogin, director of the Massachusetts-based Marine Biological Laboratory (MBL) Center for Comparative and Molecular Biology and Evolution. "This study shows we have barely scratched the surface. The number of different kinds of bacteria in the oceans could eclipse five to 10 million."[228]

Furthermore, one liter of sea water is said to contain no less than 10 billion viruses of very simple organisms, like single-celled algae, called (bacterio)phages;[229] umpteen times as many viruses (phages) as bacteria. Both of these discoveries—the long development time and their universal existence—argue clearly that nature, which constantly strives for balance, lives in symbiosis with these viruses.

Luckily, the phages' omnipresence has flown below the radar of prevailing medical viral research—otherwise there would probably be regulations against bathing in the sea without full-body condoms or epidemic-protection suits, and only under the condition that we first take prophylactic antiviral medications. Or, why not try to disinfect large bodies of seawater.

We are already well on the way to this kind of thinking, since phages are already being presented as super villains that "work using wily tricks."[230] But there is no real proof here either.

We'd be wise to remember times in which the ruling dogma of viral killers was (freely and openly) sharply attacked and dismissed as pure "belief."[231] Indeed, there were many prominent microbiologists who insisted that bacteriophages just aren't viruses, but rather products "endogenously" produced, i.e. by bacteria themselves.[232] Robert Doerr, editor of the *Handbook of Virology*, published by Springer in 1938, even held the idea that not only phages, but also other "viruses" were the product of cells.[233]

Let's look at one of their arguments: bacteriophages cannot be living entities that become active independently, since phages themselves cannot be destroyed by temperatures as high as 120 degrees Celsius.[234] "And it would probably be of use to recall the history of this decade-long dispute," says Dutch microbiologist Ton van Helvoort, "for controversies and finding consensus are at the heart of scientific research."[235]

Chapter 2

The Microbe Hunters Seize Power

*"The doctor of the future will give no medicine, but will interest his patients
in the care of the human frame, in diet, and in the cause and prevention of
disease."*[236]
Thomas Edison (1847-1931), inventor legend

*"The conclusion is unavoidable: Pasteur deliberately deceived the public, in-
cluding especially those scientists most familiar with his published work."*[237]
Gerald Geison, medical historian

*"[Modern detection methods like PCR] tell little or nothing about how a
virus multiplies, which animals carry it, [or] how it makes people sick. [It
is] like trying to say whether somebody has bad breath by looking at his
fingerprint."*[238]
Appeal from 14 top virologists of the "old guard" to the new
biomedical research generation in *Science,* 6 July 2001

*"Biology is limitless, and our experiments are only drops out of an ocean that
changes its shape with every rolling wave."*
Erwin Chargaff, co-founder of biochemical research
"The Heraclitean Fire" (1978)

Pasteur and Koch: Two of Many Scientific Cheats

The elevated status Louis Pasteur enjoyed during his lifetime is made clear by a quo-
tation from physician Auguste Lutaud in 1887 (eight years before Pasteur's death): "In
France, one can be an anarchist, a communist or a nihilist, but not an anti-Pasteurian."[239]
In truth, however, Pasteur was no paragon with a divinely pure clean slate, but rather a
researcher addicted to fame acting on false assumptions and "he misled the world and
his fellow scientists about the research behind two of his most famous experiments," as
the journal *The Lancet* stated in 2004.[240]

In his downright fanatical hate of microbes, Pasteur actually came from the ludicrous equation that healthy (tissue) equals a sterile (germ-free) environment.[241] He believed in all earnestness that bacteria could not be found in a healthy body,[242] and that microbes flying through the air on dust particles were responsible for all possible diseases.[243] At 45 years of age, he "was basking in his fame," as bacteriologist Paul de Kruif writes in his book "Microbe Hunters," "and trumpeted his hopes out into the world: 'it must lie within human power to eliminate all diseases caused by parasites [microbes] from the face of the earth.'"[244]

Flaws in Pasteur's theories were shown long ago in the first half of the 20th century by experiments in which animals were kept completely germ-free. Their birth even took place by Cesarean section; after that, they were locked in microbe-free cages and given sterile food—after a few days, all the animals were dead.[245] In rats reared germ-free, the appendix was abnormally enlarged, filled with mucus, which would normally have been broken down by microbes.[246] This made it apparent that "contamination" by exogenous bacteria is abolutely essential to their lives.[247]

In the early 1960s, scientists succeeded for the first time in keeping germ-free mice alive for more than a fews days, namely for several weeks. Seminal research on these germ-free rodents was performed by Morris Pollard in Notre-Dame, Indiana.
However, this does not undermine the fact that germs are essential for life. Mice under natural conditions have a life span of three years, which is much longer than the average life span of these germ-free lab animals.[248]

The ability to keep germ-free animals such as mice or rats alive for a longer time requires highly artifical lab conditions in which the animals are synthetically fed with vitamin supplements and extra calories, conditions that do not exist in nature. These specially de-signed liquid diets are needed because under normal rearing conditions, animals harbor populations of microorganisms in the digestive tract.[249]

These microorganisms generate various organic nutrients as products or by-products of metabolism, including various water-soluble vitamins and amino acids. In the rat and mouse, most of the microbial activity is in the colon, and many of the microbially pro-duced nutrients are not available in germ-free animals. This alters microbial nutrient synthesis and, thereby, influence dietary requirements. Adjustments in nutrient concentrations, the kinds of ingredients, and methods of preparation must be considered when formulating diets for laboratory animals reared in germ-free environments or environments free of specific microbes.[250] [251]

One important goal in administering these artificial diets is to avoid the accumulation of metabolic pruducts in the large intestine. However, it has been observed that already after a short time the appendix or cecum of these germ-free reared rodents increased in weight and eventually became abnormally enlarged and filled with mucus, that is normally broken down by microbes.[252] Furthermore, in germ-free conditions rodents typically die of kidney failure[253]—a sign that the kidneys are overworked in their function as an excretion organ if the large intestine has been artificially crippled. In any case, it shows that germ-free mice would not be able to survive and reproduce while staying healthy in realistic conditions, which can never be duplicated by researchers artificially, not even approximately.

Apart from this, it is not clear that these germ-free animals have been truly 100 percent germ-free. Obviously not all tissues and certainly not every single cell could have been checked for germs. Nobody can know that these animals are absolutely germ-free, especially if one keeps in mind that germs such as Chlamydia trachomatis may "hide" so deeply in the cells that they persist there even after treatment with penicillin.[254]

Furthermore, even if the specimens of so-called germ-free animals are maintained under optimum conditions—assumed to be perfectly sterile—their tissues do, nevertheless, decay after a time, forming "spontaneous" bacteria. But how do we explain these "spontaneous" bacteria? They cannot come from nothing, so logic allows only one conclusion: the bacteria must have already been present in the so-called "germ-free" mice.

If nature wanted us bacteria-free, nature would have created us bacteria-free. Germ-free animals, which apparently aren't really germ-free, can only exist under artificial lab conditions, not in nature. The ecosystems of animals living under natural conditions—be it rodents or be it human beings—depend heavily upon the activities of bacteria, and this arrangement must have a purpose.

But back to "Tricky Louis"[255] who deliberately lied, even in his vaccination experiments, which provided him a seat on the Mount Olympus of research gods. In 1881, Pasteur asserted that he had successfully vaccinated sheep against anthrax. But not only does nobody know how Pasteur's open land tests outside the Paris gates really proceeded, but the national hero of *la grande Nation*, as he would later be called, had in fact clandestinely lifted the vaccine mixture from fellow researcher Jean-Joseph Toussaint,[256] whose career he had earlier ruined through public verbal attacks.[257]

And what about Pasteur's purportedly highly successful experiments with a rabies vaccine in 1885? Only much later did the research community learn that they did not satisfy scientific standards at all, and were thus unfit to back up the chorus of praise for his vaccine-mixture. Pasteur's super-vaccine "might have caused rather than prevented rabies," writes scientific historian Horace Judson.[258]

These experiments weren't debated for decades largely due to the fastidious secretiveness of the famous Frenchman. During his lifetime, Pasteur permitted absolutely no one — not even his closest co-workers — to inspect his notes. And "Tricky Louis" arranged with his family for the books to remain closed to all even after his death.[259] In the late 20th century, Gerald Geison, medical historian at Princeton University, was first given the opportunity to go through Pasteur's records meticulously, and he made the fraud public in 1995.[260]

That it became so controversial shouldn't be particularly surprising, for sound science thrives in a transparent environment so that other researchers can verify the conclusions made.[261]

Secretiveness has an oppositional goal: shutting out independent monitoring and verification. When external inspection and verification by independent experts are shut out of the process, the floodgates are open to fraud.[262] Of course, we observe this lack of transparency everywhere, be it in politics, in organizations like the international Football association FIFA, and also in "scientific communities [that] believe that public funding is their right, but so is freedom from public control," according to Judson.[263] With this, mainstream research has actually managed to seal off their scientific buildings from public scrutiny.

This set-up lacks critical checks and balances, so no one is ultimately in the position to scrutinize the work of researchers and make sure research is conducted in an honest way. We are left to simply trust that they go about it truthfully.[264] But, a survey taken by scientists and published in a 2005 issue of *Nature* showed that a third of researchers admitted they would not avoid deceptive activities, and would simply brush to the side, any data that did not suit their purposes.[265] A crucial aspect of science has also been lost; few researchers now trouble themselves to verify data and conclusions presented by fellow researchers.

Such quality checkups are equated with a waste of time and money and for that reason are also not financed. Instead medical researchers are completely occupied with chasing after the next big high-profit discovery. And many of today's experiments are constructed in such a complicated manner that they cannot be reconstructed and precisely verified at all.[266] This makes it very easy for researchers to ask themselves, without having to fear any consequences: why shouldn't I cheat?

In his 2005 paper "Why most published research findings are false," Stanford University Professor John Ioannidas says that most published research does not meet good scientific standards of evidence. Ioannidas also describes how many scientific studies are difficult or even impossible to reproduce. And he states, "the greater the financial and other interests and prejudices in a scientific field, the less likely the research findings are to be true."[267]

One would hope that the so-called peer review system largely eliminates fraud. It is still commonly considered a holy pillar of the temple of science, promising adherence to quality standards.[268] But the decades-long practice of peer review is rotten to the core.[269] [270] It functions like this: experts ("peers") who remain anonymous examine (review) research proposals and journal articles submitted by their scientific competitors.

These so-called experts then decide if the proposals should be approved or the articles printed in scientific publications. There are said to be around 50,000 such peer reviewed publications,[271] and all the best known journals such as *Nature, Science, New England Journal of Medicine, British Medical Journal and The Lancet*, are peer reviewed.

There is, however, a fundamental problem: peer reviewing, in its current form, is dangerously flawed. If researchers in other fields conducted studies and published results using this process, what would happen? If their current methods were common in the car industry, for example, BMW's competitors could decide, through an anonymous process, whether or not BMW would be permitted to develop a new car model and bring it to the market. Clearly this would stifle innovation and invite conflicts of interest and fraud.

Chapter 2

"Peer review is slow, expensive, a profligate of academic time, highly selective, prone to bias, easily abused, poor at detecting gross defects, and almost useless for detecting fraud," says Richard Smith, former Editor in Chief of the *British Medical Journal*.[272] No wonder, then, that all the cases of fraud which scientific historian Judson outlines in his 2004 book *The Great Betrayal: Fraud in Science* were not uncovered by the peer review system, but rather by pure coincidence.[273] And next to Pasteur in the pantheon of scientific fraudsters appear such illustrious names as Sigmund Freud and David Baltimore, one of the best-known recipients of the Nobel Prize for medicine[274] (we'll discuss Baltimore in more detail later in this chapter).

The other shining light of modern medicine, German doctor Robert Koch (1843-1910) was also an enterprising swindler. At the "10th International Medical Congress" in Berlin in 1890, the microbe hunter "with the oversized ego"[275] pronounced that he had developed a miracle substance against tuberculosis.[276]

And in the *German Weekly Medical Journal* (*Deutsche Medizinische Wochenzeitschrift*), Koch even claimed his tests on guinea pigs had proved that it was possible "to bring the disease completely to a halt without damaging the body in other ways."[277]

The reaction of the world-at-large to this alleged miracle drug "Tuberkulin" was at first so overwhelming that in Berlin, Koch's domain, sanatoria shot out of the ground like mushrooms.[278] Sick people from all over the world turned the German capital into a sort of pilgrimage site.[279] But soon enough, Tuberkulin was found to be a catastrophic failure. Long-term cures did not emerge, and instead one hearse after another drove up to the sanatoria. And newspapers such as the New Year's edition of the satirical *Der wahre Jakob* (*The Real McCoy*) jeered: "Herr Professor Koch! Would you like to reveal a remedy for dizziness bacteria!"[280]

In the style of Pasteur, Koch had also kept the contents of his alleged miracle substance strictly confidential at first. But as death rates soared, a closer inspection of the drug's properties revealed that Tuberkulin was nothing more than a bacillus culture killed off by heat; even with the best of intentions, no one could have assumed that it would have helped tuberculosis patients suffering from severe illness. On the contrary, all individuals—be it the test patients or the ones who were given it later as an alleged cure—experienced dramatic adverse reactions: chills, high fever, and death.[281]

64

Finally, Koch's critics, including another medical authority of that time, Rudolf Virchow, succeeded in proving that Tuberkulin could not stop tuberculosis. Rather, it was feared, according to the later scathing criticisms, that it made the disease's progress even worse. Authorities demanded that Koch brings forth evidence for his famous guinea pig tests— but he could not.[282]

Historian Christoph Gradmann said that Koch "cleverly staged" Tuberkulin's launch. Everything seemed to have been planned well in advance. In late October 1890, during the first wave of Tuberkulin euphoria, Koch had taken leave of his hygiene professorship. In confidential letters, he requested his own institute—modeled on the Institut Pasteur in Paris—from the Prussian state in order to be able to research his Tuberkulin extensively.

Professor Koch calculated the expected profit on the basis of a "daily production of 500 portions of Tuberkulin at 4.5 million marks annually." On the reliability of his prognosis, he dryly observed: "Out of a million people, one can reckon, on average, with 6,000 to 8,000 who suffer from pulmonary tuberculosis. In a country with a population of 30 million, then, there are at least 180,000 phthisics (tubercular people)." Koch's announcement in the *German Weekly Medical Journal* (*Deutsche Medizinische Wochenzeitschrift*) appeared simultaneously with excessively positive field reports by his confidantes, according to Gradmann, served "for the verification of Tuberkulin just as much as for its propaganda."[283]

Scurvy, Beriberi and Pellagra: The Microbe Hunters' Many Defeats

At the end of the 19th century, when Pasteur and Koch became celebrities despite their scams, the general public had hardly a chance to brace itself against microbe propaganda. Medical authorities, who adhered to the microbes = lethal enemies theory, and the rising pharmaceutical industry already had the reins of power and public opinion firmly in their hands. With this, the course was set for the establishment of clinical studies using laboratory animals, with the goal of developing (alleged) miracle pills against very specific diseases.

The scheme was so effective that even a substance like Tuberkulin, which caused such a fatal disaster, was highly profitable. Koch never even admitted that his Tuberkulin had been a failure. And Hoechst, a dye factory looking for a cheap entry into pharmaceutical research, got into Tuberkulin manufacturing. Koch's student Arnold Libbertz was to supervise production, with close cooperation from Koch's institute, and the rising pharmaceutical industry were decisively spurred on.[284]

From this point on, scientists tried to squeeze virtually everything into the model "one disease – one cause (pathogen) – one miracle cure," something that prompted one failure after another. For example, for a long time, the prevailing medical establishment asserted that diseases like scurvy (seamen's disease), pellagra (rough skin), or beriberi (miners' and prisoners' disease) were caused by germs. The orthodoxy finally admitted, through gritted teeth, that vitamin deficiencies were the true cause.

With beriberi, for instance, it was decades before the dispute over what caused the degenerative neural disease took its decisive turn when vitamin B1 (thiamine) was isolated in 1911 – a vitamin that was absent in refined foods like white rice. Robert R. Williams, one of the discoverers of thiamine, noted that, through the work of Koch and Pasteur, "all young physicians were so imbued with the idea of infection as the cause of disease that it presently came to be accepted as almost axiomatic that disease could have no other cause [than microbes]. The preoccupation of physicians with infection as a cause of disease was doubtless responsible for many digressions from attention to food as the causal factor of beriberi."[285]

Hippocrates, von Pettenkofer, Bircher-Benner: The Wisdom of the Body

The idea that certain microbes – above all fungi, bacteria and viruses – are our great opponents in battle, causing certain diseases that must be fought with special chemical bombs, has buried itself deep into the collective conscience. But a dig through history reveals that the Western world has only been dominated by the medical dogma of "one disease, one cause, one miracle pill" since the end of the 19th century, with the emergence of the pharmaceutical industry. Prior to that, we had a very different mindset, and even today, there are still traces everywhere of this different consciousness.[286]

"Since the time of the ancient Greeks, people did not 'catch' a disease, they slipped into it. To catch something meant that there was something to catch, and until the germ theory of disease became accepted, there was nothing to catch," writes previously mentioned biology professor Edward Golub in his work, *The Limits of Medicine: How Science Shapes Our Hope for the Cure*.[287] Hippocrates, who is said to have lived around 400 B.C., and Galen (one of the most significant physicians of his day; born in 130 A.D.), represented the view that an individual was, for the most part, in the driver's seat in terms of maintaining health with appropriate behavior and lifestyle choices.

"Most disease [according to ancient philosophy] was due to deviation from a good life," says Golub. "[And when diseases occur] they could most often be set aright by changes in diet—[which] shows dramatically how 1,500 years after Hippocrates and 950 years after Galen, the concepts of health and disease, and the medicines of Europe, had not changed" far into the 19th century.[288]

Even into the 1850s, the idea that diseases are contagious held hardly any support in medical and scientific circles. One of the most significant medical authorities of the time was the German Max von Pettenkofer (1818-1901), who tried to comprehend things as wholes, and so incorporated various factors into his considerations about the onset of diseases, including individual behavior and social conditions. To von Pettenkofer, the microbe-theoreticians' oversimplified, monocausal hypothesis seemed naive, something that turned him into a proper "anticontagionist."[289]

In view of the then-emerging division of medicine into many separate specialized disciplines, the scientist, later appointed rector of the University of Munich, jeered: "Bacteriologists are people who don't look further than their steam boilers, incubators and microscopes."[290]

Ultimately, it was von Pettenkofer who at this time led the discussion on the treatment of cholera, a disease so typical to rising industrial nations in the 19th century. He held the same position that the famous doctor François Magendie (1783-1855) had adopted back in 1831, when he reported to the French Academy of Sciences that cholera was not imported, nor contagious, but rather it was caused by excessive dirt as a result of catastrophic living conditions.[291] Correspondingly, the poorest quarters in centers like London were, as a rule, also the ones most afflicted by cholera.[292]

Von Pettenkofer identified drinking water as the main cause. There were no treatment plants in those days and water was often so visibly and severely contaminated with industrial chemicals and human excrement that people regularly complained about its stink and discoloration. Studies also showed that households with access to clean water had few to no cholera cases at all.[293] Although von Pettenkofer certainly didn't deny the presence of microbes in this cesspool, he argued that these organisms could contribute to the disease's course, but only when the biological terrain was primed so they could thrive.[294]

Unfortunately, von Pettenkofer's authority could not prevent adherents of the microbe theory from taking matters into their own hands. By the end of the 19th century, they squeezed cholera into their narrow explanatory concept as well. So a microbe (in this case the bacterium Vibrio cholerae or its excretions) was branded as the sole culprit—and Pasteurian microbe theory was falsely decorated for having repelled cholera. Golub was left shouting into the void: "Why does Pasteur get the credit for that which the sanitation movement and public health were primarily responsible?"[295]

The 1,500-year history of a holistic view of health and disease was much too connect-ed with life and its monstrous complexities to disappear altogether at the spur of the moment. Yet, it virtually disappeared from the collective conscience. Geneticist Barbara McClintock was of the opinion that the concepts that have since posed as sound sci-ence cannot sufficiently describe the enormous multi-layered complexities of all forms of natural life, and with that, their secrets. Organisms, according to the Nobel Prize winner for medicine, lead their own lives and comply with an order that can only be partially fathomed by science. No model that we conceive of can even rudimentarily do justice to these organisms' incredible capability to find ways and means of securing their own survival.[296]

By the beginning of the 1970s, Nobel laureate for medicine, Sir Frank Macfarlane Burnet had also become very skeptical about "the 'usefulness' of molecular biology, [especially because of] the impossible complexity of living structure and particularly of the infor-mational machinery of the cell. [Certainly, molecular biologists are] rightly proud of their achievements and equally rightly feel that they have won the right to go on with their research. But their money comes from politicians, bankers, foundations, who are not ca-pable of recognizing the nature of a scientist's attitude to science and who still feel, as I felt myself 30 years ago, that medical research is concerned only in preventing or curing human disease. So our scientists say what is expected of them, their grants are renewed

and both sides are uneasily aware that it has all been a dishonest piece of play-acting—
but then most public functions are."[297]

Certainly not all doctors have clamored for roles on the medical industrial stage and
some were key players in keeping the holistic health viewpoint alive. Swiss doctor Max-
imilian Bircher-Benner (1867-1939) directed his attention to the advantages of nutrition
after treating his own jaundice with a raw foods diet, as well as a patient suffering from
severe gastric problems. In 1891, long before the significance of vitamins and dietary
fiber to the human body had been recognized, Bircher-Benner took over a small city
practice in Zürich, where he developed his nutritional therapy based on a raw foods diet.

By 1897, only a few years later, the practice had grown into a small private clinic, where
he also treated in patients. There was strong interest in his vegetarian raw food diet from
all over the world, so, Bircher-Benner erected a four-story private sanatorium in 1904
called "Lebendige Kraft" (living force). Aside from a raw foods diet, Bircher-Benner (whose
name has been immortalized in Bircher-Muesli) promoted natural healing factors like
sun-baths, pure water, exercise and psychological health.[298] With this, he supported treatments that had become increasingly neglected with the appearance of machines and,
particularly, pharmaceuticals: attention to the natural healing powers of the body and the
body's cells, which possess their own sort of sensitivity and intelligence.[299]

Walter Cannon, professor of physiology at Harvard, also made holistic health his central
theme, in his 1932 work *The Wisdom of the Body*. Here, he describes the concept of ho-
meostasis, and underlines that occurrences in the body are connected with each other
and self-regulating in an extremely complex way.[300] "'Wisdom of the Body' is an attribute of living organisms," wrote Israeli medical researcher Gershom Zajicek in a 1999
issue of the journal *Medical Hypotheses*. "It directs growing plants toward sunshine,
guides amoebas away from noxious agents, and determines the behavior of higher
animals. The main task of the wisdom of the body is to maintain health, and improve its
quality. The wisdom of the body has its own language and should be considered when
examining patients."[301]

The words of biologist Gregory Bateson from 1970 are certainly still valid today: "[Walter]
Cannon wrote a book on the Wisdom of the Body; but nobody has written a book on the
wisdom of medical science, because that is precisely the thing it lacks."[302]

Clustering: How to Make an Epidemic
Out of One Infected Patient

After World War II, diseases such as tuberculosis, measles, diphtheria and pneumonia no longer triggered mass fatalities in industrialized nations such as affluent America. This became a huge problem for institutions like the Centers for Disease Control (CDC), the American epidemic authorities, as redundancy threatened.[303] In fact, in 1949, a majority voted to eliminate the CDC completely.[304] Instead of bowing out of a potentially very lucrative industry, the CDC went on an arduous search for viruses.[305] But, how to find an epidemic where there isn't any? You do "clustering."

This involves a quick scan of your environment — hospitals, daycares, local bars, etc. — to locate one, two, or a few individuals with the same or similar symptoms. This is apparently completely sufficient for virus hunters to declare an impending epidemic. It doesn't matter if these individuals have never had close contact with each other, or even that they've been ill at intervals of weeks or even months. So, clusters can deliver no key clues or provide actual proof of an existing or imminent microbial epidemic.

Even the fact that there are a few individuals having the same clinical picture does not necessarily mean that a virus is at work. It can mean all sorts of things including that afflicted individuals had the same unhealthy diet or that they had to fight against the same unhealthy environmental conditions (chemical toxins etc.). Even an assumption that an infectious germ is at work could indicate that certain groups of people are susceptible to a certain ailment, while many other people who are likewise exposed to the microbe remain healthy.[306]

For this reason, epidemics rarely occur in affluent societies, because these societies offer conditions (sufficient nutrition, clean drinking water, etc.) which allow many people to keep their immune systems so fit that microbes simply do not have a chance to multiply abnormally (although antibiotics are also massively deployed against bacteria; and people who overuse antibiotics and other drugs that affect the immune system are even at greater risk).

Just how ineffective clustering is in finding epidemics becomes evident, moreover, if we look more closely at cases where clustering has been used as a tool to sniff out (allegedly impending) epidemics. This happened with the search for the causes of scurvy, beriberi and pellagra at the beginning of the 20th century. But, as illustrated, it proved groundless to assume that these are infectious diseases with epidemic potential.

The most important example in recent times is the HIV=AIDS dogma because it laid the foundation for making even the corona/COVID-19 insanity a reality. At the beginning of the 1980s, a few doctors tried to construct a purely viral epidemic out of a few patients who had cultivated a drug-taking lifestyle that destroyed the immune system. We'll discuss how virus authorities manufactured this epidemic in chapter 3. For now, we'll quote CDC officer Bruce Evatt, who admitted that, the CDC went to the public with statements for which there was "almost no evidence. We did not have proof it was a contagious agent."[307]

Unfortunately, the world ignores all kinds of statements like this. So talk of the "AIDS virus" has since kept the world in epidemic fear and virus hunters are now the masters of the medical arena. Every cold, every seasonal influenza, every hepatitis disease, or whatever other syndrome has become an inexhaustible source for epidemic hunters armed with their clustering methods to declare ever new epidemics that pose threats to the world.

In 1995, allegedly, "the microbe from hell came to England," according to media scientist Michael Tracey, who was then active in Great Britain and collected media headlines like, "Killer Bug Ate My Face," "Flesh Bug Ate My Brother in 18 Hours," and "Flesh Eating Bug Killed My Mother in 20 Minutes." Tracey writes, "*The Star* was particularly subtle in its subsidiary headline, 'it starts with a sore throat but you can die within 24 hours.'" Yet the bacterium, known to the medical world as Streptococcus A, was anything but new. "Usually only a few people die from it each year," says Tracey. "In that year in England and Wales just 11 people. The chances of getting infected were infinitesimally small but that didn't bother the media at all. A classic example of bad journalism triggering a panic."[308]

In the same year, the US CDC sounded the alarm, warning insistently of an imminent Ebola virus pandemic. With the assistance of cluster methods, several fever cases in Kikwit, in the Democratic Republic of Congo, were separated out and declared as an outbreak of the Ebola epidemic. In their addiction to sensation the media reported worldwide that a deadly killer virus was about to leave its jungle lair and descend on Europe and the USA.[309]

Time magazine showed spectacular pictures of CDC "detectives" in spacesuits impermeable to germs and colorful photographs in which the dangerous pathogen could ostensibly be seen.[310] The director of the UN AIDS program made the horror tangible by imagining: "It is theoretically possible that an infected person from Kikwit makes it to the capital, Kinshasa, climbs into a plane to New York, gets sick and then poses a risk to the USA." Within a month, however, Ebola was no longer a problem in Africa, and not one single case was ever reported in Europe or North America.[311] And a publication in which the ebola virus has been properly proven is still nowhere to be found.

Polio: Pesticides Such as DDT and Heavy Metals under Suspicion

Practically all of the illnesses that affected people in industrialized countries in the decades before World War II (tuberculosis etc.) ceased to cause problems after 1945. For a few years, the major exception was polio (infantile paralysis), which continues to be called an infectious disease. In the 1950s, the number of polio cases in developed countries fell drastically—and epidemic authorities attributed this success to their vaccination campaigns. But a look at the statistics reveals that the number of polio victims had already fallen drastically when vaccination activities started (see diagram 2).

Many pieces of evidence justify the suspicion that the cause of infantile paralysis (polio) is not a virus. Many experts, like American physician Benjamin Sandler, believe a decisive factor is a high consumption of refined foods such as granulated sugar.[312] Others cite mass vaccinations. Indeed, since the beginning of the 20th century, it has been known that the paralysis so typical of polio have often appeared at the site where an injection has been given.[313] Additionally, the number of polio cases increased drastically after mass vaccinations against diphtheria and whooping cough in the 1940s, as documented in *the Lancet* and other publications.[314] [315] [316]

Polio, like most diseases, may be conditional on various factors. It makes particular sense, however, to take poisoning by industrial and agricultural pollution into consideration, to explain why this nervous disease first appeared in the 19th century, in the course of industrialization. It spread like wildfire in the industrialized West in the first half of the 20th century, while in developing countries, in contrast, there was no outbreak.
In the 19th century, the disease was named *poliomyelitis*, referring to degeneration of spinal column nerves (myelitis is a disease of the spinal cord) typical of polio.[317] Orthodox

medical literature can offer no evidence that the poliovirus was anything other than be-nign until the first polio epidemic, which occurred in Sweden in 1887. This was 13 years after the invention of DDT in Germany (in 1874) and 14 years after the invention of the first mechanical crop sprayer, which was used to spray formulations of water, kerosene, soap and arsenic.

"The epidemic also occurred immediately following an unprecedented flurry of pesticide innovations," says Jim West of New York, who has extensively investigated the subject of polio and pesticides. "This is not to say that DDT was the actual cause of the first polio epidemic, as arsenic was then in widespread use and DDT is said to have been merely an

Diagram 2   Die Polio death rates began to decline long before major inoculation campaigns were started

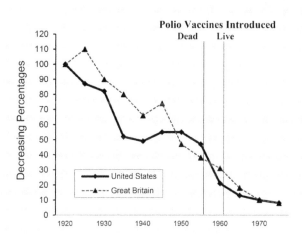

From 1923 to 1953, long before large-scale polio vaccinations began to be carried out in the mid-1950s, mortalities attributed to polio had already decreased substantially: in the USA by 47 percent; in Great Britain by 55 percent; in other European countries, the statistics are comparable. This diagram was reproduced with permission from the following book: Vaccines: Are They Really Safe and Effective? © Neil Z. Miller. Alle Rechte vorbehalten.

academic exercise. However, DDT or any of several neurotoxic organochlorines already discovered could have caused the first polio epidemic if they had been used experimentally as
a pesticide. DDT's absence from early literature is little assurance that it was not used."[318]

Nearly ten years before, in 1878, Alfred Vulpian, a neurologist, had provided experimental evidence for the poisoning thesis when he discovered that dogs poisoned by
lead suffered from the same symptoms as human polio victims. In 1883, the Russian
Miezeyeski Popow showed that the same paralysis could be produced with arsenic.
These studies should have aroused the scientific community, considering that the arse-
nic-based pesticide Paris green had been widely used in agriculture to fight "pests" like
caterpillars since 1870.[319]

"But instead of prohibiting the insecticide Paris green, it was replaced by the even more
toxic pesticide: lead arsenate, which likewise contained heavy metals, in the state of
Massachusetts in 1892," according to a 2004 article in the British magazine *The Ecologist*.[320] Indeed, a polio epidemic broke out in Massachusetts two years later. Dr. Charles
Caverly, who was responsible for the tests, maintained that a toxin was more likely the
culprit than a virus, stating emphatically that, "we are very certainly not dealing with a
contagious disease."

Within a short time, however, lead arsenate became the most important pesticide in
the industrialized world's fruit cultivation. It was not the only toxic substance used in
agricultural industries.[321] In 1907, for example, calcium arsenate was introduced in Massachusetts[322] and was used in cotton fields and factories. Months later, 69 children who
lived downstream from three cotton factories suddenly became sick and suffered from
paralysis. Meanwhile, lead arsenate was also being sprayed on the fruit trees in their
gardens.[323] But microbe hunters ignored these legitimate "cluster" factors, and instead
continued searching for a "responsible" virus.[324]

A cornerstone for the polio-as-virus theory was laid down in 1908 by scientists Karl Landsteiner and Erwin Popper, both working in Austria.[325] [326] The World Health Organization
calls their experiments one of the "milestones in the obliteration of polio."[327] That year,
another polio epidemic occurred and once again there was clear evidence that toxic
pesticides were at play. But, astoundingly, instead of following up this evidence, medical authorities viewed the pesticides as weapons in the battle against the arch enemy

microbes. They even neglected to give the children suffering from lameness treatments to alleviate the pesticide poisoning and, thus establish whether their health could be improved this way.[328] (In 1951, Irwin Eskwith did exactly that and succeeded in curing a child suffering cranial nerve damage – bulbar paralysis, a particularly severe form of po- lio[329] – with dimercaprol, a detoxification substance that binds heavy metals like arsenic and lead).[330] [331] [332]

Landsteiner and Popper instead chose to take a diseased piece of spinal marrow from a lame nine-year-old boy, chopped it up, dissolved it in water and injected one or two whole cups of it intraperitoneally (into the abdominal cavities) of two test monkeys: one died and the other became permanently paralyzed.[333] [334] Their studies were plagued by a mind-boggling range of basic problems. First, the "glop" they poured into the animals was not even infectious, since the paralysis didn't appear in the monkeys and guinea pigs given the alleged "virus soup" to drink, or in those that had it injected into their extremities.[335]

Shortly after, researchers Simon Flexner and Paul Lewis experimented with a comparable mixture, injecting it into monkeys' brains.[336] Next, they brewed a new soup from the brains of these monkeys and put the mix into another monkey's head. This monkey did indeed become ill. In 1911, Flexner even boasted in a press release, that they had already found out how polio could be prevented, adding, of course, that they were close to developing a cure.[337]

But this experiment shows no proof of a viral infection. The glop used cannot be termed an isolated virus, even with all the will in the world. Nobody could have seen any virus, as the electron microscope wasn't invented until 1931. Also, Flexner and Lewis did not disclose the ingredients of their "injection soup." By 1948, it was still unknown "how the polio virus invades humans," as expert John Paul of Yale University stated at an interna- tional poliomyelitis congress in New York City.[338]

Apart from that, it is very probable that the injection of foreign tissues in the monkeys' craniums triggered their polio-like symptoms (see Chapter 5: BSE). And when one consid- ers the amount of injected material, it can hardly be surprising that the animals became ill. Controlled trials weren't even carried out – that is, they neglected to inject a control group of monkeys with healthy spinal cord tissue. Neither did they assess the effects of chemical toxins like heavy metals injected directly into the brain.[339] [340] All of these factors make the experiments virtually worthless.

Although many scientific factors spoke against the possibility that polio was an infectious viral disease,[341] these studies would become the starting point of a decade-long fight, which concentrated exclusively on an imaginary polio virus.[342] Anything and everything, like brain parts, feces, and even flies were placed into the monkeys' brains in an attempt to establish a viral connection. Later these monkeys were even captured *en masse* in the Indian wilderness and transported overseas to the experimental laboratories—with the single aim of producing paralysis. And where virus hunters were working, vaccine manufacturers were not far away.

By the end of the 1930s, vaccine researchers had allegedly discovered a whole range of virus isolates. But these could not have been real isolates. The same holds for the photograph from 1953 that was said to be the first electron microscopic depiction of a polio virus. But the photograph shows nothing but white dots. In order to call these dots polio viruses with any certainty, the particles would have had to be purified, isolated, imaged with an electron microscope and precisely biochemically characterized. But no scientist has ever undertaken this, not even the so-called pioneers of polio research at the beginning of the 20th century, such as Karl Landsteiner, Erwin Popper, Simon Flexner and Paul Lewis; nor, decades later, Renato Dulbecco, Gilbert Dalldorf and Grace Sickles; nor Nobel laureates John Enders, Thomas Weller and Frederick Robbins.

The researchers did enthusiastically claim that they had "isolated" a virus; but in truth, they had done nothing more than take a sample of spinal tissue or even feces from a person or animal affected by polio, and inject this mix (which could have been laced with all sorts of things) into the brains of test animals. If the animals ultimately became ill, the researchers just assumed that a virus was responsible. But whatever made the animals ill; there was no proof that it was due to a virus, because the basic requirement of virus isolation (as described above) simply has not been fulfilled.[343]

And another problem cropped up along the way: the monkeys didn't get sick when they were orally administered the "glop." These researchers could only produce paralysis by injecting into the brain large amounts of substrates of unknown contents.[344] In 1941, the polio virus hunters had to accept a bitter setback, when experts reported in the scientific journal *Archives of Pediatrics* that, "Human poliomyelitis has not been shown conclusively to be a contagious disease." Neither has the experimental animal disease, produced by the so-called poliomyelitis virus, been shown to be communicable. In 1921, Rosenau stated that "monkeys have so far never been known to contract the disease 'spontaneously' even though they are kept in intimate association with infected monkeys."[345] This means that if this was not an infectious disease, no virus could be responsible for it, so the search for a vaccine was a redundant venture.

But virus hunters didn't even consider factors that lay outside of their virus obsession. By the middle of the 20th century, researcher Jonas Salk believed he had conclusively found the polio virus.[346] Even though he could not prove that what he called the polio virus actually triggered polio in humans, he still somehow believed he could produce a vaccine from it.[347]

Salk alone is said to have sacrificed 17,000 test monkeys (termed "the heroes" by one of Salk's co-workers) on the altar of vaccine research during the most heated phase of his research;[348] in total, the number of slaughtered monkeys reached into the hundreds-of-thousands.[349] But critics objected that what Salk termed the polio virus was simply an "artificial product of the laboratory."[350] Consequently, to this day, it is a huge challenge to find what is termed the polio virus where the patient's nerve cells are damaged, that is to say, in spinal cord tissue.[351]

In 1954, Bernice Eddy, who was responsible at that time for the US government's vaccine safety tests, also reported that the Salk vaccine had caused severe paralysis in test monkeys. Eddy was not sure what had triggered the paralysis symptoms: a virus, some other cellular debris, a chemical toxin? But it contained something that could kill. She photographed the monkeys and submitted them to her boss—but he rebuffed her concerns and criticized her for creating panic. Instead, of course, he should have taken her misgivings into account and started extensive inquiries. But Eddy was stopped by the microbe establishment and had to give up her polio research shortly before her warnings had proven themselves justified.[352]

On 12 April 1955, Salk's vaccine was celebrated nationwide as a substance that completely protected against polio outbreaks. US President Dwight Eisenhower awarded Salk a Congressional Gold Medal. American and Canadian television joined in the celebration. And on 16 April, the *Manchester Guardian* joined the party, stating that "nothing short of the overthrow of the Communist regime in the Soviet Union could bring such rejoicing to the hearths and homes in America as the historic announcement last Tuesday that the 166-year war against paralytic poliomyelitis is almost certainly at an end."[353]

But the triumph was short-lived. Medical historian Beddow Bayly wrote that "Only thirteen days after the vaccine had been acclaimed by the whole of the American Press and Radio as one of the greatest medical discoveries of the century, and two days after the English Minister of Health had announced he would go right ahead with the manufacture of the vaccine, came the first news of disaster. Children inoculated with one brand of vaccine had developed poliomyelitis. In the following days more and more cases were reported, some of them after inoculation with other brands of the vaccine."

According to Bayly, "Then came another, and wholly unlooked-for complication. The Denver Medical Officer, Dr. Florio announced the development of what he called 'satellite' polio, that is, cases of the disease in the parents or other close contacts of children who had been inoculated and after a few days illness in hospital, had returned home [and] communicated the disease to others, although not suffering from it themselves."[354]

Within only two weeks, the number of polio cases among vaccinated children had climbed to nearly 200.[355] On 6 May 1955, the *News Chronicle* quoted the US government's highest authority on viruses, Carl Eklund, who said that in the country, only vaccinated children had been afflicted by polio. And only, in fact, in areas where no polio cases had been reported for a good three-quarters of a year. At the same time, in nine out of ten cases, the paralysis appeared in the injected arm.[356]

This triggered panic in the White House. On 8 May, the American government completely halted production of the vaccine.[357] A short time later, a further 2,000 polio cases were reported in Boston, where thousands had been vaccinated. In "inoculated" New York, the number of cases doubled, in Rhode Island and Wisconsin, they jumped by 500 percent. And here as well, the lameness appeared in the inoculated arm in many children.[358]

Apart from that, an objective look at statistics would have shown that there was no reason to celebrate Salk's vaccine as the great conqueror of an alleged polio virus. "According to international mortality statistics, from 1923 to 1953, before the Salk killed-virus vaccine was introduced, the polio death rate in the United States and England had already declined on its own by 47 percent and 55 percent respectively," writes scientific journalist Neil Miller (see diagram 2).[359]

In the Philippines, only a few years before the US catastrophe, the first polio epidemic in the tropics occurred spontaneously, in fact, with the introduction of the insecticide DDT there.[360] Around the end of World War II, US troops in the Philippines had sprayed masses of DDT daily to wipe out flies. Just two years later, the well-known *Journal of the American Medical Association* reported that lameness among soldiers stationed in the Philippines could not be differentiated from polio, and it had advanced to become the second most common cause of death. Only combat exercises were said to have claimed more victims. Meantime, populations in neighboring areas, where the poison had not been sprayed, experienced no problems with paralysis.[361] [362] This is further evidence that DDT poisoning can cause the same clinical symptoms as polio (which is claimed to be conditional upon a virus).

Young people in industrialized countries are hardly acquainted with DDT anymore. It stands for dichlorodiphenyltrichloroethane, and is a highly toxic substance first synthesized in 1874, by Austrian chemist Othmar Zeidler. Paul Hermann Müller of Switzerland discovered its insect killing properties in 1939, for which he received the Nobel Prize for Medicine in 1948.[363] This resulted in its widespread use for pest control, even though there was already strong evidence that it was a severe neurotoxin and dangerous for all forms of life with associations that included the development of herpes zoster (shingles), paralysis, carcinogenesis and death.[364] [365] [366]

DDT is also problematic because it biodegrades very slowly in nature with a half-life of 10-20 years. Additionally, through the food chain, it can become concentrated in the fatty tissue of humans and animals. But this toxic substance wasn't outlawed until 1972 in the USA and even later in most other countries in the prosperous northern hemisphere. Today, its use is prohibited in a large part of the world and it one of the "dirty dozen" organic toxins that were banned worldwide at the Stockholm Convention on 22 May 2001.[367]

Industrial production of DDT started at the beginning of the 1940s. It was first used to fight malaria, and later became a sort of "all-purpose remedy" against all sorts of insects.[368] There was also military use of DDT: US army recruits were powdered with it to protect them from lice, and they additionally received DDT-sprayed shirts.[369] When the Second World War was over, DDT was sold on stock markets round the globe, even though strong warnings about its toxicity had been issued. "In the mid-40s, for example, the National Institutes of Health demonstrated that DDT evidently damaged the same part of the spinal cord as polio," writes research scientist Jim West of New York.[370] [371] [372]

The classic *Harrison's Principle of Internal Medicine* states, "Lameness resulting from heavy metal poisoning is clinically sometimes difficult to differentiate from polio."[373] Endocrinologist Morton Biskind came to the same conclusion in his research papers describing the physiological evidence of DDT poisoning that resembles polio pathology: "Particularly relevant to recent aspects of this problem are neglected studies by Lillie and his collaborators of the National Institutes of Health, published in 1944 and 1947 respectively, which showed that DDT may produce degeneration of the anterior horn cells of the spinal cord in animals. These changes do not occur regularly in exposed animals any more than they do in human beings, but they do appear often enough to be significant."[374]

Biskind concludes: "When in 1945 DDT was released for use by the general public in the United States and other countries, an impressive background of toxicological investigations had already shown beyond doubt that this compound was dangerous for all animal life from insects to mammals. It was even known by 1945 that DDT is stored in the body fat of mammals and appears in the milk. With this foreknowledge the series of catastrophic events that followed the most intensive campaign of mass poisoning in human history, should not have surprised the experts."[375]

Despite the fact that DDT is highly toxic for all types of animals, the myth has spread that it was harmless, even in very high doses. It was used in many households with a carefree lack of restraint, contaminating peoples' skin, their beds, kitchens and gardens.[376] In Biskind's opinion, the spread of polio after the Second World War was caused "by the most intensive campaign of mass poisoning in known human history."[377]

Along with DDT, the much more poisonous DDE was also used in the USA. Both toxins are known to break through the hematoencephalic ("blood-brain") barrier, which protects the brain from poisons or harmful substances. Nonetheless, housewives were urged to spray both DDT and DDE to prevent the appearance of polio. Even the wallpaper in children's rooms was soaked in DDT before it was glued on the wall.[378]

What from today's perspective seems like total blindness was at that time an everyday practice, not only in the United States. After 1945, DDT powder was used in Germany to fight a type of louse said to carry typhus.[379] And in agriculture, including fruit and vegetable cultivation, DDT was likewise lavishly dispersed for so-called plant protection. Through this, DDT gradually replaced its predecessor, lead arsenate, a pesticide containing heavy metals.[380]

A look at statistics shows that the polio epidemic in the USA reached its peak in 1952, and from then on rapidly declined. We have seen that this cannot be explained by the Salk-inoculation, since this was first introduced in 1955. There is a most striking parallel between polio development and the utilization of the severe neurotoxin DDT and other highly toxic pesticides like gamma-HCH (lindane), which is also slow to degrade and actually much more poisonous than DDT. While use of DDT was eventually drastically reduced because of its acknowledged extreme harmfulness, the use of lindane was curbed because it produced a bad taste in foods[381] (see diagrams 3 and 4).

"It is worth noting that DDT production rose dramatically in the United States after 1954," Jim West remarks, "which is primarily connected to the fact that DDT was increasingly exported to the Third World, to be used primarily in programs to fight malaria or in agriculture." As West points out, the following factors contributed to its changed use patterns in the US:

1. Legislation changes led to the use of warning labels, which in turn raised public awareness of DDT's poisonous nature.

2. Eventually, the use of DDT on dairy farms was prohibited. Earlier, Oswald Zimmerman and his fellow scientists had even advised the daily spraying of a 5 percent DDT solution directly on cattle and pigs, their feed, drinking water, and resting places.[382] In 1950, it was officially recommended to US farmers that they no longer wash cattle with DDT, but at first this advice was largely ignored. In the same year, cows' milk contained up to twice as much DDT as is necessary to trigger serious illnesses (diseases) in humans.[383]

3. In advertisements and press releases, DDT was no longer celebrated as being "good for you," "harmless," and a "miracle substance."[384]

4. From 1954, concentrated DDT was only used on crops that did not serve food production (for example, cotton).

5. DDT was used with more caution, something that caused decreased human intake of the poison through foodstuffs.

6. The use of DDT was extended to nationally sponsored forestry programs, so, for instance, entire forests were sprayed with it by airplane.

7. DDT was gradually replaced by allegedly "safe" pesticides in the form of organophosphates like malathion, but their uncertain toxicological effects and the new pesticides laws merely changed the type of neurological damage from acute paralysis to less-paralytic forms, such as chronic, slow-developing diseases which were difficult to define. This made it particularly difficult to prove in legal disputes or studies that these pesticides contributed to or directly caused the illnesses in question (see also Chapter 5, section: "BSE as an Effect of Chemical Poisoning" for more on the organophosphate phosmet).

Finally in 1962, US biologist Rachel Carson published her book, *Silent Spring*, in which she gives a vivid account of the fatal repercussions of extensive spraying of plant toxins on insects and particularly on birds, and predicts the consequence of a "silent spring" (without any songbirds). Through this, the public was made aware of the dangers of DDT.

But public reaction was slow, because 800 chemical companies reacted hysterically to Carson's book, prophesizing hunger and destruction if farmers were no longer permitted to use any pesticides. "The goal was very obviously to create panic and drive farmers into the arms of the chemical industry," as Pete Daniel, expert on the history of pesticides, writes in his 2005 book, *Toxic Drift*.[385]

In 1964, a North Carolina turkey breeder named Kenneth Lynch wrote to the Ministry of Health, stating that, since 1957, his home town of Summerville had been enveloped in a mist of DDT or malathion (an insecticide which can have wide-ranging neurotoxic and fatal effects)[386] every summer, in order to kill mosquitoes. And over the past years, his turkeys had "more or less abruptly developed advanced paralyses and, even though they had originally been in good health, died within two or three days."

At the same time, the fertility of the eggs had declined from 75 percent to 10 percent. "The evidence clearly indicated that the fog of insecticide is to blame," writes Lynch. With the help of a chemistry professor, he turned to the Public Health Service (PHS) and suggested carrying out corresponding studies. The national authorities, however, showed no interest whatsoever. "It seems to me [that the ministry's behavior] can hardly be interpreted as anything other than a case of bureaucracy being blinded by its own past mistakes," opined Clarence Cottam, a biologist honored by the National Wildlife Federation as a protector of nature.[387] [388]

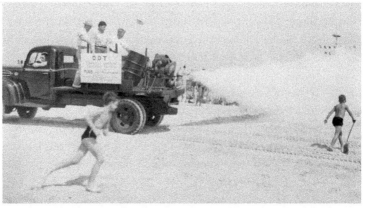

Bettmann / via Getty Images

20/20 HINDSIGHT

Even 40 years after exposure, DDT linked to breast cancer

By Justine Calma on Feb 15, 2019

On 15 February 2009, the American non-profit online magazine Grist published the article "Even 40 years after exposure, DDT linked to breast cancer." The article opened with a photo on which a pick-up truck can be seen, from which a beach with children playing is sprayed with DDT. The sign on the pick-up truck reads: "DDT—Powerful Insecticide, Harmless to Humans." The article states: "DDT was so widely used in the United States between the 1940s to 1970s that pretty much everyone at the time was exposed to some degree. The health risks associated with it were so poorly understood (and some say, overlooked) that it was sprayed directly on playing children. Author and scientist Rachel Carson called attention to growing concerns over the chemical with her seminal book, Silent Spring, published in 1962. But it would take another 10 years before DDT was banned in the U.S. ... According to a new study published this week in the Journal of the National Cancer Institute, women exposed to the pesticide DDT are still at risk for developing breast cancer four decades later. The findings are based on a 50-year longitudinal cohort of over 15,000 pregnant women, many of whom had been exposed to the pesticide before it was banned in the 1970s." Source: Screenshot from grist.org

In their refusal, political decision-makers and the chemical industry's lobbyists[389] referred primarily to the "prisoner studies" of PHS scientist Wayland Hayes.[390] In these experiments on prisoners, Hayes had aimed to show that it was completely harmless to ingest 35 milligrams of DDT per day.[391] But critics like Cottam objected that every test subject could release him/herself from the experiments at any time. And indeed, "there were a fair number who withdrew when they became a bit ill."

Since a number of prisoner test patients dropped out of the study, data on adverse effects were largely eliminated, so the study's results were worthless. Cottam points out that Hayes had most likely engaged in researcher bias to substantiate his initial views on pesticides: "Perhaps he is like many human beings who when subjected to criticism become more and more dogmatic in maintaining their initial stand." Pesti-

Diagram 3   Polio cases and DDT production in the USA, 1940-1970

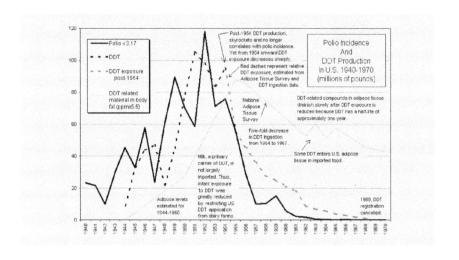

A look at statistics shows that the polio epidemic in the United States of America reached its peak in 1952, and from then on rapidly declined. We have seen that this cannot be explained by the Salk-inoculation, since this was first introduced in 1955. There is a most striking parallel between polio development and the utilization of

cide historian Pete Daniel goes a step further in saying that "[the officials in charge] knew better, but the bureaucratic imperative to protect pesticides led the division into territory alien to honesty."[392]

It would be years before the US government held a hearing on DDT and even longer until they finally prohibited it in 1972. Unfortunately, the government discussions were not widely reported, so the general public remained unaware of the connection between polio (in humans!) and pesticides, or other non-viral factors. To achieve this, in the beginning of the 1950's, ten years before Carson's *Silent Spring*, someone would have had to have written a bestseller which described the repercussions of DDT (and other toxins) in humans. Unfortunately, this was not the case; and even later on such a book has not appeared.

Diagram 4   Polio cases and pesticide production in the USA, 1940-1970

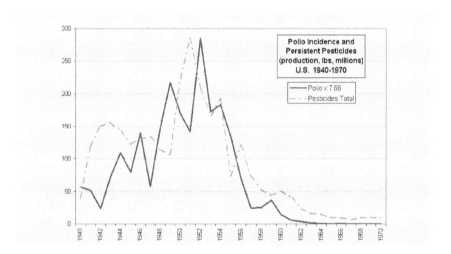

the severe neurotoxin DDT and other highly toxic pesticides. Sources: West, Jim, Pesticides *and Polio, Townsend Letter for Doctors and Patients, June 2000, p. 68-75; West, Jim, Images of Poliomyelitis; Handbook of Pesticide Toxicology, Eds.: Hayes, Wayland; Laws, Edward, Academic Press Inc., Harcourt Brace Jovanovich, Publishers, San Diego, 1991, p. 769; Historical Statistics of the US (1975), US Government Printing Office; Scobey, Ralph, Is Human Poliomyelitis Caused By An Exogenous Virus?, Archives of Pediatrics, 1954.* © Jim West

"Carson's book was good, but it was restricted to the damage to animals, whereas one looks in vain for descriptions of statistical trends or analyses in the work," says Jim West. "Even the research scientists Biskind and Scobey, who had clearly described the damage that DDT causes in humans in his 1952 study 'The Poison Cause of Poliomyelitis And Obstructions To Its Investigation,'[393] were practically unmentioned by Carson. Now who knows what kind of editorial censoring process her book had to go through before its publication." West points out that this type of censorship became the norm in future virus research: "One needs only consider that her work had been financed by the Rocke-

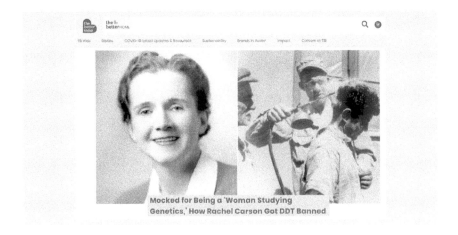

Mocked for Being a 'Woman Studying Genetics,' How Rachel Carson Got DDT Banned

On 19 August 2017, thebetterindia.com dedicated an article to "Silent Spring", published in 1962 and one of Rachel Carson's groundbreaking books that marked a new public awareness about the use of chemical pesticides, especially DDT, being published in 1962. In the article it says: "Carson was mocked and humiliated. A propaganda campaign was designed to discredit her findings, her publisher was bullied, some went as far as disregarding her qualification, only because she was a woman ... It was only in 1963, that Silent Spring gained President JF Kennedy's attention who called for a hearing to investigate and regulate the use of pesticides. An unwell Rachel prepared a 55 paged note with a list of eminent scientists who read and approved her manuscript. Her justifications and evidence, were strongly supported as right by President Kennedy's Science Advisory Committee. Silent Spring marked the beginning of an environmental movement, and DDT's agricultural use in the United States was banned in 1972. But unfortunately Rachel did not survive to see the day. She was posthumously awarded the Presidential Medal of Freedom." Source: Screenshot from thebetterindia.com

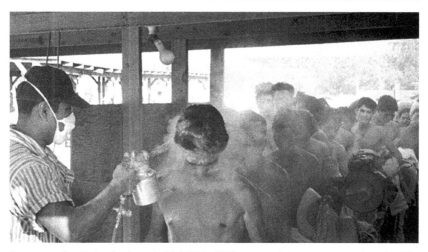

Bracero workers being fumigated with DDT in 1956 as part of the entry process into the US.
© Smithsonian Institution/Leonard Nadel

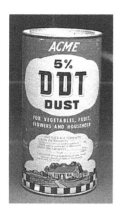

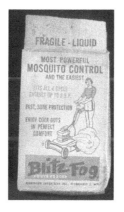

"Blitz Fog" pesticide package (1% DDT, plus the suspected carcinogens chlordane and lindane) from Northern Industries, Milwaukee, Wisconsin, USA; in gardens, the insecticide was dispersed with an atomizer ("Blitz Fog" thermalized insecticide dispenser) fastened to a motoroperated lawnmower's exhaust opening; in the early 1950s, the American chemical industry produced around 100 million pounds of DDT a year.
© From the collection of the Wisconsin Historical Museum, catalogue #1999.143.22

DDT dust "for vegetables, fruit, flowers, and household." © From the collection of the Wisconsin Historical Museum, catalogue #1999.143.20

87

feller Foundation. This makes one sit up and take notice, for the Rockefeller Foundation has supported the significant orthodox epidemic programs, including the HIV = AIDS research and numerous vaccination programs.

And William A. Rockefeller Sen. (1810-1906) had made his money by selling snake venom and pure mineral oil as anti-cancer drug. Carson's book prompted public out-cry, which contributed to DDT's ultimate prohibition. But this was a deceptive victory, which only helped to secure the public belief that democratic regulative mechanisms still functioned effectively. In actual fact, the chemical industry—because the public thought the poisonous demon had then been defeated—was able to establish its like-wise highly toxic organophosphate on the market without a problem. And, fatally, no-

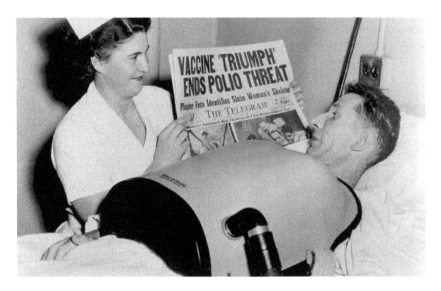

This photograph was taken on 13 April 1955 and features a beaming nurse showing a newspaper headline to a polio patient hooked up to a respirator. The caption reads: "Vaccine 'Triumph' Ends Polio Threat." In her gleefulness, the nurse entirely overlooks the psychological effect that the headline must have upon the seriously ill patient laying before her. It was too late for him to take this (purported) medical triumph, so he would have had to continue eking out his life as a paraplegic. Of course, there was, as shown, no vaccine triumph whatsoever, for the „polio spook" had largely passed before mass inoculations were finally carried out. © *March of Dimes Canada.* © March of Dimes Kanada

The Observer

Vaccines and immunisation

● This article is more than **4 years old**

A jab for Elvis helped America beat polio. Now doctors have recruited him again...

Film of Presley's 1956 publicity campaign is posted online to boost immunisation crusade against today's global threats

Robin McKie

Sun 24 Apr 2016 00.05 EST

f y ☑   387 43

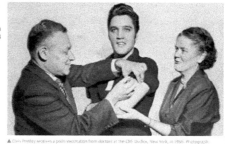

▲ Elvis Presley receives a polio vaccination from doctors at the CBS studios, New York, in 1956. Photograph:

In 1956, megastar Elvis was roped in for pushing the polio vaccine. The Observer *reported about it in 2016: "It was one of Elvis Presley's more unusual ventures. The king of rock'n'roll had just been enjoying his first taste of success with singles such as Heartbreak Hotel, and was about to appear on the Ed Sullivan Show in 1956, when he was given an unexpected medical challenge. Would he agree to be vaccinated against polio in front of the press before the show? He did. The resulting photographs were published in newspapers across the US. The publicity was part of a bid" to get more teenagers vaccinated against polio. Unfortunately,* The Observer *not only kept silent about the polio vaccine having nothing to do with the drop in polio cases, but also about the fact that test monkeys and children inoculated with the vaccine had developed the disease itself:* poliomyelitis. *Source: Screenshot from* theguardian.com

body discussed its important central topic: that poisons like DDT could cause severe damage like polio."

Gajdusek's "Slow Virus": Infinite Leeway for Explanations

The virus hunters still had many weapons to pull from their box of tricks. Such as the concept of the "slow virus": a virus capable of "sleeping" in a cell for years before striking with its pathogenic or fatal effects. The claim that a disease takes a very long time (decades) to "break out" gained popularity in the 1960s, when virus hunters convinced the medical establishment that the virus concept could even be imposed on cancer[394] [395] — that is, a disease that generally appears after years or decades.[396]

But despite a most arduous search, researchers were simply unable to find any active viruses in tumors. The disappointment and frustration was correspondingly great.[397] But a new theory was soon developed: that a virus could provoke an infection, then lie dormant in a cell for as long as it wanted—and finally, at some point, trigger cancer even when the virus is no longer present. Just as with polio earlier, the genome of a so-called slow virus has never been isolated and the particles claimed to be (slow) viruses have never been imaged with an electron microscope,[398] but the virus hunters embraced this suspect theory and adapted it to a number of modern ailments.[399]

Scientist Carleton Gajdusek prodded the slow virus concept along to serve not only an explanatory model for HIV/AIDS.[400] In the 1970s in Papua New Guinea, Gajdusek researched a sponge-like alteration in brain tissue associated with dementia, which was predominantly spread among the female population there.[401] The disease, called kuru, was only observed in two clans; they often intermarried, and, according to Gajdusek, maintained a cult of the dead ritual that involved eating the brains of their deceased (something which was later revealed as a myth).

These transmissible spongiform encephalopathies (softening of the brain), as they are called, appear sporadically and end, mostly fatally, within five years. They are generally extremely rare (approximately one case per million people), but are represented within some families with a frequency of 1 in 50, which could point to a genetic disposition.[402] Despite this Gajdusek received the Nobel Prize in 1976 for his slow virus concept. With this endorsement his idea that this spongelike alteration in brain tissue was produced by a transmissible pathogen achieved widespread acceptance as fact.

A close look at Gajdusek's trials on apes, with which he aimed to show transmissibility, should have shocked the scientific community into disbelief. But instead, they recognized these papers as proof of transmissibility and ignored the fact that neither feeding the apes brain mush, nor injecting them with it had any affect on the chimpanzees. So, Gajdusek conducted a bizarre experiment, in order to finally induce neural symptoms in the test animals.

He ground up the brain of a kuru patient into a mush full of proteins, along with a number of other substances, and poured this into the living apes by drilling holes into their skulls. This so-called disease's alleged transmissibility was founded only upon these experiments![403] How could it possibly derive proof of Gajdusek's cannibalistic hypothesis? Particularly since the hypothesis proposes that the disease could appear in humans through ingestion of infected brains, and not through direct surgical insertion into the brain.

To compound matters, Gajdusek was the only living witness of cannibalism on Papua New Guinea . He reported on these cannibalistic rites in his 1976 Nobel Prize-winning lecture, even showing photographs of the event. But in the mid-1980s, it was discovered that Gajdusek's photos, with which he aimed to document the cannibalism, actually showed pig flesh, not human flesh. An anthropological team looked into this claim and they did find stories of cannibalism, but no authentic cases.[404]

Gajdusek later had to admit that neither he himself, nor others he met had seen the cannibalistic rites.[405] Roland Scholz, professor of biochemistry and cellular biology (who died in 2011), responded to this revelation by saying that, "the scientific world seems to have been taken in by a myth."[406]

After World War II: Visible Proof of Viruses?
We Don't Need That!

Modern viral research is like Bigfoot hunting. Trackers of this legendary ape-like beast (also called Sasquatch and the Abominable Snowman) trot out the occasional questionable blurry photograph and footprint marks to claim proof of Bigfoot's existence. Based on this suspect data, they say the beast is up to ten feet tall and 440 pounds with 17-inch footprints that have even been made into plaster casts to prove its existence.[407] Virus hunters also collect dubious data, claiming to have evidence of the virus, even though an electron micrograph of the virus accompanied by an analysis its complete genetic material and virus shell is the only method of proving a virus's existence.

Bigfoot hunting, like viruses hunting, is a splendid moneymaker. Along a strip of California's Highway 101, numerous shops hawk Bigfoot-souvenirs[408] and they are popular with tourists even though it is generally accepted that Bigfoot is an invention.[409] Of course,

Bigfoot is nowhere near as lucrative as the international virus industry's multi-billion dollar business.

We must stress here that electron microscopy is fundamental to virus identification. For a long time, establishing unequivocal proof of a virus meant seeing is believing, as is the case with bacteria and fungi. The one difference is that bacteria and fungi can be seen with a light microscope, whereas viruses are so tiny that only an electron microscope (first patented in 1931) enables adequately detailed imaging to make them visible.

But, first you have to identify exactly what you're looking at, so these particles (possible viruses) must exist in a pure or purified form, in order to be able to differentiate virus particles from virus-like ones. At the beginning of the 1950s, virologists agreed that this was necessary, since, under certain conditions, even healthy cells produce a whole range of particles that could look like so-called tumor viruses (oncoviruses).[410] [411]

The importance of this process was confirmed at an international meeting of the Pasteur Institute in 1972,[412] [413] and "endured in the early 1980s," according to Val Turner, a physician and member of the Perth Group, an Australian research team.[414] "Viruses are not naked bits of RNA (or DNA). They are particles with particular sizes and shapes and other identifying features, which are obliged to replicate at the behest of living cells. They won't multiply in dead meat like bacteria. So there you have it. This predicates experiments to prove particles are a virus and that hasn't changed in a thousand years and certainly not since the 90s."

Turner uses easy-to-grasp language to describe the science: "Think of it like a paternity suit in which DNA evidence will be used and the accused is HIV and the child is a human. The crux of the case is proof that the DNA you found in the human is the same DNA you found in the accused. For the latter, you have to have rock solid proof the DNA came from the accused. Given that in cell cultures all sorts of particles appear, only some of which are viruses, you have to prove that (a) a particular particle is a virus; and (b) your DNA comes from that particle. How can you prove (a) without using electron microscopy (for many reasons) and without purification? You tell me.

"Frankly we from the Perth Group do not understand this obsession with 'old data' or 'science moves on.' Has Archimedes' principle 'moved on' that says that a body immersed in a fluid is buoyed up by a force equal to the weight of the displaced fluid—the principle applies to both floating and submerged bodies and to all fluids, i.e., liquids and gases? Do solid objects no longer displace their own volume of liquids? If everything has to be 'up to date' then in ten years nothing that is up to date now will be up to date then. Which means as long as time keeps going nothing will be right."[415] This goes for other orthodox theories as well!

By soundly characterizing the virus structure (virus purification), it is theoretically possible to irrefutably differentiate viruses themselves from virus-like particles. If this has taken place, the next step would be to get an electron micrograph of the purified virus (of course, proof that a virus exists does not automatically mean that this virus is also infectious, as had already been established in 1960, at a conference sponsored by the New York Academy of Sciences).[416] But this procedure is rarely carried out in modern viral research. Viruses that purportedly threaten to wipe out humanity (H5N1, SARS virus, etc.) have evidently never been seen by anyone.[417]

"Around 1960, before contemporary molecular biology arose, electron microscopy was held to be the best way of identifying viruses in cell cultures," writes pathology professor Etienne de Harven, a pioneer in electron microscopy and virology. De Harven's research career includes 25 years at the Sloan-Kettering Institute in New York, a private cancer research center founded in 1945, which quickly advanced to become the largest of its kind in the United States of America.[418] "For this reason, laboratories all over the world directed their efforts at this time towards observing particles in cancer cells with ever-improved methods of electron microscopy."

In 1962, the central role of electron microscopy was also recognized at the well-known Cold Spring Harbor Conference. André Lwoff, who would receive the Nobel Prize for medicine three years later, was among those who designated electron microscopy as likely the most efficient method of proving viruses' existence; he suggested investigating viruses with this procedure and dividing them into classes.[419]

A focus of medical science then (as now) was cancer. And because cancer researchers had the fixed idea that viruses were definitely cancer triggers,[420] they spent a lot of time trying to prove the presence of viruses in human cancer cells, with the help of electron microscopy. But, these efforts were unsuccessful. "One only found virus-like particles from time to time—while viruses of a certain types could never convincingly be seen," reports de Harven.[421]

Virus hunters were, once again, crushed by this scientific news. But the scientific world tends not to publicize negative results whenever possible—in scientific language, this is called, "publication bias."[422] Yet, whether the research claims promoted as evidence involve new patented drugs said to be superior to existing (cheaper) ones, or genetic markers of disease (interpreted as "risk" factors), or statistical relationships, discerning whether the claims are spurious or confirmed by clinical trials can only be ascertained by making the full body of controlled studies publicly available.

In medicine, failure to do so casts doubt on the safety and efficacy of treatments as well as undermining the integrity of the scientific literature. Scientific journals are supposed to protect the integrity of science—but they don't. As is the case with most deficient practices in medical research and practice, there is an unacknowledged financial motive. And why are scientists coy about publishing negative data? "In some cases," says Scott Kern of Johns Hopkins University and editor of the online *Journal of Negative Observations in Genetic Oncology*, "withholding them keeps rivals doing studies that rest on an erroneous premise, thus clearing the field for the team that knows that, say, gene A doesn't really cause disease B. Which goes to show that in scientific journals, no less than in supermarket tabloids, you can't believe everything you read—or shouldn't."[423] [424]

As long ago as the 1960s the established science community was coy about publishing negative data, but the cancer virus hunters' failures were so universal that it was simply inevitable that one article or another should leak out into medical publications. In 1959, the researcher Hagenaus reported in the journal *Etude du Cancer* about the difficulties identifying any typical virus particles in a wide range of breast cancer samples.[425] And in 1964, the scientists Bernhard and Leplus were unsuccessful, even with electron microscopy's assistance, in finding virus particles presumed to play a role in the development of Hodgkin's lymphoma (lymphatic cancer), lymphoid leukemia or metastases (tumors spread to various parts of the body).[426]

But these scientific studies didn't stop the virus hunters for a second. Instead of disengaging themselves from their virus tunnel vision, they grumbled about the methodology of virus determination: for example, over what are known as thin slices or thin-sections (tissue samples which are extremely precisely dissected and trimmed to size so they can be observed under the electron microscope). Thin-sections had proved effective countless times, and had also worked perfectly with mice.[427] But, the virus hunters needed a scapegoat and, instead of questioning the cancer-producing virus model, they started griping about the thin-sections. The production of the thin-sections was also thought to be too laborious and time-consuming. And who had the time for that once pharmaceutical companies began offering fast cash for quick fixes?

So, scientists turned to the much simpler and faster dye method, in which certain particles of the sample (for instance, DNA and RNA) were marked in color and then electron micrographed. But from a purely scientific perspective, the results of dye method are a disaster. Through the air-drying process that was necessary for the staining, the particles became totally deformed, so that they appeared as particles with long tails. They were full-blown artificial products of the laboratory, and they still looked exactly like so many other non-viral cellular components. This, logically, made it impossible to determine if a virus or a non-viral particle had been found.[428] [429]

A few scientists did in fact acknowledge that the dye method was dubious. But, instead of admitting defeat and returning to the thin-sections method, they began bashing electron microscopy technology! Other researchers were in turn so anxiously preoccupied with finally finding cancer viruses that they casually overlooked the worthlessness of dye method results, and theorized that the "tailed" particles were a certain type of virus. As absurd as this may sound to logical thinkers, virus hunters were even remunerated with plenty of research money for this action.

As a result, even cow's milk and mother's milk were tested for the presence of "tailed" particles in the mad rush to prove that viruses could produce cancer.[430] One well-known molecular biologist Sol Spiegelman even warned against breastfeeding in October 1971, and his message made for numerous lurid media headlines.[431] These so-called scientists brushed aside the fact that, to date, not a single retrovirus has been able to be isolated from breast cancer tissue (and probably not from human tumor tissue or blood plasma in general).[432] Shortly thereafter, Spiegelman was quoted in *Science* saying, "one can't kick off fear mongering on this scale if one doesn't exactly know if a virus particle is the cause."[433]

But mainstream viral research drifted purposefully further away from the well-established viral proof model. They latched on to Howard Temin's[434] and David Baltimore's[435] description of activity of the enzyme reverse transcriptase in connection with cancer viruses in 1970. Their research seemed so significant to the medical establishment that the two were awarded the Nobel Prize in 1975.[436]

What was so significant about this enzyme, a substance that, as a sort of catalyst, makes it possible for biochemical reactions to occur? To understand this, we must remember that, in the 1960s, scientists thought they had established that a few viruses did not possess any DNA (complete genetic information), but rather only RNA genes. This baffled the researchers since they believed viruses without any DNA (only with RNA) were not able to multiply. Until Temin and Baltimore delivered an explanation with the enzyme called reverse transcriptase. It, they said, can transform the RNA in RNA viruses (later called retroviruses because of this) into DNA, by which viruses are then able to multiply (if RNA exists alone, the conditions for replication are not met).[437]

But there was so much enthusiasm about the discovery of reverse transcriptase that virus hunters rashly assumed that reverse transcriptase was something very typical of retroviruses. They proclaimed something like this: if we observe reverse transcriptase activities in our test tubes (*in vitro*), then we can be sure that a retrovirus is present as well (even if the virus' existence has never been proven or reverse transcriptase's role hasn't been established, for instance, in the context of HIV).[438] Yet, it was presumed that the (indirectly detected) presence of reverse transcriptase was sufficient enough to prove the existence of a retrovirus, and even a viral infection of the tested cells *in vitro*.

This dogma would now become fixed in the minds of mainstream researchers and it opened the floodgates to allow indirect virus detection methods (known as surrogate markers) to take the place of direct detection procedures (virus purification and characterization as well as electron micrograph).[439]

So, in 1983, in a paper printed in *Science*, researcher Luc Montagnier of the Institute Pasteur in Paris, later celebrated as the discoverer of HIV, asserted that his research team had found a new retrovirus (which would later be named HIV).[440] This was claimed only after reverse transcriptase activity had been observed in the cell culture. But, once again, there was no scientific proof for this conclusion.

Eleven years before, in 1972, Temin and Baltimore had stated, "reverse transcriptase is a property that is innate to all cells and is not restricted to retroviruses."[441] And even Françoise Barré-Sinoussi and Jean Claude Chermann, the most important co-authors of Montagnier's 1983 *Science* paper, concluded in 1973 that reverse transcriptase is not specific to retroviruses, but rather exists in all cells.[442] In other words, if the enzyme (the surrogate marker) reverse transcriptase is found in the laboratory cultures, one cannot conclude, as Luc Montagnier did, that a retrovirus, let alone a specific strain of retrovirus has been found.

Reverse transcriptase is no longer the most significant surrogate marker, by a long shot. Now the virus hunters are fixated on antibody tests, PCR viral load tests, and helper cell counts. But these tests raise new questions, given their striking weaknesses (see chapter 3, "HIV Antibody Tests, PCR Viral Load Tests, CD4 Counts: As Informative as a Toss of a Coin"). This prompted 14 renowned virologists of the "old guard" to direct an appeal to the young high-technology-focused generation of researchers, which was published in *Science* in 2001:
"Modern methods like PCR, with which small genetic sequences are multiplied and de-tected, are marvelous [but they] tell little or nothing about how a virus multiplies, which animals carry it, how it makes people sick. It is like trying to say whether somebody has bad breath by looking at his fingerprint."[443]

No less remarkable, in this context, is an early 2006 article in the *German Medical Journal* (*Deutsches Ärzteblatt*) about a study by researchers who thought that, with the assistance of PCR, they had discovered new "exotic" bacteria. The article rightfully points out that, "only genetic traces of the pathogen are detected [with the PCR]. From this, it cannot automatically be concluded that complete bacteria exist as well."[444] [445]

The Virus Disaster of the 1970s – and HIV As Salvation in the 1980s

However, amongst the prevailing virus mania, such critical thoughts founder quickly. In the 70s, elite researchers were simply too busy channeling generous government aid into researching the possible connection between viruses and cancer. On 23 December 1971, US President Richard Nixon declared the "War on Cancer" at the behest of the medical establishment, and, with this metaphor, carried the militant tradition of the monocausal medical doctrine to the extreme, attached to the conception of viruses as the enemy. We had now become accustomed to talking about the "weapons," the "strategies," and the "arsenals" of cell-killing preparations—and weren't even taken aback when powerful people like Nixon called the new cancer war "a Christmas present for the people."[446]

To date, many hundred millions of dollars of research funds have been poured into this war (a good part of it paid by taxes)—and the results are staggering.[447] Back in 1971, a cure for cancer and a preventive vaccine were promised by 1976—but both of these are still nowhere in sight.[448] Incidentally, in the tradition of celebratory medicine, along with a trust that the public conscience and the media have short-term memory, the medical establishment rarely feels a need to keep its promises. "I am convinced that in the next decade or maybe later, we will have a medication that is just as effective against cancer … as penicillin against bacterial infections," boasted Cornelius "Dusty" Rhoads as early as 1953. He had been leader of the US Army's Department for Chemical Warfare (medical division of the US Chemical Warfare branch) during the Second World War, and was director of the Sloan-Kettering Institute for Cancer Research, founded in 1945.[449]

Death rates have meantime increased exponentially alongside skyrocketing research expenditures.[450] Today in Germany, 220,000 people die annually from cancer; in the USA, it is around 600,000. Even taking the aging of these populations into consideration, these numbers are staggering. For this reason, experts like George Miklos, one of the most renowned geneticists worldwide, criticized mainstream cancer research in *Nature Biotechnology* as "fundamentally flawed" and equated it with "voodoo science."[451]

By the late 1970s, medical experts lobbed damning critiques against mainstream cancer research. Medical scientists "had credited the retroviruses with every nasty thing—above all the triggering of cancer—and have to accept constant mockery and countless defeats," *Der Spiegel* pointed out in 1986.[452]

In addition to cancer, the concept that viruses are key causal factors has not been established with other diseases either. One notorious example is the swine flu disaster of 1976. During a march, David Lewis, a young American recruit, collapsed. Epidemic experts swooped in with their "magic wand" of clustering in their hands and claimed that they had isolated a swine flu virus from his lung. At the behest of the medical establishment, and particularly the US Centers for Disease Control (CDC), US President Gerald Ford appeared on TV and urged all Americans to get vaccinated against an imminent deadly swine flu epidemic.[453] Just like the Corona/COVID-19, the SARS and the avian flu fear mongers, Ford used the great Spanish flu pandemic of 1918 to scare the public into action.

Approximately 50 million US citizens rushed to local health centers for injections of a substance hastily thrown on the market. It produced strong side effects in 20 percent to 40 percent of recipients, including paralysis and even death. Consequent damage claims climbed to $2.7 billion. In the end, CDC director David Spencer, who had even set up a swine flu "war room" to bolster public and media support, lost his job. The ultimate bitter irony was that there were no, or only very isolated reports of swine flu.[454]

Consequently, at the end of the 1970s the US National Institutes of Health (NIH) came into unsettled political waters—just like the CDC, which was extensively restructured at the beginning of the 1980s. As a result, at the CDC and NIH, the most powerful organizations related to health politics and biomedical science, the great contemplation began. To redeem themselves, a new "war" would, of course, be the best thing.

Despite perpetual setbacks, an "infectious disease" remained the most effective way to catch public attention and open government pockets. In fact, Red Cross officer Paul Cumming told the *San Francisco Chronicle* in 1994 that "the CDC increasingly needed a major epidemic" at the beginning of the 80s "to justify its existence."[455] And the HIV/AIDS theory was a salvation for American epidemic authorities.

"All the old virus hunters from the National Cancer Institute put new signs on their doors and became AIDS researchers. [US President Ronald] Reagan sent up about a billion dollars just for starters," according to Kary Mullis, Nobel laureate for Chemistry. "And suddenly everybody who could claim to be any kind of medical scientist and who hadn't had anything much to do lately was fully employed. They still are."[456]

Among those who jumped over from cancer research to AIDS research, the best known is Robert Gallo. Along with Montagnier, Gallo who was also considered for a long time to be the discoverer of the "AIDS virus," enjoys worldwide fame, and has become a millionaire. In his previous life as a cancer researcher, on the other hand, he had almost lost his reputation, after his viral hypotheses on diseases like leukemia imploded.[457] "HIV didn't suddenly pop out of the rain forest or Haiti," writes Mullis. "It just popped into Bob Gallo's hands at a time when he needed a new career."[458]

Chapter 3

AIDS: From Spare Tire to Multibillion-Dollar Business

"If there is proof that HIV is the cause of AIDS, there should be scientific documents which either singly or collectively demonstrate that fact, at least with a high probability. There is no such document."[459]
Kary Mullis, Nobel Prize for Chemistry in1993

"Even with the greats of the AIDS establishment, Gallo does not hold back on psychiatric diagnoses. [According to Gallo,] one is a 'control freak', the next is 'uncreative' and has a 'complex' because of it, a third is – 'can I be honest?' – just plain 'crazy'. [Gallo's] impetuous anger is real when he speaks of the fight for power in the AIDS business, the fight for the money pot, the spiteful jealousy of prestige. With AIDS a lot of money is at stake – and above all fame."[460]
Der Spiegel, 29/1995

"[Freedom fighter John] Milton and Galileo would back the British Medical Journal on free speech [on HIV/AIDS]. We should never forget Galileo being put before the inquisition. It would be even worse if we allowed scientific orthodoxy to become the inquisition."[461]
Richard Smith, Editor in Chief of the *British Medical Journal* from 1991-2004, in a published letter to *Nature*

Whoever experienced the 1980's will still clearly remember: The AIDS panic picked up so quickly that there was no time for a survey of the facts. The media-stimulated fear of viruses had left behind such "traces in society," as the German weekly newspaper *Die Zeit* wrote in 1990, that "social psychologists even trace the imminent comeback of men's white underwear [as a symbol of HIV—and with that sterility right into the most intimate zones] back to the AIDS effect."[462] In 1984, *Der Spiegel*[463] announced that, by the middle of the 1990s, the last German would become ill from AIDS, dying from it two years later (as did the magazine *Bild der Wissenschaft*[464] the following year). A year earlier, the Hamburg-based magazine asked its readers: "Is a plague looming? Will AIDS come upon humanity lika an apokalyptic horseman on a black horse? ... 'Are humans also an endangered species?'" In comparison, a 1986 forecast in US magazine *Newsweek* sounded moderate: by 1991, five to 10 million Americans would be infected by HIV.[465]

In reality, no more than a few hundred Germans die annually from AIDS.[466] Moreover, these people actually die from traditional diseases (like Kaposi's sarcoma or tuberculosis), which are then redefined as AIDS (see below: "What is AIDS?"). And as for *Newsweek's* visions of horror: its prognosis was around ten times the 750,000 HIV cases identified by US authorities.[467]

750,000 is actually a cumulative number, since AIDS cases aren't tracked yearly, meaning that number represents the total number of cases since official AIDS records began in the early 1980s. Obviously, with such a method of measurement, the figures appear many times scarier than they actually are. Additionally, logic dictates that such numbers can only increase, even if the number of new cases had gone down in a given year. Incidentally, only AIDS cases are counted cumulatively.

Have you ever heard the evening news give the number of traffic accident deaths since the beginning of statistical records (and not 'just' the deaths for a given year)? Certainly not.

Strangely, the Robert Koch-Institute even admitted that they deliberately chose to record cases: "To catch the public's attention and encourage a political readiness to act, large numbers were naturally more suitable. A trick in the presentation of AIDS cases, applied internationally at the time, served to do this: in the first years, in contrast to other diseases where the number of new cases each year is given (incidence), AIDS cases were accumulated from year to year (cumulative incidence)."[468]

Anyone who impartially dives into the topic of HIV/AIDS, perpetually trips over such oddities, inconsistencies and contradictions—and searches in vain for scientific proof of the theory's basic hypotheses: that a virus called HIV, causes AIDS. At the same time, we are dealing with a very complex topic, so to make the controversies around the study of the cause of AIDS understandable, we will begin with a section which compactly explains why doubts that HIV exists and causes AIDS are justified—and why it makes sense to name factors like drug consumption or malnutrition as causes of AIDS, or better: of the many diseases grouped together under the term AIDS.

AIDS: What Exactly Is It?

Even the definition of AIDS (Acquired Immune Deficiency Syndrome) is anything but co-herent. In contrast to other diseases, there is no universal definition of AIDS that could be used as a basis for sound statistics.[469] For developing nations, for instance, the World Health Organization (WHO) introduced the "Bangui Definition" in 1986, with which many patients have been diagnosed with AIDS. According to this definition, anyone suffering from a few common and non-specific symptoms, like weight loss plus diarrhea and itch-ing, is declared an AIDS patient (without blood tests, and thereby without HIV antibody tests).[470] [471] In poor continents like Africa, where a third of the population is undernour-ished for decades, these symptoms are a well known mass phenomena.

Comparatively, in wealthy countries like the USA and Germany, people are declared to have AIDS if they have a "positive" antibody test, and simultaneously suffer from at least one of 26 — likewise well known — diseases, including the vascular tumor called Kaposi's sarcoma (KS), Hodgkin's disease, herpes zoster (shingles) or tuberculosis. If a patient has a negative antibody test and KS, they have KS. If, on the other hand, a patient tests „pos-itive" and has KS, they are an AIDS patient. But this type of definition is misleading — it is circular, since it is based on dubious, doubtful, unproven assumptions that HIV exists; that HIV can cause AIDS (or a disease like KS or herpes zoster); that a „positive" antibody test proves the existence of HIV, and so on.[472]

Where Is the Proof of HIV?

This HIV is said to belong to a certain class of viruses called retroviruses. In order to prove, then, that HIV is a specific retrovirus, it would first be necessary to isolate HIV as a pure virus, so that it can be imaged in a purified form with an electron microscope.[473] But all electron micrographs of so-called HIV taken from the mid-80s on, come, not from a patient's blood, but from "souped-up" cell cultures. In some cases the cells have been cooked up for a week in a lab Petri dish.

So-called AIDS experts didn't even try to make scientific sense of their co-culturing tech-niques until 1997, when Hans Gelderblom, of the Robert Koch-Institute in Berlin, took a stab at it.

But Gelderblom's article, published in the magazine *Virology*, leaves out the purification and characterization of the virus (merely the protein p24 was found), which does not prove that the particles are HIV. The second image of patient's blood came from the American National Cancer Institute. But the particles made visible (proteins, RNA particles) did not have morphology typical of retroviruses (let alone of a specific retrovirus).

Additionally, mainstream AIDS researchers claim that proteins like p24 and p18 are specific to HIV and they use them as HIV markers (surrogate markers), but in fact they are found in a number of so-called "uninfected" human tissue samples.[474]

Even Luc Montagnier, called the discoverer of HIV, admitted in an interview with the journal *Continuum* in 1997 that even after "Roman effort," with electron micrographs of the cell culture, with which HIV was said to have been detected, no particles were visible with "morphology typical of retroviruses."[475]

If even retrovirus-like particles cannot be recognized in these electron micrographs (let alone particles that match a retrovirus or a very particular retrovirus), this must logically mean that HIV—allegedly, a very specific retrovirus—cannot be detected. "Indeed, HIV has never been detected in a purified form," according to many renowned experts, including Etienne de Harven, the previously mentioned pioneer in electron microscopy and virology,[476] and the biologist Eleni Papadopulos and the physician Val Turner of the Australian Perth Group.[477]

Nonetheless, in 2006, it was proudly reported once again that "the structure of the world's most deadly virus had been decoded"[478] and that HIV had been photographed in "3-D quality never achieved before."[479] But a close inspection of the British-German research team's paper (published in the journal *Structure*),[480] shows that it doesn't live up to its promises:

-   Firstly, the study was supported by the Wellcome Trust,[481] and that the lead author, as well as another author, also work for the Wellcome Trust[482] that is fully in line with orthodox AIDS research and is very close to GlaxoSmithKline a pharmaceutical giant that makes multibillion dollar revenues from AIDS medications like Combivir, Trizivir and Retrovir (AZT, Azidothymidine).[483] These researchers—with clear conflicts of interest—will hardly be able to say that HIV has not been proven to exist.[484]

- Of the apparent 75 particles, the paper said that five had no well-defined core, 63 had a single core, three had a complete core plus part of a further core, while four particles had two cores; the particles with two cores were larger than those with only one.[485] "For one thing, one notices that no double-cores can be seen in the printed pictures," writes Canadian biologist and AIDS expert David Crowe, "and for another, the question arises: how can a virus have two cores at all? That would be something absolutely new!"

- In the majority of "single-cored" particles, the core was cone-shaped (morphology); in the remaining 23 particles, on the other hand, the cores were "tube-shaped" (cylindrical), triangular or simply shapeless.[486] Here as well, it is difficult to comprehend that all these particles with such different appearances could all belong to a very particular type of retrovirus (for that is what HIV is supposed to be).

- Particle sizes also varied greatly: The diameters measured by Briggs et al. ranged from 106 to 183 nanometer (one billionth of a meter). So let's compare the height of men and assume that the average man is 1.78 meters or 5.84 feet tall. If the margin measured by Briggs et al were carried over, we would get heights ranging between 1.30 and 2.25 meters (4.27 and 7.38 feet). This would hardly convince us that we were dealing exclusively with full-grown males—and that particles of such various sizes, (originating from one cell culture) are all of the same virus type.

- AIDS researcher Val Turner of the Australian Perth Group re-measured the diameters of the particles that were visible in diagram 1A of Briggs et al's paper.[487] This revealed that two of the particles (also called virions, which gives the impression that they belong to a virus that had invaded from outside) had diameters of even less than 100 nanometers.[488]

- The *Structure* article's authors themselves conceded that both printed images (which originated from one image) are "not representative" of the entire sample,[489] but that begs the question: what shapes and sizes are the particles in the pictures that were not shown? This information was not provided even when requested.

- In this context, according to relevant sources, the diameter of retrovirus particles (HIV is supposed to be a retrovirus, after all) are quoted as 100-120 nanometers,[490 491 492] something that clearly deviates from the 106-183 nanometers measured by Briggs et al.

- "It would have cleared up a lot in this context if scientists had undertaken a complete purification and characterization of the particles," as David Crowe remarks, "but this apparently did not happen." The researchers themselves say that only particles with "minimal contamination" were available.

- Not once is a virus purification method described in the *Structure* paper. In this regard, let's refer to an article by Welker et al, published in the *Journal of Virology* in 2000.[493494] They first say, remarkably, that, "it is important to have pure HIV particles" available, which confirms how important virus purification is for virus detection. However, they did not demonstrate that pure HIV had been extracted; it was also said "the electron microscopic analysis showed that the core preparations were not completely pure."

- And even if the particles were pure, the problem still arises that even after the purification process, cell components (known as microvesicles, microbubbles, and material of cellular origin) could be present, which even from an orthodox perspective are non-viral, although they may have the same size and density as so-called HIV. Unsurprisingly, we read in a paper published in the journal *Virology*: "Identification and quantization of cellular proteins associated with HIV-1 particles are complicated by the presence of nonvirion-associated cellular proteins that co-purify with virions."[495 496]

HIV = AIDS?

Is HIV the cause of AIDS? Let's allow the medical establishment to speak for itself. Reinhard Kurth, former director of the Robert Koch-Institute (one of the pillars of mainstream AIDS research), conceded in *Der Spiegel* (9 September, 2004): "We don't exactly know how HIV causes disease."[497] In the 1996 documentary *AIDS—The Doubt*, by French journalist Djamel Tahi (broadcasted on German Arte Television), Montagnier admitted to the same, saying, "there is no scientific proof that HIV causes AIDS."[498] And 12 years before, in 1984, Montagnier emphasized that, "The only way to prove that HIV causes AIDS is to show this on an animal model." But there is still no such model.[499 500]

The *California Monthly*, the UC Berkeley alumni magazine, confronted Nobel laureate Kary Mullis in an interview using a statement from another Nobelist, David Baltimore. "[Dear Mr. Mullis,] you mentioned Baltimore a moment ago. In a recent issue of *Nature*,[501] he said:

'There is no question at all that HIV is the cause of AIDS. Anyone who gets up publicly and says the opposite is encouraging people to risk their lives.'"

Whereupon Mullis replied: "I'm not a lifeguard, I'm a scientist. And I get up and say exactly what I think. I'm not going to change the facts around because I believe in something and feel like manipulating somebody's behavior by stretching what I really know. I think it's always the right thing and the safe thing for a scientist to speak one's mind from the facts. If you can't figure out why you believe something, then you'd better make it clear that you're speaking as a religious person.

"People keep asking me, 'You mean you don't believe that HIV causes AIDS?' And I say, 'Whether I believe it or not is irrelevant! I have no scientific evidence for it!' I might believe in God, and He could have told me in a dream that HIV causes AIDS. But I wouldn't stand up in front of scientists and say, 'I believe HIV causes AIDS because God told me.' I'd say, 'I have papers here in hand and experiments that have been done that can be demonstrated to others.' It's not what somebody believes, it's experimental proof that counts. And those guys [from AIDS orthodoxy] don't have that."[502]

Antibody Tests, PCR, CD4 Counts: As Uninformative as a Toss of a Coin

The most significant diagnostic tools of viral and AIDS medicine are:

1. Antibody tests (HIV tests)
2. PCR viral load tests
3. Helper cell counts (T-cells, or rather the T-cell subgroup CD4)

These are what is known as surrogate markers: alternative methods which doctors determine, on the basis of laboratory data, if someone is infected with HIV or not, and whether they have AIDS. Instead of using traditional methods for investigating whether real disease symptoms (so-called clinical endpoints) have occurred, AIDS doctors look at whether the number of CD4 cells has decreased within a certain time period; if so, the risk of contracting AIDS is said to be low. But as previously mentioned (see Chapter 2), the results given by these methods are highly dubious ways to detect viruses like HIV, the

SARS coronavirus, or the avian flu virus H5N1 and their pathogenic effects. Often enough, surrogate markers have led to misdiagnosis.[503]

Let's look first at the HIV antibody tests. They're based on an antigen-antibody theory, which assumes the immune system fights against these antigens (proteins from HIV), as they are called, which are seen by the body as foreign. Their detection triggers an immune reaction, or response, which in turn induces the formation of specifically targeted antibodies.

Now, since these so-called HIV antibody tests only prove the existence of antibodies (and not the antigen directly, which in this case would be parts of HIV), we have to assume that HIV must have been detected during the validation of the tests. Only then could one use the antigen to calibrate the antibody tests for this particular (HIV) antigen. That is, only in this way can one test whether HIV antibodies are present or not, and, if HIV has not been proven to exist, the tests cannot possibly be known definitively to react to it.

When you know this information, the antibody test manufacturer's insert isn't quite so surprising. It clearly states "there is no recognized standard for establishing the presence or absence of antibodies to HIV-1 and HIV-2 in human blood."[504] Reacting to this inter-esting fact, and in reference to a paper by the Australian Perth Group (published in the scientific journal *Nature Biotechnology*)[505] the German weekly newspaper *Die Woche* ran a headline calling it, "The AIDS Test Lottery." The article went on to say that "the antibody tests do not measure what they should: HIV infection. They also react to people who have overcome a tuberculosis infection. [Yet] the world's leading AIDS researchers at the Institute Pasteur in Paris reviewed the study before publication."[506]

But what do the tests react to, then, if not to HIV? As we've already noted with AIDS, a circular definition has also been used with the antibody tests: in the mid-1980s, the pro-teins which caused the tests to react most strongly were selected from blood samples from seriously ill AIDS patients, and used to calibrate the tests.

That these proteins have something to do with HIV, or at least are similar to a retrovirus of whatever type, has, however, never been proven.[507] And, in fact, antibody tests were not actually designed specially to detect HIV at all, as Thomas Zuck, of the American drug approval authority FDA, warned in 1986. Rather, blood tests should be screened for their resistance to false-"positive" reactions due to other germs or contaminants (something which also fits with what *Die Woche* wrote: that HIV tests "also reacted in people who had survived tuberculosis";[508] and also dozens of other symptoms, including pregnancy or simple flu, could cause a „positive" reaction).[509] [510]

But to stop using these HIV tests was "simply not practical," as Zuck admitted at a World Health Organization meeting. Now that the medical community had identified HIV as an infectious sexually transmitted virus, public pressure for an HIV test was just too strong.[511]

With HIV antibody tests, orthodox AIDS research turned traditional immunology up-side-down, by informing people who had „positive" antibody tests that they were suffering from a deadly disease. Normally, a high antibody level indicates that a person had already successfully battled against an infectious agent and is now protected from this disease. And since no HIV can be found in AIDS patients, the hunt for a vaccine is also an irrational undertaking.[512]

Even Reinhard Kurth, former director of the Robert Koch-Institute made a sobering comment in the *Spiegel* in 2004: "To tell the truth, we really don't know exactly what has to happen in a vaccine so that it protects from AIDS."[513]

Viral load measurements with the help of the polymerase chain reaction (PCR) are just as dubious and ultimately meaningless. As long as HIV has not been proven to exist, these tests cannot be calibrated for HIV—and they cannot be used to measure "HIV viral load." With the PCR method, mind you, not a complete virus, but only very fine traces of genes (DNA, RNA) may be detected and whether they come from a (certain) virus, or from some other contamination, remains unclear.[514]

Heinz Ludwig Sänger, professor of molecular biology and 1978 winner of the renowned Robert Koch Prize stated that "HIV has never been isolated, for which reason its nucleic acids cannot be used in PCR virus load tests as the standard for giving evidence of HIV." Not coincidentally, relevant studies also confirm that PCR tests are worthless in AIDS diagnosis: for example, "Misdiagnosis of HIV infections by HIV-1 viral load testing: a case series," a 1994 paper published in the *Annals of Internal Medicine*.[515]

In 2006, a study published in the *Journal of the American Medical Association* (*JAMA*) shook again the foundation of the past decade of AIDS science right to the core, inciting skepticism and anger among many HIV = AIDS advocates. A US nationwide team of orthodox AIDS researchers led by doctors Benigno Rodriguez and Michael Lederman of Case Western Reserve University in Cleveland disputed the value of viral load tests—the standard used since 1996 to assess the patient's health, predict progression to disease, and grant approval to new AIDS drugs—after their study of 2,800 "positively" tested people concluded viral load measures failed, in more than 90 percent of cases, to predict or explain immune status.

While orthodox AIDS scientists and others protest or downplay the significance of the *JAMA* article, Rodriguez's group stands by its conclusion that viral load is only able to predict progression to disease in 4 percent to 6 percent of (so-called) HIV "positives" studied, challenging much of the basis for current AIDS science and treatment policy.[516]

The same controversy plagues tests that count CD4 helper cells. Not a single study confirms the most important principle of the HIV = AIDS theory: that HIV destroys CD4 cells by means of an infection.[517] [518] Furthermore, even the most significant of all AIDS studies, the 1994 Concorde study, questions using helper cell counts as a diagnostic method for AIDS[519]—and many studies corroborate this.

One of these is the 1996 paper "Surrogate Endpoints in Clinical Studies: Are We Being Misled?" Printed in the *Annals of Internal Medicine,* this sctientific article casually concludes that CD4 count in the HIV setting is as uninformative as "a toss of a coin"—in other words, not at all.[520]

Following the news that viral load is not an accurate method of assessing or predicting immune status, the *Journal of Infectious Diseases* reported that helper cell counts may be "less reliable" measures of immune competence than the AIDS orthodoxy previously believed. The study conducted in Africa by the World Health Organization (WHO) revealed that so-called HIV negative populations can have T-cell counts below 350, a number that would, according to WHO guidelines, qualify for a diagnosis of AIDS in HIV "positive" populations.

Another "surprising" conclusion (from the point of view of the HIV = AIDS believers) from the same WHO study: HIV "positives" that started AIDS drug treatment with low helper cell counts had the same survival outcomes as HIV „positives" that began treatment with high T-cell counts![521]

"One of the most spiteful and most unhealing properties of scientific models is their capability to strike down truth and take its place," warns Erwin Chargaff, long-time professor at Columbia University's Biochemical Institute in New York. "And often, these models serve as blinkers, by limiting attention to an excessively narrow area. The exaggerated trust in models has contributed much to the affected and ingenuine character of large parts of current natural research."[522]

The biotechnology company Serono illustrates the ways in which such surrogate marker tests can be misused. The Swiss firm was suffering revenue losses with their preparation Serostim, which is supposed to counteract the weight-loss so typical of AIDS patients. So, at the end of the 1990s, Serono redefined this "AIDS wasting" and developed a computerized medical test, which would professedly determine "body cell mass." These tests were actually adopted by doctors.

And so it came about that doctors ordered Serostim when the tests showed patients had lost body cell mass, a treatment that could easily cost more than $20,000. The strange thing was that patients who, with the help of the tests, had been diagnosed with a reduced body cell mass, had in reality not lost any weight at all. On the contrary, some had even gained weight. The Serostim scheme was finally busted and, as a legal investigation showed, more than 80 percent of Serostim prescriptions had been unnecessarily ordered through the test's application. Michael Sullivan, the attorney in charge of the investigation, termed the tests "voodoo" magic, and they ultimately cost Serono more than $700 million in criminal fines. At that point, this was the third highest sum ever to be paid in such a judicial process.[523]

Illicit Drugs, Medicines and Malnutrition Lead to AIDS

There is much evidence that AIDS—that conglomerate of dozens of well known diseases—can substantially be explained by the intake of poisonous drugs and medications (antivirals, antibiotics, etc.) and by malnutrition.[524] Around 80 percent of all children declared to be AIDS patients are born to mothers who have taken intravenous drugs that destroy the immune system.[525] And the first people to be diagnosed as AIDS patients in the USA were all consumers of drugs like poppers, cocaine, LSD, heroin, ecstasy, and amphetamines, all of which have devastating effects on the immune system.[526] [527] [528] [529] [530]

The American National Institute on Drug Abuse was not alone in confirming the extreme toxicity and immunosuppressive effects of substances like heroin or poppers (nitrite inhalants) used among gay men.[531]

With poppers, the following chemical event takes place: poppers are nitrites, and when inhaled are immediately converted into nitric oxide. Through this, the blood's capability to transport oxygen is compromised; it oxidizes. The first areas to sustain damages through this oxygen deficiency are the linings of the smallest vessels (epithelia). When this damage develops malignantly it is called Kaposi's sarcoma—a vascular tumor that is diagnosed in many AIDS patients. And, as a matter of fact, tumor tissue is oxidized.[532]

This self-destructive process is particularly noticeable in the lungs, since poppers are inhaled and dead organic material is produced, which cannot be completely disposed of by the cells' weakened detoxification systems. At this point, fungi enter the game. Nature intended precisely this role for them because they ingest and metabolize all kinds of "waste." This explains why so many patients, termed AIDS cases, suffer from pneumocystis carinii pneumonia (PCP, also called pneumocystis jirovecii), a lung disease typically associated with strong fungal infestation (decay).

These patients' immune systems are weakened, which "is the common denominator for the development of PCP," according to Harrison's Principles of Internal Medicine. And the "disease [the immune deficiency upon which PCP develops] can be produced in laboratory rats by starvation or by treatment with either corticosteroids [cortisone] or cyclophosphamides."[533] In other words, with cell-inhibiting substances that are destructive to the immune system, just like AIDS therapeutics. This makes it obvious that there is no need for HIV to explain AIDS (which is nothing but a synonym for well-known diseases like Kaposi's sarcoma or PCP).

Correspondingly, the typical sufferer who is tagged as an "AIDS patient" suffers from malnutrition; particularly those affected in poor countries, but also many drug users who constitute the bulk of AIDS patients in wealthy countries. At the same time, studies show that a stress factor like drugs can trigger a new arrangement of genetic sequences (DNA) in the cells, whereby cell particles are formed—particles produced (endogenously) by the cells themselves (and interpreted by the medical industry as viruses invading from the outside, without any proof).[534] [535]

The Early 1980s: Poppers and AIDS Drugs

In 1981, five severely ill homosexual young men became the first characters in the AIDS story. American scientist Michael Gottlieb, from the Medical Center of the University of California in Los Angeles, had brought these five patients together after a search of several months, using the highly dubious clustering method (see chapter 2).[536] Gottlieb dreamed about going down in the history books as the discoverer of a new disease.[537] The afflicted patients suffered from the pulmonary disease pneumocystis carinii pneumonia (PCP). This was remarkable, because young men in their prime years do not usually suffer from this, but rather babies who come into the world with an immune deficiency, older adults, or those on immunosuppressive medication (which burdens or damages the immune system).[538]

The medical researchers apparently took no other factors into account concerning the causes, such as the patients' drug use. Instead, the medical establishment and above all the Center for Disease Control (CDC) gave the impression that the cause of PCP was completely mystifying, so the basis was set to launch a new disease. The CDC eagerly seized up Gottlieb's theses: "Hot stuff, hot stuff," cheered the CDC's James Curran.[539] It was so "hot," that, on 5 June 1981, the CDC heralded it as a red-hot piece of news in their weekly bulletin, the *Morbidity and Mortality Weekly Report* (*MMWR*), which is also a preferred information source for the media.[540]

In this *MMWR*, it was immediately conjectured that the puzzling new disease could have been caused by sexual contact, and was thus infectious. In fact, there was no evidence at all for such speculation, for the patients neither knew each other, nor had common sexual contacts or acquaintances, nor had they comparable histories of sexually transmitted diseases.

"Sex, being three billion years old, is not specific to any one group—and thus naturally does not come into question as a possible explanation for a new sort of disease," points out microbiologist Peter Duesberg of the University of California, Berkeley. "But buried in Gottlieb's paper was another common risk factor [criminally neglected by the CDC] that linked the five patients much more than specifically than sex." These risk factors included a highly toxic lifestyle and use of recreational drugs that were massively consumed in the gay scene, primarily poppers, or in medical jargon "nitrite inhalants."[541]

The term "inhalants" is used because these drugs are normally sniffed from a small bottle, and like the customary "poppers" expression the term can be traced back to the mid-19th century. In 1859, the vasodilatory effect that follows inhalation of amyl nitrite was described. This led to its first therapeutic use in 1867 as muscle relaxants for cardiac disease patients suffering from angina pectoris (chest pain). The original form of the drug was glass ampules enclosed in mesh: they were called pearls. When crushed between the fingers, they made a popping sound; hence, the colloquialism "poppers" evolved.[542]

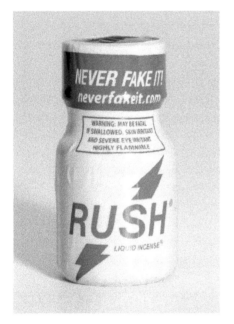

Poppers can be bought in approximately 5 cm (2 inches) high bottles. They're sold under names such as "room odorizer," "liquid aroma" or "RUSH– liquid incense"; warnings like "highly flammable" or "may be fatal if swallowed" are emblazoned in small letters on the brightly-colored vials.
© Alejandro Rodriguez

The US National Institute on Drug Abuse (NIDA) dates their use as recreational drugs from 1963.[543] From then on, the drug experienced a proper boom, assisted by the fact that in industrialized countries like the USA, drug consumption in general sharply increased in and since the 1960s and 1970s, the years of sexual and political revolution Between 1981 and 1993, the number of cocaine overdose victims delivered to hospitals jumped from 3,000 to 120,000.[544]

The gay scene made use of poppers' well-known muscle relaxant property. Taking poppers enables "the passive partner in anal intercourse to relax the anal musculature
and thereby facilitate the introduction of the penis," according to a 1975 report in the
journal *Medical Aspects of Human Sexuality*.[545] Poppers also helped prolong erection
and orgasm.[546] The substance was (and is) easy to make at home, and it is very cheap
to buy (a few dollars per vial).[547] At the same time, poppers were massively advertised
in popular gay media.[548] [549] And for promotional purposes, the drugs even had their
own comic strip spokesperson—a handsome blond hunk who promoted the (in truth,
irrational) idea that poppers make you strong and that every homosexual simply had
to take them.[550]

NIDA reported that the sale of poppers in just one US state added up to $50 million in
1976 (at $3 per vial, that equals more than 16 million bottles).[551] "By 1977, poppers had
permeated every angle of gay life," writes Harry Haverkos, who joined the CDC in 1981
and the American drug authoritiy NIDA in 1984 and who was the leading AIDS official
for both institutions. "And in 1979, more than five million people consumed poppers
more than once a week."[552]

Poppers can severely damage the immune system, genes, lungs, liver, heart, and the
brain. They can produce neural damage similar to that of multiple sclerosis, can have
carcinogenic effects, and can lead to "sudden sniffing death."[553] [554] Even the drug's label
warns it is "highly flammable; may be fatal if swallowed."[555] And the medical establishment knew about its various dangers. In the 1970s, the first popper warnings appeared
in scientific literature. In 1978, for instance, L.T. Sigell wrote in the *American Journal of
Psychiatry* that the inhaled nitrites produced nitrosamine, known for its carcinogenic
effects[556]—a warning which Thomas Haley of the Food and Drug Administration (FDA)
likewise articulated.[557]

In 1981, the *New England Journal of Medicine* (*NEJM*), one of the world's most significant
medical journals, published several articles singling out the so-called fast-lane lifestyle as a possible cause of AIDS.[558] [559] [560] This lifestyle is characterized by an extremely
poor diet and long-term intake of antibiotics and antifungal substances, which damage
the mitochondria, the cells' powerhouses (plus numerous other medicines, later primarily chemotherapy-like antiviral AIDS preparations including AZT, ddC, d4T, aciclovir
and ganciclovir).

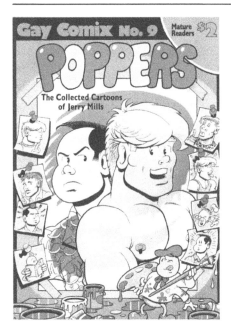

The toxic lifestyle drug poppers even got its own comic strip for promotional purposes—with a muscled and always cheerful blonde pretty boy as a hero. The character carried the message that the sex drug poppers makes one beautiful and strong and ever real gay just had to take it, which, as outlined, was simply nonsense. The image shows the cover of the gay comic "Poppers: The Collected Cartoons of Jerry Mills", number 9, winter 1986/87.

Besides poppers, many other, likewise highly toxic, drugs were on the menu, including crystal meth (methamphetamine), cocaine, crack, barbiturates, ecstasy (XTC), heroin, Librium, LSD, mandrex, MDA, MDM, mescaline, mushrooms, purple haze, Seconal, special K, tuinol, THC, PCP, STP, DMT, LDK, WDW, window pane, blotter, orange, sunshine, sweet pea, sky blue, Christmas tree, dust, Benzedrine, Dexedrine, Dexamyl, Desoxyn, clogidal, nesperan, tytch, nestex, black beauty, certyn, preludin with B12, zayl, quaalude, tuinal, Nembutal, amytal, phenobarbital, elavil, valium, darvon, mandrax, opium, stidyl, halidax, caldfyn, optimil, and drayl.[561]

David Durack asked the (still relevant) question in his lead article in the December 1981 *NEJM*: how can AIDS be so evidently new, when viruses and homosexuality are as old as history? Lifestyle drugs, according to Durack, should be considered as causes. "So-called 'recreational' drugs are one possibility. They are widely used in the large cities where most of these cases have occurred. Perhaps one or more of these recreational drugs is an immunosuppressive agent. The leading candidates are the nitrites [nitrite inhalants, poppers], which are now commonly inhaled to intensify orgasm."

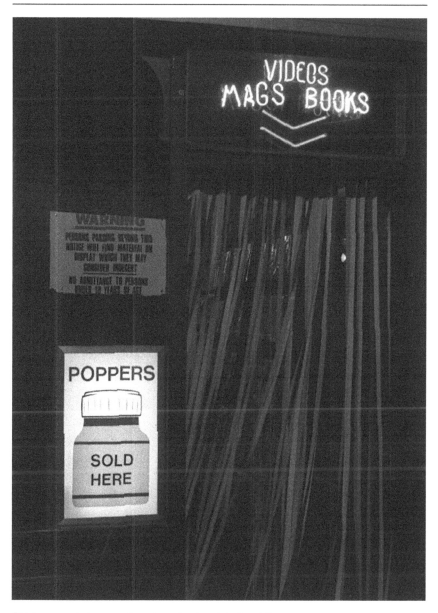

Poppers on sale in a sex shop. Source: Lauritsen, John. The AIDS War, 1993. © John Lauritsen

American author and AIDS chronicler Randy Shilts addresses this issue in his famous 1987 work *The Band Played On*: "[The poppers-AIDS starting point] would explain why the disease appeared limited to just three cities – to New York, Los Angeles and San Francisco, the three centers of the gay community,"[562] a conspicuous feature also described in the CDC's *MMWR* from 24 September, 1982.[563]

Durack additionally notes that, other than drug-using homosexuals, the only patients with AIDS symptoms were "junkies." In fact, in affluent nations like the USA or Germany, intravenous drug users have always made up a third of all AIDS patients, a fact that hasn't been acknowledged to the general public.

Immune system destruction is even more common among intravenous drug users than poppers-inhaling homosexuals. Junkies' lives are wrecked not by a virus, but (primarily) by excessive drug use over years. If the general public had known that a consistently high percentage of AIDS patients were intravenous drug addicts, perhaps the medical establishment would have been forced to study drugs as a possible cause of AIDS.

How the "Fast-Lane Lifestyle" Topic Went Out of Sight

A number of high-power organizations sought to prevent this message from getting through. First, the CDC purposely skewed their statistics. Their weekly bulletins divided AIDS patients into groups (homosexuals, intravenous drug users, racial minorities, hemophiliacs), yet they attributed a lower percentage to junkies than homosexuals. At one point, 17 percent were identified as drug users, and 73 percent were homosexuals, according to the CDC. This gave the impression that drug users were a less significant group among AIDS patients.

The CDC only admitted they played with the numbers to those who meticulously probed for more information. Journalist and Harvard-educated analyst John Lauritsen discovered that 25 percent of AIDS patients statistically labeled homosexual were also drug users. But the CDC simply lumped all of these gay drug addicts into the homosexual category. For this reason, the portion of drug users was officially 17 percent whereas in reality it should have been 35 percent (that is, more than one in three AIDS patients fits into the intravenous drug user category).[564]

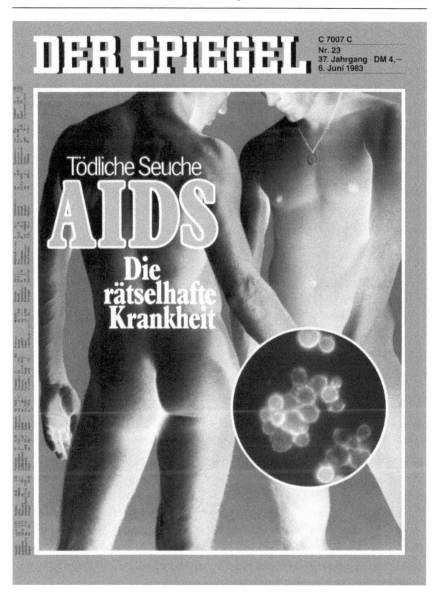

Der Spiegel 23/1983 © Der Spiegel A

Based at least in part on these skewed stats, the gay community certainly became active in the AIDS war and some became powerful gatekeepers of the AIDS establishment. "Gay men, some of them affluent and relatively privileged, found their way into private doctors' offices and prominent teaching hospitals—and from there into the pages of medical journals [and from there into the mass media]—while drug users often sickened and died with little fanfare," as sociologist Steven Epstein pointed out. And many reports in medical journals were penned by doctors who were very close to the gay scene and for that reason had treated many AIDS patients.[565]

The focus on homosexuals was so strong that, at the beginning AIDS was even called Gay-Related Immune Deficiency Syndrome (GRID).[566] Or simply, "gay-disease," primarily because clinicians, epidemiologists, and reporters perceived [the syndrome] through that filter of the 'gay men's health crisis,'" as Epstein outlines.[567]

It was also far from random that the first *Spiegel* cover on AIDS depicted two well-endowed young men, looking at each other's genitals (see picture). But with gays, the focus remained on the topic of sexual transmission, and drug use was not tied in. And so it was also said right at the beginning of the first *Spiegel* cover story in 1983: "An Epidemic That Is Just Beginning": "the gay epidemic, 'AIDS', a deadly immune deficiency, has reached Europe."[568]

These media messages quickly caused widespread belief and panic that a deadly contagious sexually transmitted epidemic was occurring, at least among gay men. Even though there was no scientific data to back these perceptions up and Gallo and Montagnier had yet to publish their 1984 papers, claiming to have discovered HIV as the cause of AIDS.

Why was the gay scene such a focus of interest? And the much more obvious connection between drugs and immune disorders ignored? Particularly since in developed countries, almost all patients said to have one of the immune deficiency diseases called AIDS have always been homosexuals and drug users. In other words, almost all AIDS patients take immunosuppressive and potentially deadly drugs and/or medications.[569]

Firstly, mainstream culture knew next to nothing about poppers and they are still used almost exclusively in the gay community. In the 1980s, gay organizations strongly objected to the idea that their much-loved drugs could play a role, particularly a decisive role, in the development of AIDS symptoms. The AIDS establishment, attached to its virus-fixation, also lured the community into their fold by creating opulently paid consulting contracts for important members of gay organizations. Pharmaceutical companies also invested money in the gay community with innumerable advertisements for AIDS medications, like a Hoffmann-La Roche ad reading, "Success creates courage," and a Wellcome ad for poppers calling amyl nitrite [i.e. poppers] "the real thing."[570]

The gay community even ignored urgent medical warnings from scientists about the dangers of poppers. Editors of *The Advocate*, a popular US magazine for homosexuals, ignored their letters, but accepted a whole series of poppers advertisements called "Blueprint for Health" from Great Lakes Products, at the time probably the largest manufacturer of sex drugs. "In this, it wrongly said that government studies had exonerated poppers from any connection to AIDS, and that poppers were harmless," writes analyst John Lauritsen, who has studied the topic of poppers and AIDS in depth.[571] These ads also suggested that poppers — just like vitamins, fresh air, exercise and sunshine — belonged to a healthy lifestyle,[572] and that they were an integral part of the gay community's "Fantasyland" and "wonderful land of drugs, parties and sex."[573]

The scene is no different today. Although certain versions of the drugs were prohibited because of high toxicity in 1988 and 1990, promotional websites for the lifestyle drug, such as bearcityweb.com or allaboutpoppers.com claimed that "poppers are the closest thing to a true aphrodisiac that exists today, and in addition they have been shown to be among the safest and most pleasurable compounds the world has ever seen."[574] [575]

Many important gay publications and organizations continue to promote poppers and censor data on adverse effects. This has had devastating consequences in society, since the gay media play an important role in informing and educating writers and journalists, who themselves deliver important messages about AIDS to the general public. "Indeed, some media organs of the AIDS movement, such as *AIDS Treatment News*, are widely recognized as agenda-setting vehicles for the circulation of scientific knowledge, and are read by activists, doctors, and researchers alike," writes Steven Epstein.[576]

A further decisive building block towards the way to the construction of the dogma that AIDS is a contagious viral disease was the behavior of the Centers for Disease Control

(CDC). From the beginning, they were unwilling to explore the drug connection.[577] [578] The CDC were set on the search for a deadly virus, without hesitating to suppress disagreeable data. In 1982, their own AIDS expert Haverkos analyzed three surveys of AIDS patients conducted by the CDC. He came to the conclusion that drugs like poppers did play a weighty role in disease onset.

But the CDC refused to publish their own high-ranking employee's study, and Haverkos transferred to the FDA in 1984 to become AIDS coordinator there.[579] The paper finally appeared in the journal *Sexually Transmitted Diseases* in 1985.[580] This prompted the *Wall Street Journal* to pen an article unambiguously stating that drug abuse was so universal among AIDS patients that this, and not the virus, must be considered the primary cause of AIDS.[581]

But such reports fell on deaf ears, for the world had already been sent down the virus road years before. Talk of drug factors ended with the CDC's second AIDS-related *MMWR* (3 July, 1981), in which further "highly unusual cases of Kaposi's sarcoma" were reported.[582] This had a viral effect upon media coverage. "When the first reports of the peculiar deadly illness from California began to wash up here, the CDC releases were our only proper source of information," remembers Hans Halter, who penned the *Spiegel*'s first cover story on AIDS. Its headline: "An epidemic that is just beginning."

Halter, himself a specialist in sexually transmitted diseases, had, as he relates, looked through the CDC data with a virologist friend. "It was clear to us," Halter claims, "that a retrovirus transmitted through sperm and blood was to blame!"[583] Halter admitted in that story that the "immune system [in homosexuals], as scientific examinations show, is also compromised through antibiotic treatment, drug consumption, and intensive use of poppers."

Yet, incomprehensibly, in the very same article, only a few paragraphs previously, Halter wrote: "First, the 'poppers' hypothesis collapsed: a control group of non-AIDS-infected homosexuals also took the stimulant, which expands blood vessels and is said to improve orgasm."[584] Not only does this contradict Halter's own understanding that a drug lifestyle damages the immune system. Also, even if the experiment Halter mentioned had actually existed, this is still a far cry from demolishing the hypothesis that poppers play a (significant) role in the onset of the disease symptoms termed AIDS.

You would think this writer must have first reviewed this study to come to such a conclusion. What exactly was being investigated? Was the paper compiled without bias or conflicts of interest? Is the argument conclusive? We don't know because no such study has ever been conducted. It's no wonder that Halter couldn't name the study upon request. Instead, he recommended looking in Shilts' book, *And the Band Played On*, adding, "maybe there are answers in it."[585] Indeed there are. According to Shilts, the poppers starting-point does offer an explanation for AIDS. "Everybody who got diseases seemed to snort poppers," writes Shilts.[586]

Of course, there will always be people who take drugs like poppers and do not get one of the AIDS diseases like lymphoma. But dosage and the length of time a person uses a drug, as well as other individual behavior patterns, living conditions, and genetic make-up always play a role. Just as a casual smoker is less likely to get lung cancer than a chronic smoker.

New York, February 2005: From Super-Drug Consumer to "Super-AIDS-Virus" Patient

On 11 February 2005, Dr. Thomas Frieden, a New York City health official, stepped up to the microphone and announced the discovery of a supposedly deadly new strain of HIV that was resistant to around 20 different AIDS medications. The world press went ballistic. German newspaper *Die Welt* headlined: "Super-AIDS in New York," and the *Süddeutsche Zeitung* speculated that the one gay male whose illness had led to Dr. Frieden's big announcement had become infected with the virus at a "bareback party," a gay sex party (bareback refers to anal sex without a condom). It was only incidentally mentioned in the article that the man had taken drugs including cocaine and crystal meth (methamphetamines) to keep him going all night long.[587]

By the end of the month, an article in the gay/lesbian magazine *San Francisco Bay Times*, points out that, "what the [mainstream] media has failed to report is that the 46-year-old patient had been on a three-month run of crystal [meth], 90 days in a row, [and] when he [finally] went to the doctor, he was just a shell of a person."[588] The man had also been a chronic drug-taker since the age of 13: first marijuana and alcohol, then later heavier drugs like cocaine and crystal meth—substances that have similarly stimulating and short-term performance-enhancing effects, and are just as toxic as poppers (which were probably also among the drug-repertoire for the man in his mid-forties).[589]

We are looking at an example of a classic AIDS patient. Let's remember here that the first AIDS patients were described as young homosexuals heavily addicted to drugs, ranging in age from 30 to mid-40s.[590] How then, could these patients possibly be helped by further chemical poisoning in the form of highly toxic medications? That the above-mentioned patient did not respond „positively" to any of the twenty AIDS medications had nothing to do with a drug-resistant virus (as is continually asserted), but rather to the fact that the already unhealthy, immuneocompromised man could not handle the highly toxic preparations.

Shortly after the news of a mutant HIV strain, a striking article appeared in *Science*, acknowledging that there was still no proof that what had been termed the "nightmare virus strain" can cause disease.[591] Jacques Normand, director of AIDS research at the US National Institute on Drug Abuse (NIDA), confirmed in an interview we got published in the weekly newspaper *Freitag*, that "the question of whether we are dealing with a super AIDS virus remains unanswered." And drugs, continued Normand, cannot be ruled out as the main cause of the 46-year old's health problems.[592]

These sentences carry even more weight when you consider that both the drug administration and specialist journals like *Science* normally stay right in line with orthodox AIDS medicine, and that real criticism or doubts on the HIV = AIDS dogma are rarely ever heard.

Gallo, 1994: Not HIV, but Sex Drugs Like Poppers Cause AIDS

At a high-level meeting of US health authorities in 1994— titled "Do Nitrites Act as a Co-Factor in Kaposi's Sarcoma?"—The best-known speaker was the National Cancer Institute's Robert Gallo, so-called co-discoverer of HIV. His statements were noteworthy. According to Gallo, HIV was surely a "catalytic factor" in Kaposi's, but even he acknowledged, "there must be something else involved." Then he added: "I don't know if I made this point clear, but I think that everybody here knows—we never found HIV DNA in tumor cells of

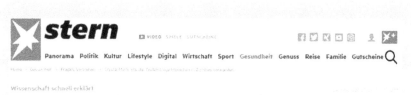

Panorama Politik Kultur Lifestyle Digital Wirtschaft Sport Gesundheit Genuss Reise Familie Gutscheine

Wissenschaft schnell erklärt

Warum Crystal Meth Menschen in Zombies verwandelt

Fast keine Substanz wirkt so stark, ist gleichzeitig extrem schädlich und macht so schnell abhängig wie Crystal Meth. Über Tschechien frisst sich die Droge nach Deutschland - und verwandelt Abhängige in körperliche Wracks.

Von Christoph Koch

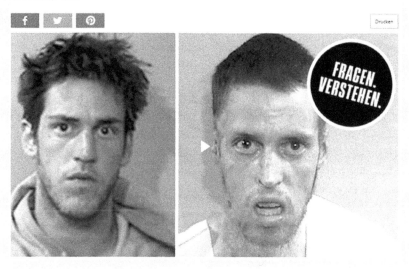

Besides poppers, many other, likewise highly toxic, drugs were on the „menu" of so-called AIDS patients. Among them: crystal meth. In February 2020, the German Stern reported: "The psychological dependency is high because meth keeps you awake and initially conveys superhero feelings. And also because many consumers experience sex much more intensely. But the supposed advantages wear out quickly—the kick goes, the greed remains. And with this a nasty addiction. The destruction is manifold: paranoia and psychoses, delusional ideas such as the obsession being populated by insects under the skin, wild aggressiveness, deterioration of memory, teeth, mucous membranes, destruction of the kidneys, emaciation. The hard consumption, often via syringe, leads to exhaustion and emaciation and ruins relaxation and sleep. Source: stern.de

KS. So this is not directly transforming. And in fact we've never found HIV DNA in T cells although we've only looked at a few. So, in other words we've never seen the role of HIV as a transforming virus in any way."

And in response to a question from Harry Haverkos, then director of the AIDS department at NIDA, who said that not a single case of KS had been reported among blood recipients where the donor had KS, Gallo allowed: "The nitrites [poppers] *could* be the primary factor."[593]

To fully appreciate Gallo's statement, we must recall that, in wealthy nations like the USA and Germany, Kaposi's sarcoma was—next to PCP—the most significant disease among patients labeled with "AIDS."[594] In 1987, for example, *Der Spiegel* described Kaposi's sarcoma patients defined as AIDS patients as the "sarcoma-covered skeletons" from the "same-sex scene."[595]

Indeed, "At present, it is accepted [even by CDC scientists] that HIV plays no role, either directly or indirectly, in the causation of Kaposi's sarcoma," writes Australian biologist and AIDS expert Eleni Papadopulos.[596] [597] [598] Given this background, it seems paradoxical that Kaposi's sarcoma is still part of the official AIDS definition in industrialized countries (anyone with KS and a „positive" test counts as an AIDS patient)—and that, contrary to the facts, even respected magazines like *The New Yorker* still assert that "Kaposi's sarcoma is a sign of AIDS"[599] (i.e. HIV causes KS).

Der Spiegel: Shabby Sensationalistic Journalism

The mass media tend to have difficulties with the facts anyway.[600] They prefer to occupy themselves with their favorite theme: sex. By the end of 1982, dozens of articles on the "mysterious new disease" had appeared in the American print media alone. Soon enough, the number jumped to hundreds per month.[601] And they constantly tossed around the idea that this virally-caused and sexually transmitted disease posed a threat to the general public. In Germany, the news magazine *Der Spiegel* took a leading role in this virus propaganda, publishing approximately 20 cover stories on HIV/AIDS since 1983, and, according to a *Spiegel*'s internal release, the magazine has reported far more on AIDS than on any other medical topic, including cancer.[602]

By late 1984, the Hamburg-based news magazine was so confident with its AIDS dossier, that they headlined, "The Bomb Is Planted" and that, in developed nations like Germany "the epidemic is breaking out of the gay-ghetto. Women are also in danger."[603] The following year, Der Spiegel explicitly expressed certainty that everyone was at risk with the cover story headline: "Promiscuity Is the Epidemic's Motor." The story goes on to state "it has become clear that the disease has started to reach out from its previous high-risk groups [homosexuals and intravenous drug users]."

The article went on to offer up the doctors' orders for curbing the spread of HIV: "Still without a cure in the fight against AIDS, doctors advise monogamy to heterosexuals and celibacy to gays." To support these theses, the magazine, which in Germany still epitomizes investigative journalism, looked to headlines from the rainbow press, including "Danger For Us All: A New People's Epidemic" from The Munich glossy Quick and "AIDS — Now the Women Are Dying" from the "master" of media warhorses, the Bild am Sonntag.[604]

The Spiegel practiced a juicy double strategy by incorporating the tabloid media's sensationalized statements into its text in such a way that they substantiated it's own theses. Yet the magazine tried to distinguish itself from the tabloids by writing that "hardly a day goes by without the boulevard press seizing up the subject [of AIDS] with headlines that go down easy." But Der Spiegel was fully invested in the game of muckraking AIDS coverage.

Particularly in the 1980s, the Spiegel had the topic sex on the brain, so articles were teeming with questions like, "Should only' homosexuals believe in it, maybe because the Lord has always had a whip waiting for them?"[605] The magazine gushed about "doing it upright" and "cock-centered routines"[606] and lamented the end of the "quickie" or the "good old one-night stand."[607] And where would tabloid journalism be without reporting on "Hollywood stars' fears of AIDS"? According to Der Spiegel, "Linda Evans, who was thoughtlessly kissed by AIDS-infected Rock Hudson on 'Dynasty', awoke night after night in terror. She cries on the telephone for help, for her nightmares show her all the stages of the disease. Burt Reynolds has to reaffirm again and again that he is neither gay, nor has AIDS."[608] Or what about this hook? "Rock-Vamp Madonna and other pop stars back off singing: 'Take your hands off me.'"[609]

Bo Derek, the sex icon of the 1970s and 1980s, "was even forbidden [by her husband] to kiss on-the-job, except with AIDS-tested film stars,"[610] according to the "Credo: 'No kiss, no AIDS.'"[611] All sorts of celebrities weighed in with their own brand of homophobic hysterics, like 'Dynasty' star Catherine Oxenberg, who said, "If I have to work with a gay in the future, I won't kiss him." *Der Spiegel* even took a jab at then US President: "30 percent of all actors are gay. Does Ronald Reagan know that?" Rock Hudson seemed to be the prime target of every AIDS-related riff: "The beasts with AIDS threaten Hollywood society. To counter the hysteria, Ed Asner, the esteemed president of the Screen Actors Guild, suggested 'striking kissing scenes from screenplays for the time being.' Now it's getting serious, by holy [Rock] Hudson!"[612]

Kissing phobia became so infectious that the CDC issued an official notice that "Kissing is not a risk factor for the transmission of AIDS."[613]

In his 1987 cover story, *Spiegel* writer Wilhelm Bittorf didn't shy away from giving his own personal views, portraying the homosexual community as a "potential pest hole," and sexual interaction with a single woman as a "necessary evil":

"A woman who I had slept with a few times, and who I found rather exciting, later told me that she was particularly proud that she had also converted gays to her charms. Gays! I felt as if someone had rammed a giant icicle into my gut. The fear that I had gotten myself infected was enormous. I have no idea why. Of course, I had earlier read, and written, a lot about AIDS, but the fear first clutched me there. The weeks leading up to the decision to take the blood test were awful. It is as if you submit yourself to an irrevocable judgment of your entire life. Then the blood test, anonymous; a week of waiting, hardly sleeping at night: one can only think of oneself. Test result: negative. But the shock is still bone deep. My sex life according to the motto 'good is what turns you on' has been over since that time. Sex afterwards, unlike beforehand, was sex with a condom, even when the girls grumbled about it. And now, months of living with just one, who I chose based on the criteria of whether she can be faithful. I live monogamously and am concentrated on just one person. I do lust after others, but I deny myself."[614]

That the *Spiegel* readers do not "know more," as the magazine is fond of saying about itself in its ads,[615] becomes clear when one looks more closely at coverage since the beginning of the 1990s. Since then, *Der Spiegel* has forced the constant interplay between fanning hopes and dashing them, continually stringing its readers along emotionally. In the 1991 story "Mother Nature Improved," "AIDS pioneer Robert Gallo" was quoted, boasting: "In ten years at most, a vaccine against AIDS will have been developed and will be ready to use";[616] and in 1995, it was optimistically reported that after the "disappointment with AZT, the new pill of hope from Basel is being generated by the kilogram in the cauldrons of the Swiss group Hoffman-La Roche: saquinavir."[617]

Then in 1996, sudden pessimism: "Since 1985, virologists, epidemic doctors, geneticists, and pharmaceutical researchers have discussed the pandemic's fatal march of victory at international AIDS congresses. The sobering result was constantly the same: AIDS can apparently not be brought under control, possibility of a cure or an effective vaccine still lies in the distant future."[618]

Only one year later, when the industry brought new active substances onto the market, *Der Spiegel* conveyed to its readers, another uplifting message: "Now, words of hope are everywhere—*Newsweek* and the *New York Times* proclaim a possible 'end of AIDS.'"[619]

Yet we're still no closer to the "end of AIDS." This did not escape the *Spiegel* either; the magazine quoted Reinhard Kurth, director of the Robert Koch-Institute, with these resigned words: "The optimism of the beginning of the 1980s is long gone," since "vaccines limiting the transmission of AIDS are the only way that promises long-term success against this most serious medical catastrophe of modern times; [but], the simplest roads to the development of an HIV vaccine are unfortunately blocked."[620]

To this, media researcher Michael Tracey writes that media coverage of AIDS "satisfied a certain kind of news value that is ignorant but loves to wallow in gore, and that readily has the ear of a public which is fascinated by the bizarre, the gruesome, the violent, the inhuman, the fearful."[621] In 1987, *Spiegel* writer Wilhelm Bittorf described, possibly without really realizing it himself, this method of shock journalism:

"AIDS has what the others are missing: nuclear death is anonymous, blind, impersonal, unimaginable even after Chernobyl, and thus dead boring. It may threaten to depopulate the earth, but that has little to do with the most private spheres of human experience. Even the worst environmental damage lies further away than the doom of infection in the erogenous zone. And if the Pershing rockets in [the German federal state] Baden-Wuerttemberg had only compromised the sex lives of the Germans, they would have been gone a long time ago."[622]

Der Spiegel generated its own "grotesque street ballads," like the story "of the Munich German teacher, infected with AIDS through mere French kissing. 'I didn't even have sex with him; the 26-year old said, bewildered. She cannot work anymore and is waiting for death." Or a woman from Düsseldorf, who purportedly destroyed her life during a holiday adventure in Portugal and lamented, "I only slept with him once."[623] These stories clearly impede the search for truth, because they suggest that the conditions illustrated are true, although nobody has verified the facts in question—and much speaks for the fact that the illustrated conditions do not represent the truth.

AIDS Is Not a Sexually-Transmitted Disease

And so, the simple and yet "politically incorrect truth is rarely spoken out loud: the dreaded heterosexual epidemic never happened," Kevin Gray, of the US magazine *Details* reported to his readers' in early 2004.[624] The "degree of epidemic" in the population of developed nations has remained practically unchanged. In the USA, for example, since 1985, the number of those termed HIV-infected has remained stable at one million people (which corresponds to a fraction of one percent of the population). But if HIV were actually a new sexually transmitted virus, there should have been an exponential rise (and fall) in case numbers.[625]

Additionally, in wealthy countries like the USA and Germany according to official statistics, poppers-consuming homosexuals have always made up around 50 percent of all AIDS patients, and intravenous drug users about 30 percent—a further seven percent are both. With this, almost all AIDS patients are men[626] who lead a self-destructive lifestyle with toxic drugs, medications, etc. In contrast, the official statistics say that in poor countries:

- A much larger proportion of the population has AIDS.
- Men and women are equally affected.
- Primarily, malnourished people suffer from AIDS.[627]

This clearly shows that AIDS symptoms are triggered by environmental factors like drugs, medications and insufficient nutrition. And it clearly speaks against the presumption that a virus is at work here "that moves like a phenomenon of globalization—just like data

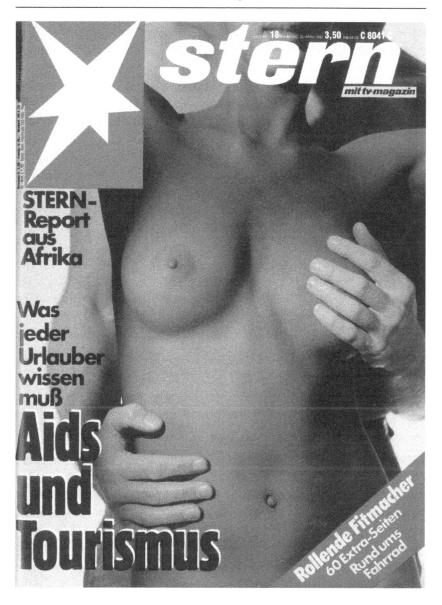

Stern 18/1987 © Stern/Picture Press

streams, financial rivers, migration waves, jet planes—fast, borderless, and incalculable," as the German weekly newspaper *Die Zeit* urgently warned on its front page in 2004.[628]

Such a pathogen would inevitably have to attack all people in all countries of the world equally: men and women, straight and gay, African and European—and not, as statistics reveal, in a racial and gender-biased way, attacking certain populations at different rates. Or as *Der Spiegel* put it in 1983 in its article "Eine Epidemie, die erst beginnt" ("An epidemic that is just beginning"): "Microorganisms do not normally distinguish between child and old person, man and woman, homosexual and heterosexual." In this context, *Details* writer Gray mentions a joke which made the rounds in the New York City Department of Health when the accumulation of AIDS statistics began: "What do you call a man who [says he] got AIDS from his girlfriend? A liar!"[629]

In fact, the largest and best-conceived studies on the subject of sex and AIDS show that AIDS is not a sexually transmitted disease. [630][631][632] The fact is glaringly obvious in the most comprehensive paper on this topic: Nancy Padian's 1997 study on seroconversion rates among couples, published in the *American Journal of Epidemiology* with an observation period of ten years (1985-1995). In it, not a single case could be uncovered in which an HIV negative partner eventually became "positive" (or "seroconverted") through sexual contact with his or her HIV „positive" partner. That is to say, the observed transmission rate was zero.[633]

23 April 1984: Gallo's TV Appearance Carves the Virus Dogma in Stone

American virologist Robert Gallo and US Health Minister Margaret Heckler stepped in front of the cameras on 23 April 1984, with an important message: "Today we add another miracle to the long honor roll of American medicine and science. Today's discovery represents the triumph of science over a dreaded disease. Those who have disparaged this scientific search—those who have said we weren't doing enough—have not understood how sound, solid, significant medical research proceeds."[634]

The media immediately passed the news on to their audiences, without questioning what kind of "medical research" had led these scientists to believe what would soon become the dogma of the AIDS establishment: that AIDS can only occur in the presence of a viral infection, and that the virus dramatically destroys the patient's helper cells (T cells). Gallo and Heckler then promised that an AIDS vaccine would be ready by 1986.[635]

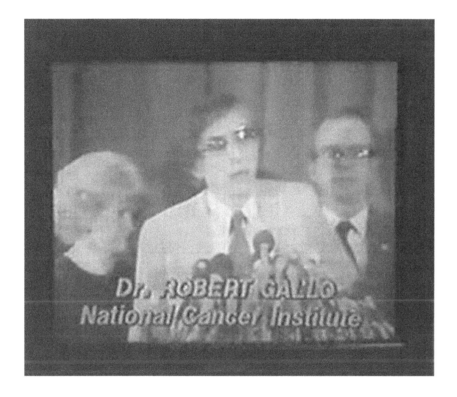

"The probable cause of AIDS has been found: a variant of a known human cancer virus," *asserted US microbiologist Robert Gallo at a press conference on 23 April 1984 (at his left,* *then American health minister Margaret Heckler). Source: TV documentary "AIDS–The* *Doubt" by Djamel Tahi, broadcasted on German ARTE Television, 14 March 1996.*

The public is still waiting for this promised vaccine. And the rest of us who have questioned the HIV = AIDS theory are still asking for evidence of Gallo's thesis that a virus is involved in the onset of AIDS symptoms like the rare cancer Kaposi's sarcoma, the lung disease PCP, herpes zoster, the deficiency-related tuberculosis, and a growing number of other diseases and disorders added to the "AIDS-related" list yearly. Neither can the AIDS establishment explain why even AIDS patients in the end-stage have very few helper cells said to be "infected" with what is termed HIV (although the orthodoxy precisely alleges that HIV attacks and kills these T cells). For this reason, the collapse of the immune system cannot be plausibly explained by the HIV = AIDS theory either. In 1985, the specialist publication *Proceedings of the National Academy of Sciences* drew attention to this helper T cell "paradox."[636]

22 years later, the *BBC* published the report „HIV infection theory challenged" about a study, led by Emory University in Atlanta and the Institute of Child Health in London. The author Jaroslav Stark is quoted with the words that „scientists have never had a full understanding of the processes by which T helper cells are depleted in HIV, and therefore they've been unable to fully explain why HIV destroys the body's supply of these cells at such a slow rate." Gallo's papers were first printed in the journal *Science* weeks after the press conference. Thus, prior to his spectacular TV appearance, and for some days afterwards, nobody was able to review his work. This presented a severe breach of professional scientific etiquette, especially as review later showed that Gallo's studies did not deliver any proof for the virus thesis.[637]

But nobody opposed these very serious breaches of public trust. Instead, Gallo cast himself— surfing on the global wave of virus panic—as an infallible researcher. And the journalists believed him, so this virus-driven AIDS plan quickly embedded itself in the media, and from this time onwards it would drive all public information on AIDS. The words "virus," "cause," and "AIDS' were inseparably linked—and the world believed that AIDS is contagious. Scientific journalists around the globe were thrilled to have a great story about a sexually transmitted epidemic, not to mention a brave medical hero and savior in Robert Gallo.

The fact that most of the world fell for Gallo's theory hook, line and sinker was confirmed in an investigation by Steven Epstein. The sociologist analyzed AIDS reports in leading specialist magazines in the opinion-shaping time from 1984-1986. It was shown that, among published texts referencing Gallo's *Science* paper, the proportion that described the virus = AIDS hypothesis as a fact jumped from 3 percent to 62 percent between 1984 and 1986.

"Expressions of doubt or skepticism [of the virus thesis]—let alone support for other hypotheses—were [in contrast] extraordinarily rare throughout this period from 1984 to 1986," Epstein argues.[638] "Findings such as these certainly support [culture critic Paula] Treichler's claim—that Gallo and his close associates established a network of citations that served to create the impression of greater certainty than Gallo's own data warranted. In circular fashion, each article points to a different one as having provided the definite proof; the buck stops nowhere."[639] This had a huge influence on the mass media (and with it on public opinion), which typically merely regurgitates information printed in *Nature, Science* or other specialist journals.[640]

New York Times: Chief Medical Reporter Altman's Cozy Relationship with Epidemic Authorities

The reports of much of the mass media also influenced the content of scientific journals, according to a study published in 1992 in the *New England Journal of Medicine*. Even top scientists trust mass media sources like the *New York Times*,[641] a paper that often serves as the measure for other mass media. That is why editors often ask American journalists pitching their story ideas, "Has the *New York Times* broken the story yet?"[642]

But, how objective and sound was the *New York Times'* coverage of AIDS? Epstein also investigated this and found that in the specialist publications between 1984 and 1986, both the proportion and the total number of articles in which it was blindly assumed HIV caused AIDS increased drastically.[643]

The chief medical reporter for the *New York Times*, Lawrence Altman, distinguished him-self as the leading media protagonist for the theory that AIDS is caused by HIV. Altman was so convinced of Gallo's assertions that within weeks of the Heckler-Gallo conference on 23 April 1984, he was using the neologisms "AIDS virus" and "AIDS test" even though Altman's 15 May 1984 article acknowledges that, "As the Red Cross and other studies progress, one of the most difficult questions that needs to be answered is: What does a „positive" blood test result mean? At this stage of AIDS research, scientists do not know if a „positive" test result means that the individual has an active infection, could transmit AIDS, had the infection at some unknown point in the past but recovered without becom-ing ill, or could still develop a fatal case at some future time."[644]

135

Yet, no mainstream media reports have since answered this "difficult" question, and soon enough, it was simply dropped from public discourse. "AIDS virus" has become a synonym for "HIV," just as "AIDS test" has replaced the more correct though still puzzling term "antibody test" even though Altman himself acknowledged some months later that "scientists have not yet fulfilled Koch's postulates for AIDS."[645]

Both terms have firmly established themselves.[646] However, this is highly problematical, however, because it allows scientific theories that have never been proven to pose as facts. In this case: That a virus called HIV causes the diseases grouped together under the term "AIDS" (Kaposi's sarcoma, shingles, tuberculosis, etc.)
That the existence of HIV antibodies can actually be proven with an HIV test

Critics have questioned Altman's objectivity and accused him of bias towards the Centers for Disease Control. In 1963, as a doctor, Altman joined the Epidemic Intelligence Service (EIS), which had been formed a few years after the Second World War. Altman was a high-ranking EIS scientist.[647] And like the CDC, which is fixated on the dangers of infections so that it has practically excluded other possible causes, such as chemical substances or toxins,[648] the EIS has always been biased towards one goal: fight the viruses.

The EIS website information proudly claims that EIS pupils had "discovered how the AIDS virus was transmitted."[649] And so that as few people as possible leave the elite squad, its own alumni association fundamentally "attempts to foster a spirit of loyalty to the EIS program through its activities."[650]

Likewise, the virus-fixated CDC, likewise, cannot be classified, in principle, as an objective information source at all. However, politicians and journalists continue to trust that any information the CDC makes public can be relied on without examination.[651] For instance, in 2005, the German *Süddeutsche Zeitung* wrote: "Worldwide, the 'Centers for Disease Control' [CDC] in the USA are considered a model of a fast and consistently acting epidemic authority."[652]

Altman, thanks to his high-level connections at the CDC, received various scoops from the epidemic officials.[653] And in 1992, he even openly admitted in *Science* that he had relied on the views of the CDC. And when "the CDC was not confident to publish" the story Altman "didn't think it was his paper's [*The New York Times*'] place to announce" it.[654] But strangely, nobody found it necessary to ask why the top medical reporter from the *New York Times,* who has a substantial influence upon the formation of public opinion, feels bound to follow the line of a federal authority.

1987: Top Experts Take the Stage as Critics of the AIDS Orthodoxy

In the mid-1980s, with "fast-lane lifestyle" theme cleared from the table to make room for the virus feast, there were no really weighty voices of opposition to the dominant views on AIDS. As social psychologist Elisabeth Noelle-Neumann fittingly argues, only members of a certain elite had the necessary influence upon people in power to decisively influence the formation of public opinion.

At the same time, "excellence must appear early before the public eye," says Noelle-Neumann.[655] And so it did, in the form of Peter Duesberg, member of the National Academy of Sciences, the USA's highest scientific committee, and one of the best-known cancer researchers in the world. A critic of the first class had entered the ring to dispute the cause of AIDS.[656] But Duesberg's first major critique did not appear until 1987, in the journal *Cancer Research* – in other words, at a time when virus panic had already bombarded the public conscience for many years.

And, as those days and years ticked by, it became less and less likely that advocates of the "AIDS virus" theory would back-pedal, since they had already heavily invested financially, personally and professionally in HIV. Be it in the *Spiegel, Die Zeit, The New York Times, Time* or *Newsweek* – the AIDS orthodoxy's theory had been championed everywhere. Researchers such as Gallo found themselves simply unable to retreat from their original claims because "stakes are too high now," notes American journalist Celia Farber. "Gallo stands to make a lot of money from patent rights on this virus. His entire reputation depends on the virus. If HIV is not the cause of AIDS, there's nothing left for Gallo. If it's not a retrovirus, Gallo would become irrelevant."

And Gallo wouldn't be the only one to sink into insignificance. Additionally, "it would be very embarrassing to say that now, maybe, the antibody [test] wasn't worth committing suicide for or burning houses for," states Farber.[657] And, in fact, numerous people, many of them completely healthy have killed themselves just because they tested HIV "positive."[658] As with the polio epidemic, with AIDS the clear toxicological connections have been completely removed from the picture in the course of virus mania. Here, we must consider that there is no money to be earned with recreational drug-related hypotheses, which emphasizes poisoning by drugs, medicines and other chemical substances like pesticides. On the contrary, prohibiting certain chemical substances would cause huge profit losses for production and processing industries as well as the pharmaceutical, chemical, auto-motive and toy industries—and also for the media, whose existence is largely dependent on proceeds from these industry's advertisements.

In contrast, the virus theory clears the way for profits in the multibillions, with the sales of vac-cines, PCR and antibody tests and antiviral medications. "In the world of biomedical research, ties to industry are pervasive but mentioning the fact is not," writes William Booth in *Science* as early as 1988.[659] Correspondingly, new viruses are constantly invented and implicated—Eb-ola, SARS, avian flu, human papillomavirus (HPV)—to keep the cash flowing.[660]

But doubts on the virus dogma were so clearly and comprehensibly formulated, that from the end of the 1980s, more and more people began to share in the criticism. Among them were several renowned scientists such as former Harvard microbiologist Charles Thom-as,[661] who founded the organization "Rethinking AIDS" at the beginning of the 1990s[662] (renamed "Reappraising AIDS" in 1994[663]—and renamed later again "Rethinking AIDS"). Thomas assembled hundreds of medical professionals, molecular biologists and other identified critics of the HIV = AIDS theory.

Among them was Harvey Bialy, co-founder of the *Nature* offshoot *Nature Biotechnolo-gy*, and Yale mathematician Serge Lang (who died in 2005); like Duesberg, Lang was a member of the National Academy of Sciences (a list of more than 2000 critics is found on Rethinking-AIDS' website, which re-formed in early 2006: www.rethinkingaids.com).

"It is good that the HIV hypothesis is being questioned," Nobel Prize winner for Chemis-try, Walter Gilbert told the *Oakland Tribune* in 1989.[664] Duesberg, Gilbert acknowledged, "is absolutely correct in saying that no one has proven that AIDS is caused by the AIDS virus. And he is absolutely correct that the virus cultured in the laboratory may not be the cause of AIDS. There is no animal model for AIDS, and where there is no animal model, you cannot establish Koch's postulates." These arguments were so convincing, according to Gilbert, that he "would not be surprised if there were another cause of AIDS and even that HIV is not involved."

Some time later, Gilbert expressed fundamental reservations in an English TV documentary critical of HIV/AIDS: "The community as a whole doesn't listen patiently to critics who adopt alternative viewpoints, although the great lesson of history is that knowledge develops through the conflict of viewpoints, that if you have simply a consensus view, it generally stultifies, it fails to see the problems of that consensus; and it depends on the existence of critics to break up that iceberg an to permit knowledge to develop."[665]

The media prefer to make this consensus argument their own, even though it's their duty to diligently research every medical claim, sort fact from theory and question even majority rule (however formed) to clarify every issue. But in 1990, for instance, even the venerable *New York Times* countered the provocative argument of alleged "solitary dissenter" Peter Duesberg when it claimed that "virtually all of the leading scientists engaged in AIDS work believe that Duesberg is wrong."

Yet, by 1990, as shown above, many renowned researchers said that mainstream research could not deliver any proof for their HIV = AIDS theory.[666]

In 2000, *Newsweek* magazine expressed its incredulity that the "consensus doesn't impress" the critics of the virus hypothesis in the article "The HIV Disbelievers." Simultaneously, the piece calls the arguments of orthodox scientists "clear-cut, exhaustive, and unambiguous." But evidence to support this statement could not be provided by *Newsweek* (not even upon request).[667]

1994: AIDS Researcher David Ho—as Convincing as a Giraffe with Sunglasses

John Maddox, the editor at *Nature* from 1966-1996 led a personal campaign against critics of the HIV = AIDS hypothesis. He even publicly censored Duesberg. On 7 November 1994 he justified this to the *Spiegel,* saying he found it "irresponsible" to say "drug consumption is the cause of AIDS."[668] Sir Maddox later contradicted this in a personal letter to Kiel internist Claus Köhnlein on 20 September 1995, saying that he had "not censored Duesberg because of his views but because of the manner in which he insists on expressing them." And Maddox added, "that a hemophiliac relative of my wife died of AIDS."[669]

But Maddox's behavior–steering a scientific discussion in such a way based on personal views–is most frivolous and unethical. By doing this, he does no justice to his responsibility as Editor in Chief of *Nature*–a publication whose contents are taken at face value by the mass media.

Maddox took advantage of the huge influence of "his" *Nature* magazine again, at the beginning of 1995, when he published a paper by AIDS researcher David Ho, who claimed to have conclusively proven that HIV alone causes AIDS.[670] But critics ripped Ho's paper to pieces.

The quality of the data and the modeling were incomprehensible and "about as convincing as a giraffe trying to sneak into a polar bears only picnic by wearing sunglasses," as Australian scientist Mark Craddock jokes in his detailed critique.[671]

In turn, Nobel laureate Kary Mullis concludes: "If Maddox seriously thinks or thought that these publications really prove that HIV causes AIDS, then he should go outside and shoot himself–because if he had had no justification before, why did he reject all my possible explanations and alternative hypotheses? Why did Maddox have such a fixed opinion? Why did the whole world have such a fixed opinion? If it had taken until 1995 to find out what produces AIDS–how could everyone have known it for ten years? The facts are now on the table, and when one examines them closely, HIV cannot be the cause of AIDS. There is no reason to believe that all these AIDS diseases have the same cause."[672]

This staggering critique eventually found public validation in November 1996, when a paper was printed in *Science* that "took the ground out from under the feet" of Ho's theses, according to journalists Kurt Langbein and Bert Ehgartner in their book *The Medicine Cartel*.[673] The *Science* paper revealed that Ho had actually found no trace at all of the annihilating battle in the body between HIV and the immune system, the connections of which the renowned scientist claimed to have discovered.[674]

The Media under the Spell of Celebrity Researchers

Unfortunately, few reporters in the mass media did the necessary homework before writing about HIV and AIDS. Instead, the papers were constantly packed with stories approved by the AIDS establishment, for which heroes and kings, traitors and villains are needed.[675] And scientific journalists are particularly prone to striking up hymns of praise.

"First came God, then came Gallo," decreed Flossie Wong-Staal, Gallo's closest collaborator and consort in the *Los Angeles Times* in 1986.[676] One year later, the *Washington Post* quoted Sam Broder, director of the American National Cancer Institute, as saying: "Einstein, Freud — I'd put him [Gallo] on a list like that, I really would."[677]

With David Ho, such excess was likewise not held back. On Christmas Day, 1996, just a few weeks after the journal *Science* had criticized the foundation of Ho's work, the German *Tageszeitung,* without any irony intended, called him the "redeemer" and "the long-awaited Messiah of the AIDS scene."[678]

The reason for such jubilation? A catchy slogan with which Ho became famous in the mid-1990s, and which at least for a few years became the global chief doctrine for AIDS therapy: "Hit HIV hard and early!" It endorsed prescribing high dosages of antiretroviral medication as early as possible, even on patients testing HIV „positive" who do not show any disease symptoms.[679]

A few days after his canonization by the *Tageszeitung,* Ho was celebrated on the cover of *Time* magazine as "Man of the Year 1996." He was portrayed as a "genius," whose "brilliance" had produced "some of the boldest yet most cogent hypotheses in the epidemic campaign against HIV. [His] spirit is startling, manifested in a passionate transcendence [that] is evident in his gestures ... [Ho] is an extraordinary American success story." The *Spiegel* didn't want to be out-of-step and soon declared Ho, thanks to his "decided optimism" to be "the new shining light in the research world."[680]

This euphoria did not last. In February 2001 even Altman had to admit in his *New York Times* that there had been an official turnaround in AIDS therapy and Ho's concept ("hit HIV hard and early") had to be abandoned. It had turned out that the medications were too toxic, causing liver and kidney damage, and that their effects were immunosuppressive, i.e. they put patients' lives in danger.[681] Yet, even this defeat didn't stop the *Süddeutsche Zeitung* from wrongly writing at in 2004 that, "Ho's maxim 'hit HIV hard and early', with which he revolutionized HIV therapy," had led to "patients having better chances of survival."[682]

AIDS Medications: The Fable of Life-Prolonging Effects

In 1987, the antiretroviral medication AZT became the first authorized AIDS medication. At the time, and for years afterwards, HIV/AIDS patients were typically given only one drug. This changed in 1995, when the multiple combination therapy (HAART) was introduced, in which, as is evident from the name, multiple substances are administered at the same time. Here, once again, the media broke out the streamers and confetti for another AIDS establishment party. For instance, *Science* declared the "new weapons against AIDS" as the "breakthrough of 1996."[683] And, it was universally reported that the antiretroviral preparations would "help people with AIDS live longer," as the *Washington Post* announced in 2004.[684]

Hans Halter from the *Spiegel* even gave concrete numbers: "Those who are under the influence of medications presently live on average 10 to 15 years. In contrast, the others who do not take any preparations only live five to ten years."[685] These drugs generated billions of dollars in excess revenue for drug-makers: in 2000, global revenue was $4 billion; by 2004, it jumped to $6.6 billion, and in 2020, it should crack the $30 billion mark. For pharmaceutical giants, the preparations are bestsellers. At Roche, for example, Fuzeon, on the market since August 2004, triggered a 25 percent increase in turnover.[686]

But claims for the lifespan-increasing effectiveness of HAART medications are untenable. A close look at Halter's comparison of survival rates, for instance, as gathered from the *Ärzteblatt* (*Medical Journal*) *for Schleswig-Holstein*, shows that the average survival time for patients taking medication was four months in 1988 and 24 months in 1997.[687] And according to CDC bulletins, it now amounts to 46 months[688] — a long way from the 15 years mentioned by Halter. But however big the increase in lifespan, one glaring omission is that everyone — doctors as well as patients — approaches the issue more carefully, because they have become ever more aware of drug toxicities.

Now, these drugs are often administered or taken with interruptions (so-called drug treatment "holidays") and also in lower doses. The earliest example of this treatment about-face happened with the first AIDS medication, AZT, which, at the end of the 1980s, was still given in doses of 1,500 mg a day. But at the beginning of the 1990s, the daily dose was reduced to 500 mg, since even mainstream medicine couldn't overlook the fact that the administration of higher doses led to much higher death rates.[689]

Apart from that, we must soberly recognize that even a remaining lifetime of 46 months is not all that long, especially when you consider that perhaps millions of these medicated people are living with serious drug side effects that adversely affect quality of life.

Diagram 5   Number of AIDS cases in the USA, 1982-1995 according to the old AIDS definition (dark bars; "classical AIDS") and according to the 1993 definition (white bars; includes CD4 cell criterion)

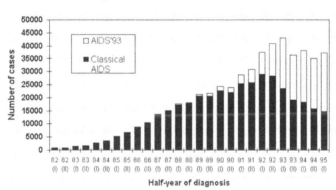

Fig.1 Incidence of AIDS in the USA

The number of AIDS cases in the USA doubled overnight as a result of the widening of the AIDS definition in 1993. This ensured the peak number of AIDS cases, and with it the mortality peak was pushed along from the early to the mid-1990s. "If public and policy makers would have realized that the epidemic of AIDS was declining, this might have resulted in reduction of budgets for AIDS research and prevention programs, including the budget of the CDC themselves," stated the research scientist Vladimir Koliadin. Source: Koliadin, Vladimir, Some Facts behind the Expansion of the Definition of AIDS in 1993, March 1998; see https://www.virusmyth.com/aids/hiv/vknewdef.htm

We must also recognize that there are these so-called long-term survivors or "non-progressors". Common to these "positive" people is the fact that they have rejected AIDS medications from the start or only took them for a short time. Many of them are or were still alive 20 years after they tested "positive."[690] [691]

The AIDS establishment now calls these HIV „positive" individuals who reject AIDS medications "elite controllers" as if they are somehow super-human.[692] The establishment now claims that 2 percent of AIDS patients may fit this category, but only a large controlled global study (which is actually missing) would be able to determine the exact number of HIV „positive" individuals who remain healthy without taking AIDS drugs. However, the number of "elite controllers" is probably much higher, yet the "vast majority of [so-called] HIV-"positives" are long-term survivors!" as Berkeley microbiologist Peter Duesberg states. "Worldwide they number many, many millions."[693]

A look at the CDC statistics before 1993[694] (and 2003 statistics from the Robert Koch-Institute)[695] shows that the number of AIDS deaths in the USA and also in Germany had already peaked in 1991, and decreased in the years following. And logically, the multiple combination therapy introduced in 1995/1996 cannot be responsible for this decrease. Newer CDC statistic, however, do show that the mortality peak lies approximately in 1995/1996. How can this be?

According to statistician Vladimir Koliadin, who analyzed the mortality data, this is due to the fact that in early 1993, AIDS in the USA was once again significantly redefined. From 1993 on, any individual testing HIV „positive" with less than 200 CD4 cells per microliter of blood was counted as an AIDS patient. If both criteria were met, a diagnosis of "AIDS defining" diseases like shingles (herpes zoster) or Kaposi's sarcoma was no longer necessary (although the old definition of, say, a „positive" HIV test + Kaposi's = AIDS was still valid).

This broadening of the AIDS definition meant that many people had the "AIDS patient" label superimposed upon them, even though they were actually not sick at all. A laboratory figure showing that an individual had less than 200 CD4 cells per microliter of blood was good enough for the AIDS establishment. But what this value ultimately means is, as discussed, anything but clear.[696] Countries such as Canada have even decided not to introduce the CD4 cell count as criteria for the AIDS definition.[697]

In any case, the number of AIDS cases in the USA doubled overnight as a result of the widening of the AIDS definition in 1993. This ensured the peak number of AIDS cases, and with it the mortality peak was pushed along (see diagram 5) from the early to the mid-1990s. "If public and policy makers would have realized that the epidemic of AIDS was declining, this might have resulted in reduction of budgets for AIDS research and prevention programs, including the budget of the CDC themselves," according to Koliadin. "Expansion of the definition of AIDS in 1993 helped to disguise the downward trend in epidemic of AIDS. It is reasonable to suppose that an essential motive behind the implementation of the new definition of AIDS just in 1993 was strong unwillingness of the CDC to reveal the declining trend of AIDS epidemic."[698]

Even if we pushed all these considerations to the side, the introduction of combination therapy (HAART) and new active substances (particularly protease inhibitors) in 1995/1996 cannot explain the reduction in AIDS mortalities anyway; when the new substances were introduced, they were not available to even a good proportion of patients.
The opposite was probably the case. A meta-analysis with data from Europe, Australia and Canada shows that in 1995, patients used combination therapy during only 0.5 percent of treatment time. In 1996, the value lay at 4.7 percent, which is still extremely low.[699] Former CDC director James Curran told CNN that, at the time, "less than 10 percent of infected Americans had access to these new therapies, or were taking them."[700]

Ten years later, while the media celebrated HAART's 10th birthday, the Lancet published a study that challenged the propaganda about HAART, showing that decreases in so-called viral load did not "translate into a decrease in mortality" for people taking these highly toxic AIDS drug combinations. The multi-center study—the largest and longest of its kind—tracked the effects of HAART on some 22,000 previously treatment naive HIV „positives" between 1995 and 2003 at 12 locations in Europe and the USA. The study's results refute popular claims that the newer HAART meds extend life and improve health.[701]

Commenting on the article, Felix de Fries of Study Group AIDS-Therapy in Zurich, Switzerland had this to say: "The Lancet study shows that after a short period of time, HAART treatment led to increases in precisely those opportunistic diseases that define AIDS from fungal infections of the lungs, skin and intestines to various mycobacterial infections." De Fries also notes that HAART has led to no sustained increases in CD4 cell counts, no reduction in AIDS-defining illness and no decrease in mortality rates; its use is also associated with a list of serious adverse events such as cardiovascular disease, lipodystrophy, lactic acidosis, liver and kidney failure, osteoporosis, thyroid dysfunction, neuropathy, and cancers among users.[702]

Yet, why even argue over pros and cons of HAART since statements about the life-pro-longing effects of the medications are impossible to verify in the first place? Statements about the life-prolonging effects of the preparations are namely impossible, because the precedent condition has not been met: placebo-controlled studies. Since if one has no comparison with a group taking an ineffective preparation (placebo), it is not possible to know if the changes (improvement or worsening in patient's health) are due to the med-ication or not. Placebo studies, however, have practically not been carried out anymore since the 1987 Fischl study published in the *NEJM*, because, as it is said, the Fischl study found AZT to be effective.[703]

For this reason, the AIDS establishment has since argued that it's no longer ethically jus-tifiable to withhold the (allegedly) lifesaving antiretroviral medication from the patients (not even in test series).

People as Guinea Pigs

There are several objections, however, to this alleged "ethical" argument. Not only do even leading orthodox AIDS scientists state that in medical science "no researcher can assess a drug's effectiveness with scientific certainty without testing it against a placebo." Also, as outlined, it was not HAART, but the huge widening of the definition of the disease as well as the drastic reductions in doses of AIDS drugs such as AZT that made the death rate from AIDS come down in the mid-1990s. Moreover, new studies show that most of the medical industry's drug promises are false. Pharmaceuticals hyped in glossy advertisements and TV commercials aren't responsible for improving test patients' health—rather, this can largely be traced back to the placebo effect.

This is particularly worth noting when you consider that no expense is spared in bringing medications onto the market: expenditures for pharmaceuticals increased by 2,500 per-cent between 1972 and 2004—from $20 billion to $500 billion annually.[704] [705]

Moreover, two studies by the American Food and Drug Administration (FDA) make a case for the general introduction of placebo controls. This makes sense, since it is fully possible that proposed new drugs will have no effect at all. Or that, compared to the placebo, they are harmful; something that is also very possible, because medications are, as a rule, often connected with side effects—even fatal ones sometimes.[706] [707]

What right does the medical industry have to preach about ethics when its own human trials sweeps mortalities and physical damage under the carpet in the lust to get authorization to market their medications to the general public? In the USA alone, 3.7 million people—mostly poor Hispanic immigrants—have registered to participate in medical trials.

Lack of transparency and conflicts of interest continue to plague these drug trials, which are sponsored by the largest pharmaceutical companies in the world.[708]

Even our most vulnerable citizens aren't protected from the machinations of the medical industrial complex, as revealed in 2004. Infants as young as a few months old were experimented upon in US clinical trials, partly financed by pharmaceutical firms like GlaxoSmithKline, involving cocktails of up to seven medications. They were mostly black and latino children from the poorest of circumstances gathered together under the auspices of institutions like the Incarnation Children's Center (ICC) in New York; the ICC was even remunerated for supplying children for the tests. "Stephen Nicholas, for example, was not only director of the ICC until 2002; he also simultaneously sat on the Pediatric Medical Advisory Panel, which was supposed to check the tests—which signifies a serious conflict of interest," criticizes Vera Sharav, president of the Alliance for Human Research Protection (AHRP), a medical industry watchdog organization.

These first-line Phase 1 and Phase 2 trials are associated with the highest health risk because they are not meant to establish efficacy, so impact on the trial participants is highly unpredictable. These early trials aren't meant to deliver an effective therapy, but rather, figure out how toxic the substance is (Phase 1) in order to then estimate if the active substance being tested has any effect at all (Phase 2). Biotechnologist Art Caplan explained that the odds are typically stacked up against the drug: if Phase 1 trials prove that a substance is useful for an individual, this would have to be termed a "miracle."[709]

"The children were suffering horribly from the side effects of the drugs tested on them," according to journalist Liam Scheff, who broke the story in early 2004, on an alternative website. "And children who didn't want the substances were even forced to take them. For this, plastic tubes were sewn through the abdominal wall by surgeons, through which the substances can be directly injected into the stomach." The result: brain and bone marrow damage, blindness, strokes—and "some children also died," according to Scheff.[710] The *New York Post* seized upon the story and ran the headline: "AIDS Tots Used as 'Guinea Pigs'"[711]—a term which the BBC also used for their television documentary "Guinea Pig Kids."[712]

In 2005, an official investigation ultimately came to the conclusion that "government-funded researchers who tested AIDS drugs on foster children over the past two decades violated federal rules designed to protect vulnerable youths."[713]

This finally prompted the *New York Times*, which is otherwise always the first on the scene on the subject of HIV/AIDS, to take up the highly explosive topic as well, with a decidedly different spin. In an article, two pediatricians were quoted as saying that, "to have withheld promising drugs from sick children just because they were in foster care would have been inhumane," and "there is impressive evidence that [the children] were helped [by the medications]."[714]

Details on this evidence, however, were never offered up. We even requested that authors of the *Times* article name the studies that prove these statements—but there was no response.[715]

This might seem incredibly shocking, but it is all-too common in AIDS research. "I have scoured the literature for evidence that the anti-HIV drugs actually prolong the lives, or at least improve the quality of the lives, of the children given these drugs—but I could not find any support for either possibility," says AIDS researcher David Rasnick. "For example, the study 'Lamivudine in HIV-infected children' by Lewis et al, not only has no control group but the authors also acknowledge that the [antiretroviral] study compound Lamivudine acts as a DNA chain terminator. And there is no data in the paper showing that the drug does anything good for the children. On the contrary, among the 90 children in the study," "11 children had to be withdrawn from the study for disease progression [in other words, it didn't work for them] and 10 because of possible Lamivudine-related toxicity, and 6 had died.'"[716]

But the AIDS orthodoxy continued along its own path, calling the clinical trials involving children so "resounding" in their success "that the tests are now being spread out to Asia and Africa," according to Annie Bayne, spokesperson for the Columbia University Medical Center, which was also involved in the trials. This is not unusual, for AIDS research often goes into poor countries to carry out its medication trials. This is also true for trials of the efficacy of so-called microbicides, which are said to prevent the sexual transmission of HIV, and from which so much is promised.

"Marvelous microbicides: [the] intravaginal vaginal gels could save millions of [human] lives," announced the *Lancet* in 2004, then qualifying their hopes by adding that, "first someone has to prove that they work." Nothing has been proven at all, yet the miracle has already been announced far and wide. Experts, as the *Lancet* continues, were of the firm opinion that "microbicides will only reach everyone who needs them [if] large pharmaceutical companies get involved. In the remotest part of Thailand you can buy a bottle of coke. We want microbicides to be available like that."

This is all the more striking if you consider that the first microbicide tests of the active substance nonoxynol-9 (n-9) ended in catastrophe. At first, n-9 was glorified by researchers as an "ideal potential microbicide because *in vitro* [test tube] studies pointed to its effectiveness."[717] 900 "sex-workers" from Benin, the Ivory Coast, South Africa and Thailand were selected for a clinical trial, which involved smearing gel laced with n-9 into their vaginas. But the gel not only had no medical efficacy, as UNAIDS admitted,[718] it also damaged the poor women's vaginal epithelial cells.[719]

AZT Study 1987: A Gigantic Botch-Up

"If there is really doubt about whether a standard treatment is effective, the FDA should require that clinical trials of new treatments have three comparison groups—new drug, old drug, and placebo," writes Marcia Angell, former Editor in Chief of the *New England Journal of Medicine*.[720] For AIDS research, this meant that placebo groups had to be introduced to medication trials, for there were justified doubts that the efficacy of AZT (the standard AIDS treatment) had really be proven with the 1987 Fischl study.

Journalist and Harvard analyst John Lauritsen, who has viewed the FDA documents on the Fischl study, came to the conclusion that the study was a "fraud";[721] the Swiss newspaper

Weltwoche termed the experiment a "gigantic botch-up"[722] and *NBC News* in New York branded the experiments, conducted across the US, as "seriously flawed."[723] However, this criticism was not to be found in the rest of the mainstream media either because the statements of the AIDS establishment are completely trusted, or because, like the *Neue Zürcher Zeitung's* scientific editorial staff, they do not even know of even such a significant study as that of Fischl et al.[724]

The Fischl experiments were, in fact, stopped after only four months, after 19 trial subjects in the placebo group (those who did not receive AZT, but rather an inactive placebo) and only one participant from the so-called verum group (those who were officially taking AZT) had died. Through this, according to the AIDS establishment, the efficacy of AZT appeared to be proven.

But the arguments don't add up. A clinical trial observation period of only four months is much too short to be informative, considering the usual practice of administering AIDS medications over years, or even a lifetime.[725] All too often long-term studies are missing in these and other medical research fields.

In the USA, for example, around $100 billion is spent annually on medical research. This figure has doubled since the mid-1990s, and almost a third of it comes from tax dollars. Yet long-term evaluations of pills and treatments are criminally neglected: just 1.6 percent of the $100 billion budget is allocated to long-term studies.[726] For patients taking medications, "this is like Russian roulette," states British doctor Robert Califf.[727]

The AZT study was financed by AZT maker Wellcome (today GlaxoSmithKline), which is clearly a conflict of interest. But somehow this, like the sloppiness of the Fischl study, didn't bother anyone, especially not the pharmaceutical groups (nor the media!), for whom AZT would become a cash cow[728] (it was actually said that AZT was worth its weight in gold).[729]

Yet, the Fischl study's double blind requirements (according to which, neither researchers nor patients were permitted to know who was taking AZT and who was taking the placebo) were violated after only a short time. In their desire to be given the alleged wonder-preparation, patients even had their pills analyzed to be sure that they were among the group receiving the medication and not the placebo; public propaganda had made test subjects believe that only AIDS medications like AZT could save them.

FDA documents also reveal that the study results were distorted, because the group that took AZT, and had to battle the adverse side effects, received more supportive medical services than the placebo subjects. For example, in the AZT group, 30 patients were kept alive through multiple blood transfusions until the end of the study—in the placebo group, on the other hand, this was only true in five cases.[730] [731]

"There was widespread tampering with the rules of the [Fischl] trial—the rules have been violated coast to coast," said lead NBC reporter Perri Peltz in 1988, adding that "if all patients with protocol violations were dropped, there wouldn't be enough" to be able to continue the study.[732]

"When preparing this report, we repeatedly tried to interview Dr. Anthony Fauci [probably the most powerful AIDS official in the USA] at the National Institutes of Health," reports Peltz. "But both Dr. Fauci and Food and Drug Administration Commissioner Frank Young declined our request for interviews."[733] These are the experiences of practically everyone who has criticized the theories of dominant AIDS medicine.[734] [735]

The renowned British doctor and epidemiologist Gordon Stewart, for instance said: "I have asked the health authorities, editors-in-chief and other experts concerned with HIV/AIDS repeatedly for proof of their theses—and I've been waiting for an answer since 1984."[736]

"Welcome to the club, Perri!" wrote John Lauritsen in his book "The AIDS War: Propaganda, Profeteering and Genocide from the Medical-Industrial Complex": "When it comes to questions of HIV or AZT, the Public Health Service bureaucrats and 'scientists' won't speak to me either; they have also refused to speak to the BBC, *Canadian Broadcasting Corporation Radio*, *Channel 4 television* from London, Italian television, *The New Scientist*, and Jack Anderson."

The same happened to one of the authors of this book, Torsten Engelbrecht, in 2017 when he sent Fauci, and his NIAID, questions regarding the Fischl study. To this day he has not received any answer.[737]

Of course, Fauci was willing to talk—in media that did not ask critical questions and only let him pray down his advertising messages. On February 19, 1988, Fauci appeared on the televisioin program *Good Morning America*, as Lauritsen writes in his book. And he was asked why only one drug, AZT, had been made available. He replied: "The reason why only one drug has been made available—AZT—is because it's the only drug that has been shown in scientifically controlled trials to be safe and effective."

But "this brief statement contains several outstanding falsehoods," as Lauritsen points out. "First, there have been no 'scientifically controlled trials' of AZT; to refer to the FDA-conducted AZT trials as 'scientifically controlled' is equivalent to referring to garbage as la haute cuisine. Second, AZT is not 'safe': it is a highly toxic drug—the FDA analyst who reviewed the toxicology data on AZT recommended that it should not be approved. Third, AZT is not known objectively to be 'effective' for anything, except perhaps for destroying bone marrow."[738]

Nevertheless, Fauci did not get tired of spreading factually unsubstantiated statements about AZT throughout the world. Even in 2020, at the end of April, Fauci was not afraid of promulgating the untruth about AZT during a White House meeting about Gilead's drug remdesivir, by saying "the first randomized placebo-controlled trial with AZT ... turned out to give an effect that was modest"[739] (more on remdesivir see chapter 12).

Harvey Bialy, co-founder of *Nature Biotechnology*, said: "I am very tired of hearing AIDS establishment scientists tell me they are 'too busy saving lives' to sit down and refute Peter Duesberg's arguments although each one assures me they could 'do it in a minute if they had to.'"[740]

We also contacted leading mainstream mass media and specialist journals including the *New York Times, Time, Der Spiegel, Die Zeit, Stern, Tageszeitung, Weltwoche, Neue Zürcher Zeitung, Nature, Science, Spektrum der Wissenschaft*, asking them to send us clear evidence:

- That the existence of HIV has been proven
- That so-called HIV antibody tests and PCR viral load tests as well as the CD4 helper cell count specifically diagnose HIV/AIDS
- That HIV is the sole or primary cause of the diseases grouped together as AIDS
- That HIV is contagious and can be transmitted through sexual contact or blood
- That antiretroviral preparations are effective and prolong lifetime
- That the AIDS statistics proclaimed by the WHO and UNAIDS are sound
- That non-viral factors such as drugs, medications and malnutrition can be ruled out as primary causes[741]

But to date, not a single study has been revealed to us, not even from any of the many orthodox scientists and journalists we queried. This includes *Nature* writer Declan Butler, who wrote in the world-renowned journal in 2003: "Most [mainstream] AIDS researchers strongly dispute these statements" that there is no proof that HIV causes AIDS, that HIV is contagious, and so on. But Butler failed to respond to our request that he provide evidence of this in the form of relevant studies.[742]

We also contacted John Moore of Cornell University in New York, who was quoted in Butler's *Nature* piece, and who thinks "revisionists are best ignored. [They are leading] an unwinnable debate based on faith not fact."[743] But when we asked Moore if he could name the factual evidence for his HIV = AIDS = death-sentence theory, he responded by calling these critics the "HIV-is-a-pussycat-fraction" and charged them with "pure stupidity and malice."[744]

Scientific historian Horace Judson writes that, "Central to the problem of misconduct is the response of institutions when charges erupt. Again and again the actions of senior scientists and administrators have been the very model of how not to respond. They have tried to smother the fire. Such flawed responses are altogether typical of misconduct cases."[745]

These opinions were never known by the Fischl trial subjects. After four years, 80 percent of them had died; a short while later, all of them were dead. This is shocking but not really surprising, considering that AZT is an extremely poisonous chemotherapy-like medication, invented by researcher Jerome Horwitz in the 1960s. Horwitz's goal had been to develop a DNA blocker, which inhibits cell replication, to kill cancer cells. But, his test mice perished from the extreme toxicities of AZT.[746]

"On paper, [Horwitz's] logic was impeccable, [but] in reality, it simply didn't work," summarizes *BusinessWeek* journalist Bruce Nussbaum in his book "Good Intentions—How Big Business and the Medical Establishment are Corrupting the Fight against AIDS, Alzheimer's, Cancer and More." Nussbaum: "When the experiment ended in failure, so, in a way, had the first half of Horwitz's life. Disgusted, he turned on AZT." Horwitz himself said he was so cloyed with the drug that he "dumped it on the junk pile. I didn't [even] keep the notebooks." AZT was "so worthless" to him that he "even didn't think it was worth patenting."[747]

The AIDS Therapy Dilemma

AZT was in fact stored away instead of being dumped as toxic waste, and when AIDS mania surfaced in the 1980s, it was pulled out of the cupboard again. And the "AIDS virus" hypothesis, just like the many other virus theories for serious illnesses like leukemia, breast cancer and multiple sclerosis, would probably have disintegrated long ago, if not for AZT. In 1987, it became the AIDS "therapy" even though, in the recommended dosage, it was just fatal.[748] The medical community ignored the possibility that AZT-poisoning was the cause of death because they still had stuck in their minds the pictures of the first AIDS patients in the beginning of the 1980s, who certainly looked as if they'd been struck down and carried off by a deadly virus.

So, when doctors looked at these AZT patients in 1987, they refused to make any connection with the highly toxic antiviral AZT. Their belief in the deadliness of HIV was so firm that they weren't even shocked when all patients died within a short time. And so, with the Fischl study published in the *NEJM*, these doctors believed it worked and still allege to have tangible proof of AZT's efficacy.

A kind of "big bang" for this HIV=AIDS dogma was the story of Hollywood actor Rock Hudson. Born in 1925, the 1.96-meter tall man died in October 1985 and was presented to the world as the first megastar the "AIDS virus" took down. Hudson gave AIDS "a face" and the virus hunters godlike status, although there was and is no justification for drawing the conclusion that a virus killed him (to do justice to the significance of this event we sketch this deceptive AIDS legacy of Rock Hudson in the epilog at the end of this book).

HIV mania appears to cause its own range of symptoms: primarily a strong bias against the facts, including that chemical substances like drugs or prescription medications (particularly antiviral) are extremely toxic and can trigger precisely the observed symptoms (also mentioned on package labels) which they aim to prevent: destruction of mitochondria, anemia, bone marrow, and consequently immune system damage, etc.[750]

In the end, a vicious circle arises. Virologists have no proof of their thesis that a virus triggers the diseases grouped together under the term AIDS. So they consider proof to be collecting subjective information from clinicians who assert that the medications are

Viramune HIV Infant Prophylaxis Safe

–

by Michael Smith, North American Correspondent, MedPage Today   2011-12-22

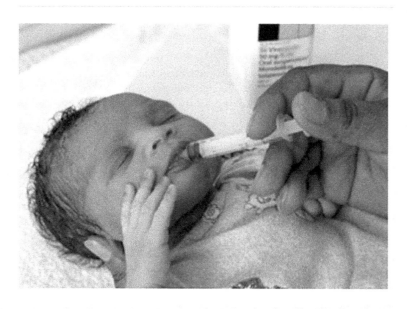

This photo shows an African newborn, being administered a dose of Viramune (nevirapine), for the purpose of so-called HIV prevention (for Viramune's side effects, see Table 2). But what Medpage Today reported in 2011—that Viramune is "safe"—is not correct. „Viramune has a dangerous toxicity,“ as South African advocate and Viramune-expert Anthony Brink points out. "However, on the basis of HIVNET 012, an American study conducted in Uganda in the late 1990s, nevirapine is given to HIV „positive" mothers in labour and to their newborn babies in dozens of developing countries—where the manufacturer Boehringer Ingelheim gives the drug away free to establish its future market."[749] Revelations in December 2004 by a top-ranking US National Institutes of Health whistleblower, Jonathan Fishbein, exposed not only the extremely sloppy manner in which the study was conducted, but also the NIH's deliberate, fraudulent suppression of serious adverse event data in the trial, including unreported deaths. Source: Screenshot from Medpage Today effective. But, in industrialized countries, doctors very often treat patients not because they are sick (a large proportion have no physical complaints whatsoever), but rather because they have tested "positive," they show only a certain number of helper cells or a slight so-called viral load has been measured via PCR.

Virologists tell general practitioners that patients are carrying the deadly HIV. The medications available for this, however, are highly toxic; their use produces an immune deficiency syndrome—and exactly fulfils the predictions of the virus hypothesis (that people

Table 2   Retrovir (AZT), Viramune (Nevirapine)
Toxicity and therapeutic value of two AIDS medications
(altogether, there are more than two dozen AIDS drugs)

Medication Manufacturer	Known Toxicities (manufacturer's label)	Therapeutic Value (manufacturer's label)
Retrovir (AZT Glaxo-SmithKline	"Retrovir (AZT) has been associated with hematologic toxicity [blood toxicity], including neutropenia [anemia] and severe anemia" "Prolonged use of Retrovir has been associated with symptomatic myopathy [muscle wasting]" "Lactic acidosis and severe hepatomegaly [liver swelling] with steatosis [fat degeneration], including fatal cases, have been reported with the use of nucleoside analogues [Retrovir, Epivir, Zerit] alone or in combination"	"Retrovir is not a cure for HIV infection" "The long-term effects of Retrovir are unknown at this time" "The long-term consequences of in utero and infant exposure to Retrovir are unknown, including the possible risk of cancer"
Viramune (Nevirapine) Boehringer-Ingelheim	"Patients should be informed of: the possibility of severe liver disease or skin reactions associated with Viramune that may result in death" "Severe, life-threatening and in some cases fatal hepatotoxicity [liver damage], including hepatic necrosis [liver death] and hepatic failure, has been reported in patients treated with Viramune" "Severe, life-threatening skin reactions, including fatal cases ... have included cases of Stevens-Johnson syndrome, toxic epidermal necrolysis [skin death]"	"Viramune is not a cure for HIV-1 infection"

Source: Scheff, Liam, The House That AIDS Built, see www.altheal.org/toxicity/house.htm, package inserts

will become severely ill and die). Healthy people are "treated" and worsening health is then attributed to the viral illness, which the drug therapy cannot counter.

Ultimately, if the medication doesn't have any health-stimulating effects, this is also attributed to HIV's alleged craftiness; the virus itself is said to cause "treatment-resistant viral mutations." The patient dies with typical AIDS symptoms like dementia, wasting (weight loss), and neural damage. In their virus fixation, nobody imagines that the patient dies, not of AIDS, but of the very medical endeavors meant to heal.

Some HIV patients who are really sick do respond to antiretroviral medications. But this is because most of these patients suffer from what are called opportunistic infections (infections that occur as a result of an immunological/physical weakness, which in turn can have many non-viral causes).

This means that they are infested by bacteria or fungi. In this context, antiretroviral treatment works like a shotgun therapy, destroying everything bound to DNA— including fungi, tubercle bacteria (Mycobacterium tuberculosis) and other microbes.

However, those who take protease inhibitors may face serious consequences in the long term, because these drugs can also cause liver failure (see livertox.nih.org). Hence, the side effects should therefore not be underestimated for any antiviral medication that is used for treatin so-called AIDS patients. A study published in *Nature Genetics* in 2011 warned of the "of irreversible long-term effects of the drugs on mtDNA mutations raising the specter of progressive iatrogenic mitochondrial genetic disease emerging over the next decade."[751]

Especially the smallest earthlings are not immune to such consequences. For example, the German journal *Deutsches Ärzteblatt* reported in 2002 that "clinical data have shown that serious undesirable side effects for the child can be expected when using antiviral combination therapies in pregnancy."[752]

And in an overview analysis of the topic from 2013 it says with regard to possible birth defects caused by AZT (AZT is still often part of a HAART) that there are "increasing concerns about congenital malformations, including potential cancer, mitochondrial defects, heart abnormalities, abnormalities in the blood and urinary system and sexual apparatus."[753]

Even Goethe knew that medicines could kill. Faust says:[754]

"Here was the medicine, the patients died and nobody asked who convalesced. So we ravaged with hellish electuaries [medicine] worse than the pestilence in these valleys, these mountains. I myself administered the poison to thousands; they withered, I had to witness that the brazen murderers were praised."

All on AZT: The Deaths of Freddie Mercury, Rudolph Nureyev and Arthur Ashe

Even celebrities fall for the theory that antiretroviral substances like AZT are the only hope in the battle against AIDS. Take, for example, Freddie Mercury, former front man of British rock band Queen, who was bisexual and had himself tested during the general AIDS panic at the end of the 1980s. The result: "positive." Mercury was terrified and took his doctor's advice to begin taking AZT. Mercury belonged to the first generation of patients, who received the full AZT load (1500 mg a day). At the end, he looked like a bone rack, and he died in London on 24 November 1991 at the age of 45.[755]

Rudolf Nureyev, of Tatar origin and held by many to be the greatest ballet dancer of all time, also began taking AZT at the end of the 1980s. Nureyev was HIV "positive," but otherwise he was completely healthy. His personal physician, Michel Canesi, recognized the deadly effects of AZT and even warned him about the drug. But Nureyev proclaimed, "I want that drug!" Ultimately, he died in Paris in 1993[756] – the same year that former Wimbledon champion Arthur Ashe met his maker at the age of 49, after he had been declared HIV „positive" in 1988 and his doctor prescribed for him an extremely high AZT dose.[757]

At one point, Ashe did discuss AZT's toxicity. In October 1992, he wrote a column for the *Washington Post.* "The confusion for AIDS patients like me is that there is a growing school of thought that HIV may not be the sole cause of AIDS, and that standard treatments such as AZT actually make matters worse," Ashe acknowledged, adding, "there may very well be unknown co-factors, but that the medical establishment is too rigid to change the direction of basic research and/or clinical trials."[758] Ashe wanted to stop taking AZT, but he didn't dare: "What will I tell my doctors?" he asked the *New York Daily News.*[759] In our article "Das trügerische AIDS-Erbe von Rock Hudson" ("The Deceptive AIDS Legacy of Rock Hudson"), published on World AIDS Day (December 1) in 2017 in the online magazine *Rubikon*, we go into more detail about the sad fates of these three megastars and especially that of Rock Hudson (about Rock Hudson, see the epilog at the end of this book).

"Magic" Johnson: "There Is No Magic in AZT, and No AZT in 'Magic'"

What American tennis legend Ashe didn't have the heart to do—resist the pressure of prevailing AIDS medicine and decide against taking AZT—apparently saved the life of basketball megastar Earvin "Magic" Johnson. At the end of 1991, Magic shocked the world with the news he had tested HIV "positive." "It can happen to anybody, even Magic Johnson," said *Time* magazine on 18 November 1991.[760] A few days later, *Time* wrote that the basketball player had "put the risk of heterosexual transmission squarely in center court." But what was the basis of this assumption? Nothing at all, for the American magazine—just like the rest of the media world—simply referred to Johnson's mere conjecture that he had "picked up the AIDS virus heterosexually," that is to say through sex with a woman.[761]

Evidence to support this statement is not available. Magic Johnson had tested positive, but at the same time, he was the picture of health—until "AIDS ruler" Anthony Fauci and his personal doctor, the New York AIDS researcher David Ho, insistently advised him to take AZT. Johnson followed their advice. But Magic's health rapidly deteriorated,[762] so much, in fact, that he felt "like vomiting almost every day," according to a 1991 *National Enquirer* story "Magic Reeling as Worst Nightmare Comes True—He's Getting Sicker."[763] But virus mania was by then so dominant that nobody thought that the extremely toxic medications could have caused Magic's serious health problems.

There was not a lot of time to think about it anyway, as Johnson's symptoms suddenly disappeared after a short time. In the summer of 1992, after the media announced his retirement from basketball in late 1991[764], he even led the US basketball team to the gold medal at the Olympic Games in Barcelona.[765] This was a grandiose achievement,

and had he still been under the influence of AZT, there was no way he could have accomplished such a thing.

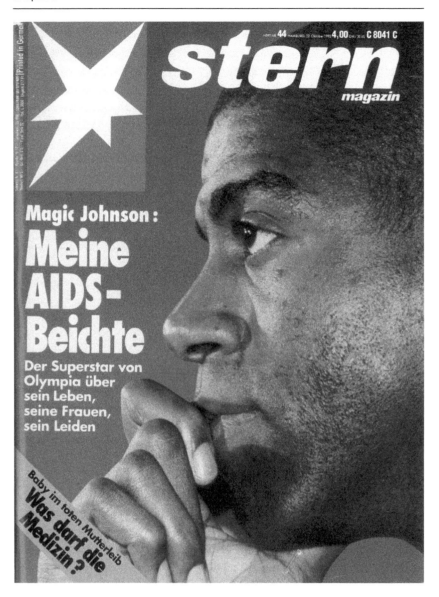

Stern 44/1992 © Stern/Picture Press

One assumes, then, that Magic only took AZT for a very short time; when he discontinued the medication with the deadly side effects, his complaints likewise disappeared. Indeed, years later, in 1995, he admitted in a personal conversation in Florida that he had only taken AZT for a very short time. The medications were connected with far too severe side effects. And so came the saying, "There is no magic in AZT, and no AZT in 'Magic.'"[766]

But AIDS drug manufacturers also play a highly competitive game in an marketing-driven industry. For several years GlaxoSmithKline (GSK) used "Magic" Johnson to spread its miracle cure messages especially among urban blacks. The basketball star's image is splashed on billboards, subway posters and full-page ads in newspapers and magazines. The ads picture a robust-looking Johnson and feature messages such as, "Staying healthy is about a few basic things: A positive attitude, partnering with my doctor, taking my medicine every day."[767]

Those ads are now gone because Johnson got a better offer from Abbott and is now promoting another combination AIDS drug, Kaletra.

However, this does not necessarily mean that Johnson himself is taking these highly toxic drugs. As outlined, the opposite is obviously true. Magic is the poster boy for HIV „positive" heterosexuals and he's a spokesman for a drug manufacturer, so he has a financial conflict of interest that may disallow him from revealing if he is really taking GSK's Combivir or Abbott's Kaletra and, if so, how much drug he's really taking. "Johnson has not directly confirmed that he is taking the drugs he pushes," says AIDS drugs researcher David Rasnick.

In October 2004, we approached the Magic Johnson Foundation to ask if the basketball player has taken any AIDS medications since the Olympic triumph in 1992, and, if so, for how long. But, as of today, we have not received a response.

Hemophiliacs and AIDS

The publication of the Darby study in September 1995 in the world's most important science magazine *Nature* also contributed to the cementing of the belief that AIDS is a viral disease. In it, death rates of hemophiliacs in England who had tested HIV „positive" were compared with those of their HIV negative hemophiliac counterparts over a period from 1985-1992. The printed graph showed that the death rate of „positive"-tested hemophiliacs began to rise from about 1986; in 1987 it rose even more sharply. In comparison, the graph showing HIV negative hemophiliacs remained practically unchanged (see diagram 6). Orthodox medicine claimed that this was proof that these deaths were caused by HIV.[768] [769]

But this study stirred up sharp criticism. Previously mentioned Australian researcher Mark Craddock, for example, penned a decisive paper and submitted it to the science journal *Nature*. But it was rejected—along with papers by Peter Duesberg[770] or with one of the Australian Perth Group[771]— even though the logic behind their critiques is impressive.

Hemophiliacs lack coagulation factor VIII and a replacement has been available since the 1960s causing hemophiliacs' life expectancy to continuously rise until 1985, right when HIV antibody tests were introduced. This is a decisive factor, negligently missing from the Darby study.

The HIV antibody tests introduced in 1985 were immediately and massively deployed. At the same time, the whole world memorized the formula: „positive" test = HIV infection = AIDS = death sentence. Because of this, the rise in hemophiliacs' death rates is alternatively explainable. Those who received a „positive" test result were put into a state of shock and many committed suicide. The rest, regardless of their health status, were automatically treated as AIDS patients.

Researchers and doctors tried out all sorts of toxic substances on them, administering them long-term, including antifungal medications and Eusaprim, an antibiotic that hinders cell division. This also involved hemophiliacs who had tested „positive" but otherwise didn't have any health problems—until they started taking the toxic AIDS medications.

We can't be sure exactly which medications were administered to those declared AIDS patients, since they weren't listed in detail, as *Nature* editor John Maddox confirmed in 1995.[773] But, the *Spiegel* reported in 1985 that, "more than a dozen different medications are in clinical trials in the United States alone—all of them have shown little success so far, and are burdened with severe side effects.

Diagram 6   Death rates of hemophiliacs in Great Britain with a high degree of clotting factor deficiency (upper graphic) and of hemophiliacs in Great Britain with light to moderate clotting factor (lower graphic), from 1976 to 1992

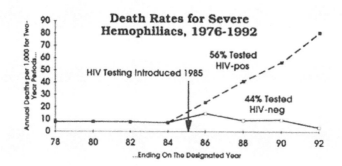

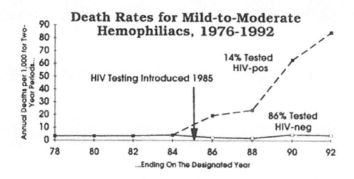

Hemophiliac mortality increased only after the introduction of HIV medicine in 1985. Since about half of Darby's 2,037 severe hemophiliacs were already so-called HIV „positive" by this time, surely HIV-caused mortality should have exerted a detectable influence prior to 1985 in this group. Hence, "only one theory can explain why the explosion of hemophiliac mortality should occur only on the heels of HIV testing: the increased mortality was caused by the pharmaceutical drugs", as biologist Paul Philpott in his article "Darby Debunked: Pro-HIV he-mophiliac study actually points towards non-contagious AIDS".[772] Source: Duesberg, Peter; Koehnlein, Claus; Rasnick, David, The Chemical Bases of the Various AIDS Epidemics: Recreational Drugs, Anti-Viral Chemotherapy and Malnutrition, Journal of Biosciences, June 2003, pp. 396-398

Even 'HPA-23', the substance favored by French scientists and developed at the Louis Pasteur Institute, and with which Rock Hudson was treated last autumn, has its difficulties. In Paris, a clinical study of 'HPA-23' is being carried out on 33 subjects; but, the medication had to be discontinued with numerous patients because of extreme blood and liver damage."[774]

In 1987, AZT burst onto the market and all „positive" patients, including hemophiliacs, immediately received the medication associated with fatal side effects—which suggests why hemophiliacs' death rates sharply increased from this point onward. Incidentally, Rock Hudson died in 1985, officially of AIDS. Less well-known is the fact that Hudson's male partner had tested "negative" and had no AIDS symptoms—something which clearly speaks against AIDS being a viral disease (see also the epilog in this book).

In the mid-1990s, American congressman Gil Gutknecht became aware of this and all the other inconsistencies and shortcomings of the HIV = AIDS hypothesis. He confronted the AIDS establishment's highest operatives with a whole range of critical questions, including: "Where is the proof that clearly shows that AIDS is a contagious disease?" But Gutknecht never got a real answer either.[775]

Incidentally, hemophiliacs are given blood plasma which is freeze-dried before it's administered, often for long periods. If you hypothetically assume that this virus does exist, it would not survive such extreme conditions, as mainstream medicine admits.

The Centers for Disease Control states that this drying process of "human blood or other body fluids reduces the theoretical risk of environmental transmission to that which has been observed—essentially zero. Incorrect interpretation of conclusions drawn from laboratory studies have unnecessarily alarmed some people."[776]

No surprise, then, that in specialist literature, there is not a single clear-cut case of HIV infection among health care workers who typically deal with blood on a daily basis.[777]

Africa: How Well-Known Diseases Are Redefined as AIDS

As statistics on HIV infection remain stable or decrease in developed nations, the AIDS establishment and the media turn their focus to Africa. Headlines and TV news stories are scary: millions of Africans have died and will die from HIV/AIDS. But in reality, these are computer-generated estimates from the World Health Organization (WHO), based on a highly questionable data pool. And they seem grotesquely exaggerated when one compares them with the population statistics of precisely those countries where depopulation has been predicted for many, many years.

"Botswana has just concluded a census that shows population growing at about 2.7 per cent a year, in spite of what is usually described as the worst AIDS problem on the planet," writes South African author Rian Malan in a cover story for the British news magazine *The Spectator*: "Africa Isn't Dying of AIDS." Malan points out that "there is similar bad news for the doomsayers in Tanzania's new census, which shows population growing at 2.9 per cent a year. Professional pessimists will be particularly discomforted by developments in the swamplands west of Lake Victoria, where HIV first emerged, and where the de-populated villages of popular mythology are supposedly located. Here, in the district of Kagera, the population grew at 2.7 per cent a year before 1988, only to accelerate to 3.1 per cent even as the AIDS epidemic was supposedly peaking. Uganda's latest census tells a broadly similar story, as does South Africa's."[778] [779]

"AIDS is a huge business, possibly the biggest in Africa," says James Shikwati, founder of Inter Region Economic Network, a society for economic promotion in Nairobi (Kenya). In a 2005 interview with *Spiegel* editor Thilo Thielke, Shikwati added that, "nothing else gets people to fork out money like shocking AIDS figures. AIDS is a political disease here: we should be very skeptical."[780] But the people in the control centers of politics, science and media aren't suspicious, so they ignore the extreme discrepancy evident between perpetual predictions of horror ("Africa will be depopulated by AIDS") and actual population increases.

It is still firmly assumed that the HIV antibody tests, which are an important basis for the WHO's AIDS projections, are reliable measurement instruments. But let's take a closer look back to 1994. At that time, the *Journal of Infectious Diseases* published a paper on HIV tests with lepers in Zaire, compiled by no less than Max Essex, who is said to be one of the founding fathers of orthodox AIDS science, and of the theory that HIV or AIDS originally comes from Africa.

Essex observed that lepers reacted "positively" to the HIV test. For this reason, Essex points out that the results of the tests should be taken with a grain of salt—above all for patients suffering from diseases like leprosy or tuberculosis. And in places where these diseases are so widespread, particularly in central African cities, antibody tests are probably insufficient to define an HIV infection without any doubt. Essex thought it best to let this observation count for all African countries.[781]

Neville Hodgkinson, then medical correspondent for the *Sunday Times* jumped on the topic and spent weeks traveling through Africa. "When I asked people what disease they

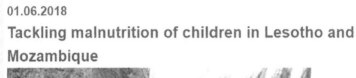

01.06.2018
Tackling malnutrition of children in Lesotho and Mozambique

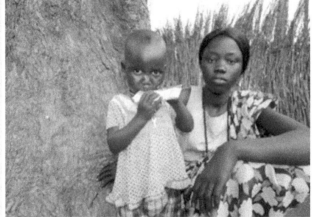

SolidarMed

In 2018, the organization Medicus Mundi Schweiz reported that in African countries such as Mozambique "it is estimated that 45 percent of deaths among children are linked to malnutrition." That was in 2018—more than 30 years after the HIV/AIDS insanity was "launched." And while politics has done everything possible to push an unproven and highly contradictory HIV = AIDS thesis in these more than 30 years, it has criminally neglected to do what is absolutely necessary: provide social structures to ensure that young children are not suffering and dying from miserable starvation. Source: Screenshot from plone.medicusmundi.ch were dying of, they replied: 'from AIDS.' Whereupon I inquired: 'but from which disease in particular?' To this they said: 'This patient has tuberculosis, that one chronic diarrhea, this one malaria and that one leprosy'—all diseases that have been known in Africa for ages. But then everything was rediagnosed as AIDS—out of fear of AIDS."[782]

In this context, Joan Shenton, British filmmaker and known critic of the official HIV=AIDS dogma, tells the following insightful story in her book "Positively False: Exposing the Myths Around HIV and AIDS": "Lucy tested so-called HIV 'positive' in Bukoba (Tanzania), with a single, unconfirmed blood test (wealthier countries typically test twice). From this time, Lucy was considered an AIDS patient, whereupon a certain Philippe Krynen and his wife Evelyne took her in. They were convinced that, if people like Lucy were properly treated (without toxic medications), they could achieve stable health again.

This is exactly what happened with Lucy. The Krynens took the young African women out of her village and helped her get a more stable stone house and a better job. "And so it came that, within the next four or five months, Lucy began to recover, and also gained back weight," says Philippe Krynen.

Her old friends saw her with new eyes, and let go of their fear that Lucy could infect them. At the same time, they began to wonder if Lucy really had AIDS. At any rate, the AIDS stigma had been imposed upon Lucy, something which often leads to isolation. But now Lucy was doing fantastically without medication. And indeed, she never developed symptoms of any of the many well-known diseases that have been redefined under the term AIDS."[783]

Nobel laureate Kary Mullis added that, "They got some big numbers for HIV positive people [in Africa] before they realized that antibodies to malaria—which everyone in Africa has—show up as 'HIV positive' on tests."[784] And not only malaria, but dozens of other typical illnesses like chronic fever, weight loss, diarrhea and tuberculosis also cause „positive" test results.

The HIV/AIDS epidemic is actually a smorgasbord of well-known diseases, many of which correlate closely with poverty.[785] [786] You can't speak concisely about AIDS in Africa without featuring the subject of poverty. Yet, this is still criminally neglected in a region where a third of the population is malnourished and more than 30 percent of babies are born underweight.[787] As we know, malnutrition has devastating effects upon health, and is a decisive factor in many diseases such as tuberculosis.

At least *The Lancet* took on this topic in 2004 and printed an article titled: "Preventing HIV/AIDS Through Poverty Reduction." This document praised Thabo Mbeki who was South Africa's president from 1999 till 2008 and who was generally sharply scolded for his critical position towards the AIDS establishment, by pointing out that "Mbeki has highlighted poverty as a factor contributing to the spread of the epidemic, [and] it is useful to consider the role of poverty as a factor contributing to it, and the implications of this for prevention efforts."[788]

Chapter 4

Hepatitis C: Toxins Such as Alcohol, Heroin, and Medical Drugs Suffice as Explanation

"Where is the hepatitis C virus? Has anybody seen it?"[789]
Michael Houghton, alleged co-discoverer of the
hepatitis C virus at the 8th Intern. HCV Congress
in Paris in 2001

"Toxic shocks like smoking or alcohol consumption can traumatize the liver,
causing genetic instabilities. The human cell itself, then, can produce the
genetic particles which are fished out by orthodox researchers with their
PCR tests and simply interpreted as exogenous viruses. But before jumping
on the virus bandwagon, one must have closely analyzed if these really are
viruses—which has not happened with hepatitis C."
Richard Strohman
Professor of Molecular and Cellular Biology

Still in 1997, Liver Diseases Were Seen to Avoid Drug Therapy

Hepatitis C is commonly known as a liver infection caused by a virus (the so-called hepatitis C virus: HCV for short). According to theories, the disease is primarily transmitted through blood and blood products. In the 1970s, American researcher Jay Hoofnagle attempted to combat hepatitis C with medications. In 1978, he joined the US National Institutes of Health (NIH) to continue his research on treating liver diseases.

At this time, leading experts in this area, the hepatologists and even the pharmaceutical companies were still of the opinion that treatment of hepatitis C patients with antiviral medications was too difficult and too dangerous, since these substances were so full of side effects, and, directly after ingestion, they landed in the organ that was stricken anyway: the liver. For that reason, advances in medication therapy could hardly be observed.

There were experiments with the antiviral interferon, which was tested on cancer pa-tients. But these trials were anything but a success. Hoofnagle was of the opinion, how-ever, that the antiviral preparations had the potential to fight hepatitis C, even though mainstream researchers didn't share Hoofnagle's optimism.

"The idea of treating a liver disease [with medications] went against the grain," Hoofna-gle told the medical journal *The Lancet* in 1997. "Liver disease was considered to be a good reason to avoid drug therapies."[790]

This is no surprise, since substances like interferon ultimately work like chemotherapy and for that reason can severely affect more than just the liver.[791] It was also observed that, after interferon administration, herpes developed, or the number of white blood cells (leukocytes) decreased, something that signals a weakening in the immune system. Interferons could also influence the nervous system, causing psychological alterations like depression and confusion.[792]

The side effects of HCV medications are frequently so strong that treatment has to be stopped. "We need medications that are more effective and tolerable than current treat-ment forms with the active substances interferon-alpha and ribavirin," stated Raffaele DeFrancesco, scientific director of the biochemical department at the Instituto Ricerche Biologia Moleculare in Rome. But DeFrancesco only meant that new medications should be developed to defeat the alleged virus.[793]

The virus mania pattern of thought had also infected theories about hepatitis. And so, all at once, the opinion was *en vogue* that liver diseases could, even must, be treated by antiviral medications.[794]

The damage to the human body and particularly to the liver caused by medications is typically less drastic than in the case of — still too often life-long — antiviral AIDS treatments. But, mainly because most patients diagnosed with hepatitis C have just a temporary treatment, with medications such as interferon and ribavirin.

And even this frequently leads to severe anemia and high fever. Also a risk of cancer cannot be ruled out with ribavirin either, because it has effects similar to chemother-apy which is potentially fatal.

How to Create a Hepatitis C Virus

Mainstream science says that, based on their studies, hepatitis C is a virus with contagious potential. But the experiments carried out to prove this theory are highly questionable going back to 1978 and a paper published in *The Lancet*. Researchers took blood from four patients; it was assumed that they had obtained their non-A, non-B hepatitis (this is what hepatitis C was called until the late 1980s) through a viral infection via blood transfusion. They also drew blood from a blood donor who had been mixed up in two hepatitis cases. Then, this blood serum was injected into the bloodstreams of five chimpanzees that had originally been caught in the wilderness of Sierra Leone in Africa.

But none of the animals contracted hepatitis (that is to say, they did not get liver disease). Around the 14th week, liver values were slightly raised for a few days, which can be interpreted as an immune reaction to foreign blood (and not a viral infection). To rule out the possibility that this was an immune reaction, the researchers should have taken a control group of chimpanzees and injected the same amounts of blood from healthy people. But this did not happen. Instead, an animal was simply locked in a separate room and observed, without having been injected with anything at all. These experiments, then, cannot be interpreted as proof that there is a hepatitis virus with infectious potential.[795]

The hepatitis C virus was then created in 1987, by a team of scientists, including Michael Houghton, of the Californian biotechnological company Chiron, and Daniel Bradley of the CDC, whose task was to find a virus that constitutes hepatitis C.[796] [797] This found virus was then supposed to serve as the basis (antigen) for an antibody test calibrated for hepatitis C virus. Since they couldn't find a complete virus, they decided to forage around for the tiniest traces of a virus, for fragments of genes (nucleic acid sequences) presumed to represent a virus. With the help of a special laboratory process, the polymerase chain reaction (PCR), a tiny piece of a gene was taken from a particle that didn't appear to belong to the host's genetic code. From this, the virus hunters concluded that they were dealing with foreign genetic material from a not-yet-discovered virus.

But for the reasons repeatedly mentioned in this book, we must seriously doubt that a hepatitis C virus had actually been found.[798] PCR is much too sensitive. It detects gene-fragments (DNA or RNA particles) which in themselves do not constitute a virus—

but which are claimed to be parts of a virus that has not been identified. In any case, nobody has yet managed to detect a corresponding virus structure in the blood serum of so-called hepatitis C patients. As with HIV, the virus purification necessary for a clear identification has not taken place. And there is no paper showing that a so-called high viral load correlates with viruses visible through an electron microscope (viral load is the laboratory parameter measured with PCR—the surrogate marker—upon which basis doctors decide whether to prescribe medications or not).

This even led Michael Houghton, said to be a co-discoverer of the virus, to put forward the key question before a large audience at a major hepatitis C congress in Paris in 2001: "Where is the hepatitis C virus? Has anybody seen it?"[799]

Apart from this, the genetic snippets built up into the hepatitis C virus existed in the apes' liver tissue in such small quantities that they should not have been considered a cause of a liver disease. But Chiron saw an entirely different picture: there was the evil hepatitis C virus (HCV). And so, on the basis of these gene parts, they began to build their HCV antibody test. The Procleix test alone, with which blood tubes are said to be tested for these so-called HCV antibodies, now brings in more than $60 million per quarter for Chiron.[800]

Even blatant contradictions are gladly overlooked in this context. This piece of a gene said to come from HCV can only be found in about half of so-called hepatitis patients.[801] And a 1997 study printed in the *European Journal of Clinical Chemistry* (later *Clinical Chemistry and Laboratory Medicine)* showed that the gene sequences officially classified as belonging to the hepatitis C virus can also been found in those who had "negative" HCV antibody tests. Generally, researchers contend that there is still no convincing evidence that the gene-snippets are indeed specific to a pathogenic hepatitis C virus.[802] [803]

The virus theory does not fulfill any of Koch's first three postulates, which must be established to show a causative relationship between microbe (e.g. virus) and disease. The first postulate requires that a truly pathogenic virus can be found in large quantities in every patient suffering from the disease (this is not even close to the case). The second postulate is that the virus can be isolated and made to grow (but a hepatitis C virus has never been found in an intact form). And the third postulate says that this isolated pathogen must be able to trigger the same disease in animal models like chimpanzees.

In this case, though, no isolated virus was transmitted, but rather blood; and there was no proper control group either (in which animals would be given blood—but without the suspected pathogen).[804]

Some researchers have proposed a "reconsideration" of Koch's postulates as they consider them obsolete due to their (misplaced) faith in nucleic acid based microbial detection methods (such as PCR tests) and the difficulty of isolating viruses.[805] But we can already see from our discussion above about the inconsistent presence of purported HCV gene sequences that even these slackened criteria would not be fulfilled.

Nonetheless, the virus hunters assert that the hepatitis C virus is passed on from junkies through contaminated needles (the CDC even blamed this for most HCV infections in the USA).[806] But a 1999 study published in the *American Journal of Epidemiology* gives us another picture. The paper's goal was namely to find out if needle exchange programs, through which drug addicts are provided with clean needles, help to prevent HCV transmission.

The experiment couldn't confirm this theory. Junkies who used these needle exchange programs tested „positive" more often than "injecting drug users" (IDU's) who had no access to the programs. The researchers concluded that these programs do not help to prevent a so-called HCV infection.[807] [808] In other words, even when junkies constantly use clean needles so-called HCV antibody tests nonetheless (or with this specific study, in particular) still come out „positive." Nevertheless, the hepatitis C antibody tests have been widely used (the blood test was developed in 1990).

The 2020 Nobel Prize in Medicine—Scientific Failure Reloaded

But instead of facing up to these fundamental shortcomings of the hypothesis that hepatitis C is a viral disease and doing the only logical thing, namely throwing this hypothesis overboard, the Nobel Prize was also misused in this case to establish a dogma (see also chapter 10, subchapter "Nobel Prizes in Medicine for the Solidification of Dogmas").

In fact, in October 2020, the Nobel Committee announced that Harvey J. Alter, Charles M. Rice and Michael Houghton—the one who asked "Where is the hepatitis C virus? Has anybody seen it?"—would be awarded the Nobel Prize in Medicine for their "seminal discoveries that led to the identification of a novel virus, hepatitis C virus. Prior to their work, the discovery of the hepatitis A and B viruses had been critical steps forward, but the majority of blood-borne hepatitis cases remained unexplained. The discovery of hepatitis C virus revealed the cause of the remaining cases of chronic hepatitis and made possible blood tests and new medicines that have saved millions of lives." That sounds downright fairytale—and it is, at least when you get down to the truth of the matter.

Really fact is however that the world had a hepatitis C test epidemic to contend with. Patients who test „positive" are stamped as "HCV positive" and it's hammered into their heads that they are carriers of a liver-destroying virus, which allegedly, after a dormant phase of around 30 years, triggers liver cirrhosis (the end-stage of liver damage). The patients are consequently bombarded over a long period with medications, which ultimately damages the very organ in which chemicals are metabolized: the liver.

Most HCV „positive" patients have no disease symptoms at all, not even in the liver.[809] Nevertheless, they are treated with toxic medications that destroy liver cells, while the livers of patients in whom the detoxification organ is already affected are additionally damaged with medications. The tragic end result of such a treatment was made clear by a study, conducted by Jay Hoofnagle and published in the *NEJM* in 1995. The active substance fialuridine (brand name Fiau) was tried out on hepatitis B patients. Five patients died and two could only be saved by liver transplants.[810] It is well worth noting that none of the patients had any physical (clinical) complaints before the medication was started.

Those who still believe that medications are active in some way should know that in hepatitis C research there are no placebo-controlled randomized double-blind studies with clinical endpoints. This means that, as with AIDS or cancer research, no hepatitis C clinical trials look at two groups of subjects randomly assigned to receive either the active substance or an inactive preparation (placebo). Neither doctor nor test subject (double blind) should know who's taking the active substance and who's taking the placebo. The trials should run for long periods (for hepatitis C around 30 years) and be oriented on clinical endpoints (e.g., death). Only then can it be shown whether patients treated with the medications actually live longer. But without such placebo studies, statements on the effectiveness or a medication's life-prolonging effects are impossible.

Hepatitis C Can Also Be Explained Without a Virus

Just as with HIV/AIDS, there are numerous peculiarities in the theory that a virus triggers hepatitis C. There are patients whose elevated liver values can be observed using tradition-al blood tests, but they test negative on the antibody test. This prompts some virus-fixated researchers to speculate wildly that these could be "occult" hepatitis C viruses[811]—instead of suspecting that perhaps there's no evil virus at work here whatsoever.

There are further inconsistencies. As studies show, it's not uncommon for HCV „positive" individuals to later, incomprehensibly, test negative, as if by magic, without having gone through any treatment.[812]

Most HCV „positive" patients don't even suffer from any symptoms. And, as is the rule, they only have real liver damage if they have consumed alcohol and drugs. Here, there is a very conspicuous overlap: almost 80 percent of drug addicts are HCV „positive."[813] To this Rainer Laufs, director of the Institute of Microbiology at the University of Hamburg and one of the leading advocates of the view that hepatitis C is caused by a virus, says: "It is worth noting that intravenous drug abuse plays such a large role in the spread of HCV infection."[814]

Mainstream medicine should ask whether the monocausal virus model for hepatitis C really makes sense. Especially considering that if hepatitis C is indeed a contagious viral disease, the number of cases would show a bell shape: at the beginning a rise in the number of hepatitis infections and—once people have built up immunity against the allegedly evil agent—a following decline. But this is not the case. Rather, the number of those officially declared HCV patients in Germany, for example, has remained at 400,000 to 500,000 for a long time.[815]

Another worthy investigation would be to look as whether toxins like alcohol, heroin or medications are, at the very least, co-factors for what is called hepatitis C, if not the fundamental cause. It's fully justifiable to assume that substances like alcohol damage liver cells, cause the production of the genetic snippets on a cellular level, and are then picked up by PCR tests and falsely interpreted as HCV particles by orthodox researchers.

Last but certainly not least, no virus is necessary whatsoever to explain the 30 years that it takes on average until the affected patient's liver gives up the ghost (liver cirrhosis). Sooner or later, toxic chemical substances like alcohol, heroin or cocaine take care of this on their own (without viral help), by gradually unleashing their destructive effects.

Unfortunately, these simple truths are words in the wind, ignored by the virus hunters. Since the 1980s, hepatitis doctors have been so fixated on antiviral medications that the headlines in the newspapers sound like advertisements for pharmaceutical companies: "Hepatitis C – the underestimated danger"; "Hepatitis C – the unrecognized danger"; "Hepatitis C – the new major epidemic. It's coming silently but violently."

In a Northern German city called Itzehoe, the media luridly reported that a HCV „positive" surgeon had infected many of his patients with HCV. HCV screening took place with antibody tests and a few patients were HCV „positive." So, the conclusion was drawn that they had been infected by the surgeon, even though there was no evidence that a viral infection had even really taken place – not least because many people are living with what is called the hepatitis C virus; the tests must come out „positive" in approximately 2 percent of cases. 2,000 tests could garner 40 "positives." So, a doctor could spark a hepatitis C epidemic simply by carrying out the so-called HCV antibody tests on all his patients.

From time to time, media headlines have been a bit more critical, like: "Hepatitis C danger overestimated?" But these articles are the exception to the rule, which is puzzling since anyone who weighs up the various risks of an antiviral hepatitis C therapy would come to the conclusion that no medications should be prescribed. Mainstream medical research has shown that there is "no lasting success" to be attained with the medications.[816] Nevertheless, the virus hunters are tireless and continue to claim that antiviral hepatitis medication produces significant improvements by referring to various studies, such as the one by Hadziyannis et al.[817] [818]

But all these studies are irrelevant because they prove that the medications do not heal and, even worse, that they cause harm.[819] In 2000, a large American study was published in the *Annals of Internal Medicine*.[820] Blood serums from the subjects had been drawn and frozen between 1948 and 1954, and was then being tested for hepatitis C. The researchers found that there was practically no difference in subsequent liver disease between HCV „positive" and HCV „negative" patients. Simultaneously, among HCV „positive" subjects, little liver damage was found and few mortalities could be traced back to liver disease.

The researchers concluded that mainstream research had highly overestimated the risk that a healthy individual who tested „positive" for HCV later comes down with liver cirrhosis. At the same time, it is plausible to assume that substances like alcohol and drugs (including several hundred medications known to have damaging effects on the liver)[821] could be the main causes. There is no reason, then, to treat HCV „positive" patients with antiviral active substances.

"My experience as a physician is that a „positive" hepatitis C test could indicate liver damage, rather than a viral infection," says Seattle-based naturopath John Ruhland. "The patients I have seen with hepatitis C had liver damage that had primary causes such as alcohol and drug abuse. To truly understand what is causing this hepatitis C 'epidemic', follow the money trail. Millions of dollars are being made by selling drugs and treating people for an often non-existing problem."[822]

Ruhland adds that the human body has a tremendous capacity to heal itself. This principle, known as the healing powers of nature, is the foundation of naturopathic philosophy. Ruhland's goal as a naturopathic physician is to help restore balance to the body, the mind, and the spirit. An intermediate-range goal may be to focus on preventing specific future illnesses. The long-term goal is to work with the patient to improve his or her health, not just by eliminating illness, but also by promoting wellness.[823]

Pamela Anderson: The Virus Industry's Poster Girl

Unfortunately, an objective examination of the subjec of hepatitis C is thwarted time and time again by publications in specialist journals and the mass media, which dwell upon the disease's alleged infectious and epidemic potential. The best-known hepatitis C case is probably that of American actress and former "Baywatch" nymph Pamela Anderson. Anderson announced in 2002, when she was 34 years old, that she had been diagnosed with hepatitis C, which elicited global consternation.

The Canadian-born megastar disclosed that she believed she had been infected by her ex-husband, drummer Tommy Lee, when they were tattooing each other.[824] The following year the Hollywood star announced that her doctors had told her she had a maximum of ten years to live.[825]

Proof of this does not exist. But, the global media had a sensational story to boost circulation and audience ratings—and virus hunters had a global platform to claim that HCV is caused by a life-threatening virus. All of a sudden, after leading a quiet existence for so long, hepatitis C was known all over the world. Just a short time later, Anderson even became a kind of a poster girl for the American Liver Foundation, which promotes antiviral therapy. The blonde bombshell made for an effective in-your-face advertisement of medication that had never been proven and certainly its potential damage had never been ruled out.

'I am CURED' Pamela Anderson posts nude snap as she celebrates being free of Hepatitis C

SHE announced back in 2002 that she had contracted Hepatitis C, but now Pamela Anderson is celebrating being free of the disease.

By KIRSTY MCCORMACK
PUBLISHED: 12:03, Wed, Nov 4 2015 | UPDATED: 12:09, Wed, Nov 4 2015

SHARE f TWEET in

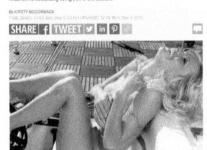

Pamela Anderson is celebrating being free of Hepatitis C

Source: Screenshot from www.express.co.uk

In 2015, the 1990s sex symbol capped it all off by posting a photo on Instagram showing her unclothed and being in high spirits, accompanied with the following message: "I'm cured. I don't have hepatitis C anymore. I pray that everyone living with hepatitis C can afford treatment" (see screenshot). There could hardly be a better advertisement for these drugs, whose potentially lethal effects have been adequately demonstrated, but whose benefits have not.

Chapter 5

BSE: The Epidemic that Never Was

"The assumption that BSE is an epidemic caused by an infectious agent called a prion in meat and bone meal has not been proven. To prove this, at least one controlled feed experiment with cattle herds would be necessary. But this has not been done. A feasible alternative hypothesis is that the BSE epidemic in England was caused by a combination of factors: a genetic defect in the gene-pool of a few cattle herds, which was bred into frequency in pursuit of the best-possible efficiency in milk production, poisoning from insecticides and heavy metals, copper deficiency and/or autoimmune reactions."[826]

Roland Scholz, Professor of Biochemistry and Cellular Biology

Sievert Lorenzen

Professor of Zoology and author

of the book *Phantom BSE Danger*, 2005

BSE: Prophecies of Horror and Wastes of Money

The hysteria caused by the alleged bovine epidemic BSE (Bovine Spongiform Encephalopathy which is a spongelike brain disease) reached its peak in 2001 and caused people to fear that they could contract the so-called deadly new variant Creutzfeldt-Jakob disease (nvCJD or vCJD) by simply tucking into a juicy steak. Scientists and politicians alike initiated the strangest safety procedures, like killing masses of cattle.

"An apocalyptical spirit ruled the country," cried the German *Frankfurter Allgemeine Sonntagszeitung* in 2002. "Hundreds of thousands of BSE cattle will be discovered in the coming years, predicted serious scientists and self-proclaimed experts. There was talk of thousands, even tens of thousands of expected deaths – human, not bovine – caused by a new form of Creutzfeldt-Jakob disease [induced, according to theories, by ingestion of BSE-infected beef]. Reports of the allegedly impending new plague of humanity were everywhere. Two ministers had to resign."[827]

The horror scenarios have not proved true. Not a single German has died from this variant of Creutzfeldt-Jakob disease (nvCJD or just vCJD), although at the end of the 1990s, there was still talk of a "time bomb effect" and the death of up to ten million people was still held as a possibility.[828] But in 2001, the *British Medical Journal* called it "Creutzfeldt-Jakob disease: the epidemic that never was,"[829] and at the beginning of 2005, a British research team gave the all-clear and reported: "Creutzfeldt-Jakob Disease Is Cancelled."[830]

In reality, a giant BSE bureaucracy was erected, "which registers every twitch in the stable and tests every one of the butcher's slices," according to the *Frankfurter Allgemeine Sonntagszeitung*. The program came with a hefty economic price; "BSE hysteria has cost Germany at least €1.5 billion to date," said Sucharit Bhakdi, Director of the Institute of Microbiology and Hygiene at the University of Mainz (his comments appeared in 2002, it is worth noting). And yet, the obligatory BSE tests on cattle were "completely pointless" and "a pure waste of money."

Among the 5.1 million tested cattle, just 200 sick animals were found. And these 200 "BSE cattle" could have "infected three people at most, and that over the next 30 years," states Bhakdi. His advice: do nothing. It is completely sufficient to do just that when (so-called) infected animals are taken away.[831]

The Dogma of the Infectious Disease BSE

Since then, virus mania has continued to plague the beef industry. Companies like the Swiss firm Prionics, which controls 50 percent of the world market for BSE tests,[832] continue to make millions (ultimately at a cost to the consumer). The belief that an infectious particle, or more precisely a prion (proteinaceous infectious protein) makes cattle sick is still firmly anchored in the public conscience. And yet, since the beginning of the 1990s, data has been diligently collected and published—but despite all efforts, there is still no real proof of the hypothesis that a deformed protein (prion) has infectious properties and is capable of causing brain-softening (spongiform encephalopathy): BSE in cattle, and the new variant Creutzfeldt-Jakob disease (vCJD) in humans.

The atomic structure of these allegedly infectious prion proteins isn't even known.[833] "BSE is termed an epidemic, but this is wrong—just as the presumption that BSE is contagious is also wrong," writes Anton Mayr, Chair of Microbiology and Epidemiology at the University of Munich. "And even BSE's transmissibility to humans, neither with classical Creutzfeldt-Jakob disease (CJD for short) nor the new current form, new variant CJD or nvCJD, has not been proven."[834]

"Depending on the spirit of the times and which authorities are in power, one dogma or another dominates the scientific scene, often with an exclusivity that does not admit any other possibilities and hinders new ideas," writes Roland Scholz, Professor of Biochemistry and Cellular Biology in Munich, and a critic of the dominant BSE theory. "And in the BSE drama, this dogma is infection."[835] Here, Nobel Prizes can play a controlling and unhealthy role. On the one hand, these awards usually follow the spirit of the times, i.e. along conventional lines of thought. On the other, they can cement paradigms.

Into the 1960s, scientists were of the opinion that encephalopathy in sheep (known as Scrapie, because the animals constantly scratch themselves) only occurred endemically, that is, only within certain flocks. In which case, up to 30 percent of a herd can be afflicted. Scrapie [sheep disease] is said to be a genetic disease that can be eliminated by establishing adequate breeding protocols, according to research done by Herbert Parry in 1962.[836]

But after the awarding of the Nobel Prize in 1976 to the previously mentioned researcher Carleton Gajdusek (see Chapter 2), Scrapie, like all spongiform encephalopathies (softening of the brain), was redefined as an infectious disease. It was reclassified after Gajdusek's 1970s research on dementia observed in the population of Papua New Guinea; he declared this spongelike brain disease (spongiform encephalopathy; BSE is also classified as one) to be a viral disease transmitted through food.

The sneaky virus culprit, however, could not be found. Nonetheless, microbe-obsessed research continued to hold tight to its pathogen theory. Virus hunters were desperate to impose the contagion theory onto dementia as well.

The work of Stanley Prusiner served as a basis for this theory. In 1982, he succeeded in identifying plaques (accumulations) in the brain, which are characteristic of a brain suffering from neural damage—and which are said to be the cause. In these plaques, certain proteins called prions are found, which primarily build up on neurons, in an abnormally altered structure (the β-pleated sheet structure). Whereas, the normal (healthy native) prion protein shows predominantly spiral-shaped α-helix structures and hardly any "abnormal" β-pleated sheet structures.

The speculative plaque development model implies, then, that prion proteins with an abnormally altered β-pleated sheet structure are the source of plaque formation. The idea is that, as particles foreign to the body, they succeed in getting into the host. Upon arrival, they impose their deformed β-pleated sheet structure upon the normal protein with its a-helix form. And this b-structure makes it easier for prion proteins to clump together, so plaques accumulate on the neurons and jam neural receptors.

These plaques can then only be degraded with difficulty. This process gradually leads to a build-up of "molecular waste" in the brain, causing the death of increasing numbers of neurons. The holes that develop through this, as well as the deposits between cells (vacuoles), give the brain the spongelike appearance so typical of the disease (the term "spongiform encephalopathy" comes from the Latin *spongia* = sponge).

In 1987, Prusiner succumbed to temptation and brought his till then largely ignored "prions" into the epidemic game, something that brought him an enormous degree of recognition. Ten years later, in 1997, he was even "ennobled" with the Nobel Prize, as the *Deutsche Ärtzteblatt* wrote.[837] With this, the infection topic had been cemented. The "Prusiner prion" was declared to be the trigger for spongiform brain diseases, and was said to be more dangerous than all previous infectious agents.

So dangerous that it is allegedly impossible to deactivate a prion by the usual means (heat, radiation, chemical substances). It was the first time that a protein alone was branded as infectious evil-doer. It was said to be especially dangerous because the immune system can't fight it off, since it occurs naturally in the body and is not a foreign substance.

Note that, according to this theory, plaque formation is initiated by abnormally structured prion proteins from a foreign organism; these then clump together with healthy prion proteins in the new organism to form plaques; these plaques and the prions found in them are composed of proteins occurring naturally in the body.

Diagram 7   Prusiner's speculative and unproven plaque-formation model

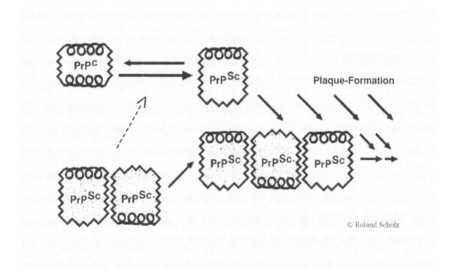

The illustration describes the model of the alleged infectiousness of the prion protein (PrP), with „c" standing for „cellular" and „Sc" standing for „Scrapie" (the membrane protein which is found in as an aggregate in Scrapie sheep). If the protein aggregates that have developed in a spongiform-altered brain are injected directly into a healthy brain, they trigger an accelerated aggregation process in similar proteins in this brain. Through protein-protein interaction, the aggregate causes membrane protein molecules to be rearranged from the "healthy" or "normal" helical into the pleated sheet form, and allows them to accumulate on the aggregate, which gradually grows to the size of a plaque. Prusiner first called this "amplification," but not long later he (falsely) renamed it "infection," because it sounded dangerous.

But the scientific community just parrots his theory without analyzing how the "infection" arises, or whether a simple immune reaction against foreign proteins might not possibly have left its histological traces (as researcher Alan Ebringer claims, this phenomenon has been known as "Experimental, Autoimmune, Encephalomyelitis", in short EAE, for decades).
Apart from that, the aggregate shown in this diagram, which is said to have entered the brain as an infectious agent, did not enter the body orally (i.e. through food), but rather through an intracerebral injection (directly into the brain). And this is clearly not the way that animals in the wild or humans could become „infected."

Activism Feigned for Safety

In 1986, as the BSE epidemic hysteria began in Great Britain, health authorities believed it was an infection involving a pathogen transmitted through feed. Without having any detailed evidence at hand they speculated that prions were present in the sheep suffering from brain-softening (Scrapie). These prions were said to have subsequently managed to reach cattle by way of the meat and bone meal (which contained waste from slaughtered sheep) used as cattle feed.

Through this, it was said, the cattle became sick.[838] And so a mere conjecture quickly became a hypothesis that was blown up into a threatening scenario in the interplay between the media and certain scientific circles.

"The media plays a fatal role, because, in its tendency to come to short-term sensationalistic clear statements, it often feigns a clarity—or a threat, that really is not supported by scientific findings," said Jürgen Krönig, then England correspondent for German weekly newspaper *Die Zeit,* in criticism of his own profession.[839] The media had decisively contributed to hysterical public reactions, which in turn brought the political and scientific establishment to hasty action. Pictures of stumbling cattle and of cow carcasses being shoved into incinerators further fueled the flames of hysteria. Prions became the "horsemen of the apocalypse" that threaten humanity.

But with a little critical analysis, we see the deep rift between truth and illusion. The food industry has conveyed to the public an incredibly distorted picture of food production since the 19th century, through advertisements and public relations. Truth matters little in this spin doctoring, and is massively impeded by the attempts of all sorts of cliques and interest groups to get maximum profit.

"I think that primarily to blame [in the BSE disaster] are the agricultural ministers, who have a sort of symbiotic relationship to agro-business: to the large corporations, not just the meat feed manufacturers, but the chemical groups as well," says Krönig. "Through this, research was contaminated from the onset: this means the experts were directed too much by their interests. The research was not carried out openly. This has to change, for only when there is absolute clarity over the reasons, can something sensible really be undertaken."[840]

How tightly research and big business are interwoven can also be seen in the example of Nobel Prize-winner Prusiner, who has developed his own BSE quick test and promoted it far and wide through an article published in the scientific journal *Spektrum der Wissenschaft* in early 2005. Prusiner did not hesitate to emphasize that the test could possibly also be suitable for testing human blood for BSE—something that, if it became reality, would mean that the test manufacturers had the equivalent of a money tree in their hands. One can only agree with Prusiner when he himself writes in his article: "One may suspect that I propagate the thorough CDI test [Prusiner's quick test] in my own interests."[841]

The Infection Hypothesis Is Founded on Dubious Experiments

So the theory goes that prions have spread across the borders of species (for example from sheep to cow). And researchers concluded that if prions can manage the jump from sheep to cow, then humans could also become infected from beef products.

The problem: There are numerous flaws in the experiments upon which these hypotheses are based. Extracts from the brains of animals with neural diseases were directly injected into the brains of test animals. When, after a year, they detected the existence of the nerve-damaging accumulations (plaques) and holes in the brains, it was taken as proof that a prion had caused an infection, which in turn had caused the development of the plaque.

But the alterations in the brain could also have another cause. They could be consequences of an immune reaction, for instance, with which the body defends itself against foreign proteins (in this case the foreign prion proteins). However, researchers didn't consider this at all, even though a 1998 study by immunologist Alan Ebringer of King's College, London pointed out the possibility that many experiments involving injecting brain material from animals suffering from encephalopathies into the brains of healthy animals didn't necessarily cause the transmission of Scrapie or BSE (as is held to be the case); even if these animals did later develop neurological symptoms and plaques were found in their brains.[842] [843]

We must also remember that laboratory experiments in which cerebral matter is directly transmitted from one brain to another proves nothing in terms of infection, since this is supposed to occur via the mouth (orally). When was the last time your brain came into contact with someone else's brain mass?

Ebringer: "The Prion-research workers do something that is not allowed. They inject brain tissue homogenates into experimental animals, and when neurological symptoms appear they say they have transmitted BSE. However, they have done nothing of the sort, because what they are doing is producing experimental allergic encephalomyelitis (EAE). I think all prion experiments involve production of EAE and not transmission of BSE."[844]

An additional mind-boggler is that the prion experiments involved no proper control experiments (involving a comparative group of animals that are injected with something that can be compared to what the original test subjects receive).

In 2004, a paper was published in *Science* claiming to have produced a sort of irrefutable proof for the prion infection = brain-softening theory. In the experiment, brain extracts from infected animals were not injected directly into the brains of the test mice. Instead, a deformed prion with a β-pleated structure was artificially produced, and it was assumed that this structure would give the prion an infectious property. Then this prion protein with the β-pleated structure was injected into mouse brains. After one to two years, the mice developed neurological disorders.[845]

But, once again, the experiments have no scientific value. Not only because neurophysiology and immunology differ between mice and humans, so that results can be fundamentally misleading.[846] Also, as with many experiments conducted by the guild of prion researchers, there were no control experiments involving an extract that can be compared to the originally administered fluid. The salt solution alone, which was injected into the brains of the control animals, is not a true control. The researchers should have taken at least one other solution containing a protein and have introduced it into the brains of the test mice. Or, even better, a genetically engineered prion protein that did not have the β-pleated structure, but rather the "healthy/normal" a-helix form.[847]

Defendants of the "prions in meat and bone meal hypothesis" also refer to tests in which raw brain material is fed to laboratory animals. But raw brain that comes from brain-diseased animals cannot be equated with animal feed meal, since these substances have completely different contents. Here as well, the test results cannot be carried over to reality. Furthermore, adequate control groups are missing from these experiments as well (groups of animals that are fed healthy cow brain).

For this reason, it cannot be asserted that a certain constituent in the brain material fed to the mice (a deformed prion, for example), had produced alterations in their brains after a year or more — or if the brain material itself had not been responsible.[848] For this reason, the observed symptoms can also be interpreted as portraying the results of an immune reaction.[849]

Of course, experimental games and speculation are perfectly suitable for impressing gullible research colleagues, politicians, journalists and the public. But, they are scientifically worthless. "For no controlled feeding experiments in the field exist — studies that anyone with a healthy dose of common sense would require, and which everyone believes have long been carried out by inventors of the meat and bone meal hypothesis," criticizes Roland Scholz.

This means, a large herd should have been separated into two halves: one group receives meat and bone meal and the other doesn't receive this feed. Since this has been neglected, however, the conclusion is evident: it has not yet been shown that cattle become infected with BSE by being fed meat and bone meal. That an infectious protein in meat and bone meal triggers BSE is still an unproven conjecture.

Incidentally, it would have been even more informative, if a controlled experiment had been carried out with specifically manufactured meat and bone meals (consisting of material from Scrapie sheep or BSE cattle), something that, incidentally, could still be done. Then one could figure out whether the meat and bone meal is a trigger at all — and if so, what kind of infectious agent it was — or if a change in the animal meal's manufacturing process could possibly have been the cause.[850]

BSE: A Genetic Defect Due To Inbreeding

Due to the lack of proof for the thesis that prions in meat and bone meal can trigger the bovine disease BSE, it seems particularly advisable to keep an eye out for other attempts at explanation as well. It could very well be that a defect in the genetic make-up of cattle from a few British herds was multiplied to such an extent through overbreeding that the animals became ill.

BSE manifests primarily in young cattle aged two to five years (cattle can live up to 25 years), while most diseases comparable to BSE tend to appear at an advanced age. With the rare disease called "mad cow disease," the animals were considerably older. With humans as well, these spongiform encephalopathies (brain-softening) that do not appear within families are typically age-related diseases. But children and adolescents also come down with the spongiform encephalopathies, which can be frequently observed within families.

With modern high-performance cattle breeding, most cows are descended from only a few bulls that are often related to each other. Thanks to artificial insemination, the semen of a single bull is said to guarantee high-performance cows as daughters and can supply an entire region. Incest should be avoided, but with breeding geared only towards high performance—in England, a cow provides 60-70 liters of milk daily—this rule is usually not observed. "A single bull in a region's insemination institute could then be the father of many of a district's cattle herds, and simultaneously also their grandfather," writes Roland Scholz. "With this, what has been usual in flocks of sheep for centuries has arrived in cattle herds over the past few decades."

With spongiform encephalopathies, the paradigm shift from infection to genetics could have been executed with Prusiner. In his investigations into the cause of SE on a molecular level, he found that a certain membrane protein on neurons (prion) had a tendency to reshape from the functional/sound β-helix form into the functionless β-pleated sheet form.

These β-pleated sheet proteins shaped like corrugated metal tend to clump together with other proteins that likewise feature a β-pleated sheet structure. The aggregates grow, develop the plaques (clumps) on the nerve cells typical of brain-softening, and can then force other prion proteins to re-shape: first on the same cell, then on neighboring cells, so that the process spreads throughout a brain area (like a row of falling dominoes after the first one has been knocked over).[851] Prusiner called the plaques, which multiply autocatalytically (driving themselves on) prions. He originally termed the process the "amplification" (replication) of a protein that had an abnormally altered structure—something that was later confused with infection.[852]

This amplification process is considerably accelerated when an amino acid is substituted at a critical point through a mutation in the respective gene. For example, in carriers
in a family, in which a certain type of encephalopathy frequently appeared, the base
thymine was substituted for cytosine in the gene codon 102, which usually encodes the

Diagram 8   No connection: BSE in the South vs. vCJD
                   in the North of England

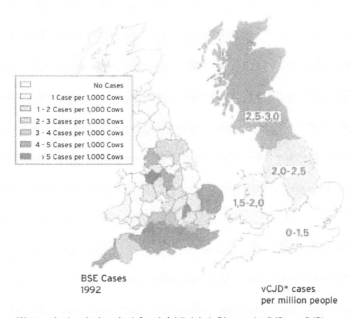

BSE Cases
1992   vCJD* cases
                                                        per million people

*New variant or just variant Creutzfeldt-Jakob-Disease (nvCJD or vCJD)

*Apart from the fact that the few cases of the Creutzfeld-Jakob disease (CJD) variant hardly
provide sufficient material for serious epidemiological analyses, it is generally overlooked
that there was a South-North divide in BSE cases in Great Britain (left depiction of GB),
whereas with the new variant CJD (vCJD) it was exactly the other way around; here, a
North-South divide existed (right depiction of GB). This contradicts the assertion that
ingesting BSE meat can trigger vCJD.*

amino acid leucine. The consequence is that this codon 102 gene no longer encodes leucine, but rather the amino acid proline. Proline, however, is known as a "helix breaker." By 1995, 18 different mutations had been discovered in SE families (in which spongiform encephalopathies or brain-softening conspicuously frequently occurred). Time of occurrence, degree of severity and the course of disease were dependant upon mutation type and position.[853]

BSE as an Effect of Chemical Poisoning

The general acceptance of the hypothesis that BSE is an epidemic (triggered by feeding animals meat and bone meal in which infectious prions can be found) means that no attention is paid to the fact that BSE's epidemiology does not correspond with the feeding of meat and bone meal at all. As an article in *The Lancet* shows, within Great Britain, most cases of Creutzfeldt-Jakob disease (CJD) were observed in people in northern Scotland,[854] while most cattle with BSE were to be found in southern England, as shown in a paper printed in *Nature* (see diagram 8).[855] But according to the mainstream BSE theory, consumption of BSE meat triggers Creutzfeldt-Jakob disease (a theory that, to stress one more time, is completely unproven), but, this could only be explained if the meat from the BSE-infected cattle from the south of England was only eaten in the north of Scotland. This, however, is practically impossible.[856]

In 1985, a law was passed in England forcing British farmers to apply phosmet to the necks of their cattle (see image with the cow).[857] Phosmet is what is known as an organophosphate, and the highly toxic insecticide, which causes severe neural damage, is used against warble flies. Only in Great Britain, Northern Ireland and Switzerland was phosmet used in such high concentrations—the countries where almost all BSE cases have occurred.[858] A British organic farmer by the name of Mark Purdey noticed that his cows did not come down with BSE, ecologically-kept cows did not come down with BSE, although they had been feed meat and bone meal—but had not been treated with organophosphates.[859]

The British government knew about these connections. And so, at the beginning of the 1990s, the law requiring phosmet application to cattle necks was repealed, since there was a likely connection between the organophosphate and the appearance of BSE. At the same time, from 1993 on, there was also a drastic reduction in BSE cases. The British BSE investigative board also admitted that organophosphate was evidently a co-factor in the onset of BSE. And it has been known for a long time that chronic organophosphate poisoning "leads to a polyneuropathy [severe neural damage]," according to toxicologist Heinz Lüllmann.[860]

This was confirmed by the research results of neuroscientist Stephen Whatley, from the London Institute of Psychiatry. According to this research, financed through private donations,[861] phosmet could be the trigger for BSE diseases.[862] Whatley wanted to pursue the subject more thoroughly and requested additional experiment funds from governmental institutions. But the authorities rejected Whatley's application – something which seems all the more baffling considering Whatley's emphasis that "there is no contradictory data," that is to say there is still no scientific paper that refutes his conclusions."[863]

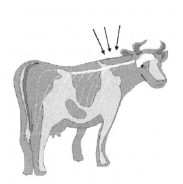

In 1985, a law was passed in England which forced British farmers to apply phosmet to the necks of their cattle (see arrows). Phosmet is an organophosphate, and the highly toxic insecticide, which can cause severe neurological damage, is used against warble flies. The illustration shows the place (neck) where phosmet is applied. The toxin penetrates through the skin into the bloodstream and thus damages the central nervous system. © Dr. med. Günther Zick

In this context, why don't all cows that are treated with organophosphates come down with BSE? One may think that the dose makes the poison (from the Latin: *dosis venenum facit*). However, even if all cattle received the same toxin dose, they would not react the same way, since the cattle have individual genetic makeups. Furthermore the amount of phosmet applied by each farmer could also vary significantly. If a toxin can accelerate the outbreak of a disease (as alcohol can liver disease), then it can also be the lone cause.

If, however, it was officially verified that phosmet was a cause of BSE, compensation claims worth billions would be filed, not only against the British government, but also the insecticide manufacturers. This is certainly not a desirable outcome for the powers that be, and, so, clear connections are allowed to disappear into a fog of prions.

Incidentally, the poisoning or intoxication hypotheses are easy to test, and, in contrast to the virus or prion hypotheses, they are confutable, meaning proof that a theory is right or wrong through toxicologic and epidemiologic verification. But unfortunately, these tests have not been carried out.[864]

Regrettably, for about ten years, the trend has increasingly been towards the scaling down of toxicological institutes, while pharmaceutical institutes gain ever more significance. Through this, the critical aspects of toxicology (poisonous nature of medications and other chemical substances) increasingly disappear into the background, because the primary focus is researching medications.

Besides phosmet, other poisonous substances could impair the health of the cattle, such as poisoning by the heavy metal manganese. In factory farming, high amounts of manganese are fed to chickens, whereupon, by way of the processing of the chicken droppings, the heavy metal gets into the meat and bone meal and into the cattle.[865]

Experts also refer to a possible copper deficiency, which could have attacked the cattle's nerves. Such copper deficiencies can produce severe neurological defects and have been seen for a long time in grazing animal. Among experts, these are described as "endemic ataxia."[866] [867]

BSE Is Not an Infectious Disease

The assumption that BSE is an epidemic in Great Britain, caused by an infectious agent called a prion in meat and bone meal has not been proven. To prove this, at least a controlled feed experiment with cattle herds would have been necessary. But this wasn't done. "According to published data on the epidemic's appearance and spread, a plausible alternative hypothesis could be that a recessive genetic defect had accumulated in a few cattle herds," states Scholz. "The cause would be the excessive breeding in the pursuit of the best possible efficiency in milk production, in which, as a negative result of breeding, an increased predisposition to contract BSE was coincidentally bred-in without being noticed for a long time."

But, it's more likely that the BSE epidemic in England was precipitated by a genetically determined predisposition combined with other stresses (poisoning with insecticides or heavy metals, copper deficiency or autoimmune reaction), to which BSE-prone animals are particularly sensitive and, thus, get sick earlier. Or exposure to toxins like phosmet could be responsible. All of these theories bring us to this conclusion: BSE is *not* an infectious disease.

If there is no reason to assume that this disease is transmitted from animal to animal and from species to species, it makes no sense to fight it by exterminating healthy animals or entire herds.

The assertion that human health is endangered by BSE derives from the unproven "prions in meat and bone meal" hypothesis. This claim based on a conjecture is nothing but pure speculation.

vCJD (the new variant Creutzfeldt-Jakob disease) is not a new disease, but rather a once-rare diagnosis that has recently become more common (even if 1 in 5 million is still very rare). The risk of contracting vCJD through the ingestion of beef products (including the brain, declared to be the risk material) is minimal in comparison to the numerous risks of everyday life.[868]

Chapter 6

SARS: Hysteria on the Heels of AIDS and BSE

"A universal human problem is: if after a long search and painful uncertainty, we finally believe we can explain a certain issue. The emotional commitment that we have made can be so large that we prefer to declare undeniable facts that contradict our explanation to be untrue or insubstantial, instead of adapting our explanation to these facts. That such retouching of reality could have considerable consequences for our adaptation to reality goes without saying."[869]
Paul Watzlawick (From his book *How Real Is Real?*)

*"What I believe and what I can prove,
those are two different pairs of boots"*
Columbo
TV series, *Columbo* (Episode "Murder Among Brothers," 1995)

First 9/11, Next the War in Iraq—and then SARS?

If one believes the media, the world has repeatedly been devastated by large new epidemics over the last two decades. At the beginning of the 1980s, AIDS appeared, a few years later came hepatitis C, followed by BSE in the 1990s and by 2003, SARS (Severe Acute Respiratory Syndrome). But these new epidemics differ from epidemics of the past on one decisive point: while whole populations have been decimated in the wake of the plague, cholera and typhoid fever (although it has not been proven at all that a virus has raged here), the number of those actually affected by the new epidemics is comparatively small.

According to the Robert Koch-Institute, just a few hundred people die from AIDS each year in Germany. As for hepatitis C, we are still waiting for the liver cirrhosis epidemic. And the BSE epidemic has not presented most countries with a single clinical case, but rather only „positively" tested animals.

195

Although death from so-called infectious diseases is increasingly becoming a rarity (here in Germany less than 1 percent of all mortalities), our modern world is plagued by epidemic fear. How else could a few cases of pneumonia – and that is what it was all about with the SARS patients – invoke such fear in Chinese citizens that, en masse, in large cities like Hong Kong and Singapore,[870] they put surgical masks over their mouths? Such masks could be found on every desk in the Chinese province of Ningbo?[871] The Industrial and Commercial Bank of China and the City Commercial Bank of China decided to stash bank notes away for 24 hours before bringing them back into circulation (in the hope that the SARS virus would waste away on the notes during this time?) and even went as far as sterilizing money by exposing it to ultraviolet light for four hours and by treating it with disinfectants.[872]

The German sporting goods manufacturer Adidas, which produces more than half of its worldwide-sold sneakers in China, reacted with emergency response plans. It even considered relocating production to Indonesia. Although inititally, activism on a smaller scale was practiced when a strike force distributed a hygiene regulations leaflet to factory workers asking if all workers wore protective masks and regularly washed their hands.

German chemical giant BASF reported, meanwhile, that they had experienced an outbreak in their office, when a Chinese secretary became ill over a weekend. But luckily, all 250 employees already knew about this come Monday: after the first reports on SARS, BASF had ordered every employee to carry a card with the telephone numbers of three colleagues in their pockets, so that in case of an emergency, everyone was required to call the colleagues immediately. By that weekend, the news had gone viral via phone lines and 20 people who worked closely with the ill secretary were ordered to stay at home. Simultaneously, the entire floor where the secretary worked was disinfected for two days, and from that time toilets were scrubbed many times daily. A BASF spokesman expressed his satisfaction: "The crisis management has worked."

Lufthansa, in contrast, was completely caught off-guard by the crisis. The German airline lost more than €300 million in the first quarter of 2003 after many airplanes were grounded. And then the group announced that another 15 planes had to be quarantined bringing the total number of grounded planes to 70. "First the 11 September [with the terrorist attacks in New York], then the war in Iraq and now SARS – it's the worst crisis in decades," said German newspaper Die Zeit about the Lufthansa situation.[873]

In the hysteria, everyone completely overlooked the fact that people constantly contract pulmonary infections and die. Over the first nine months of the "epidemic," which began at the end of 2002, the World Health Organization alleged that there were just less than 800 "probable SARS fatalities,"—and this was in China, it is worth noting, with its more than 1 billion people,[874] as well as in Hong Kong and Taiwan.[875] To put this in perspective, these few hundred mortalities are so few that they only make up a fraction of the pneumonia cases constantly at hand.

SARS "counts among the very rare diseases," as the *Deutsches Ärzteblatt* emphasized in April 2003.[876] And three years later, in July 2006, they reported that the (presumably existing) SARS-Coronavirus "is clinically irrelevant."[877]

Why such mass panic? Even the rock band The Rolling Stones felt compelled to avoid Hong Kong and Singapore,[878] and the head of the University of California at Berkeley forbade hundreds of incoming Asian students from coming to the elite institute.[879] It was even surmised that Asia's economy and stock markets stood on the brink of collapse.[880] And how could the tsunami catastrophe over the New Year 2004-2005 damage the Asian economy less than SARS, even though, according to WHO estimates, the giant tidal wave claimed more than 200,000 victims within a short time (easily a hundred times as many people lost their lives than those who officially died from SARS)?[881]

The "scratched windshield" theory described by philosopher Paul Watzlawick in his book "How Real Is Real?" offers an explanation for such mass phenomena:

"Around the end of the 1950s, a strange epidemic broke out in the city of Seattle: increasing numbers of car owners observed that their windshields were littered with small crater-like scratches. This phenomenon gained the upper hand so quickly that President Eisenhower, at the request of Washington State Governor Rosollini, sent a group of experts from the American board of standards to clear up the mystery. According to Jackson, who later summarized the process, the committee very quickly found that, two theories about the windshields were circulating among the city's inhabitants.

"On the basis of one, the so-called 'Fallout' theory, recently held Russian nuclear tests had contaminated the atmosphere, and the radioactive deposit caused by this had been transformed into a glass-corrosive dew in Seattle's damp climate. The 'asphalt theoreticians,' on the other hand, were convinced that the long stretches of freshly paved freeways, which Governor Rosollini's ambitious roadwork program had generated, sprayed acid drops against the previously untouched windshields, also influenced by Seattle's damp atmosphere. Instead of investigating these theories, the men from the board of standards concentrated on a much more tangible fact and found that in all of Seattle, no increase in scratched windshields could be observed.

"In truth, rather, it had come to a mass phenomenon. When reports of crater-scarred wind-shields began accumulating, more drivers began investigating their cars. Most of them did this by leaning over the glass outside and checking them up close, instead of doing it from inside and *looking through* the windshield from the normal angle as usual.

From this unusual perspective, pits were found which are usually there (but unnoticed) in a car that is being used. What had arisen in Seattle, then, was an epidemic not of dam-aged windscreens, but rather of *stared-at* ones. This simple explanation, however, was so deflating that the whole episode went the way of many sensation-causing reports: which the mass media first dish up as sensations, but the mundane explanations of which are kept quiet, leading to the immortalization of a state of disinformation."[882]

With SARS, doctors all over the world, likewise, suddenly looked at pulmonary infections from another angle—namely from the perspective of a dangerous new virus and a new laboratory test (SARS antibody test).

Critical Thoughts on SARS Epidemiology: How Did Carlo Urbani Really Die?

An article in the journal *MMW Fortschritte der Medizin* (*Advances in Medicine*) describes SARS' suspected "route of infection":

"On 21 February 2003, a doctor from [China's gigantic industrial province] Guangdong brought the virus by bus to Hong Kong, a city of seven million, where he was to attend a wedding. Already seriously ill, he booked into a hotel and allegedly infected a further sev-en people there, including the index patients for Canada and Vietnam [index patients are the first patients, through whom an epidemic is said to be triggered]. After his condition

MARCHE

La moglie di Carlo Urbani, il medico della Sars: «La sua lezione utile a tutto il mondo, ma compresa solo a metà»

MARCHE

Sabato 28 Marzo 2020 di Lorenzo Sconocchini

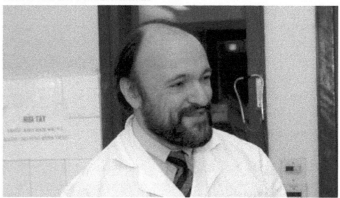

At the end of March 2020, the Italian newspaper Corriere Adriatico *recalled the story of medical doctor Carlos Urbani, who died shortly after he created the term SARS on March 29, 2003. The headline of the article reads: "Carlo Urbani's wife, the SARS doctor: 'His lesson is useful for the whole world, but only half understood.'" Indeed, much of the world didn't understand the lesson, which, of course, is different from what Urbani's wife meant. The real lesson is that one should not blindly trust a few promoted virologists and that no virus tunnel vision should not be attached to the research into the causes of diseases.*
Source: *Screenshot from* corriereadriatico.it

had rapidly deteriorated, he was taken to a hospital where he infected more patients and died ten days later. The Vietnamese index patient flew to Hanoi. There, he was treated by an Italian WHO infection specialist, Carlo Urbani, who gave the syndrome its name: Severe Acute Respiratory Syndrome (SARS). On 29 March, Urbani himself died from the infection."[883]

And yet, every attempt had been made to protect Urbani and the patients from the evil, pathogenic microbes. As the *New England Journal of Medicine* (*NEJM*) reports, "a four-hour discussion led the government to take the extraordinary steps of quarantining the Vietnam French Hospital, introducing new infection-control procedures in other hospitals, and issuing an international appeal for expert assistance.

Additional specialists from the WHO and the Centers for Disease Control and Prevention (CDC) arrived on the scene, and Médecins sans Frontières (MSF, or Doctors without Borders) responded with staff members as well as infection-control suits and kits that were previously stocked for outbreaks of Ebola virus."

The fear went so deep that, to shield Urbani from viral attacks, an "isolation room" was spontaneously set up, in which the expert "fought SARS for 18 days in a Bangkok hospital."[884] At the same time, guidelines for dealings with patients were published: patients should be kept in isolation and, if possible, they should lie in "negative pressure rooms," rooms where the air allegedly "contaminated" by the virus cannot leak out.[885]

But none of this helped; the patients died, and so did Urbani on 29 March 2003. A new causative agent—the SARS virus—was allegedly to blame. The *New York Times'* leading medical journalist, Lawrence Altman, rushed to the scene immediately. Shortly after Urbani's passing, he wrote about the dangers of SARS infection: "It can affect anyone who has the bad luck to be in the way of a contaminated sneeze or cough. SARS can be so explosive that scores of family members and health workers can be infected from a cough from one patient."[886] There is, however, no proof of this scenario. And if this were really true, then it should have come to an exponential increase in disease cases, and the number of infected patients should have reached dizzying heights. But this did not happen, and SARS should never have been feared at any point.

A virus should also have attacked all age groups. But "SARS has largely spared children"—for "unknown reasons," Altman remarked with surprise (without having given this important central fact any attention). Furthermore, the *NEJM* stated "no new [SARS] cases in health care workers have been reported."[887]

In fact, no epidemic took place whatsoever—and certainly not one among health care workers. This also clearly argues against the possibility that a highly contagious virus is at work, since nurses, caregivers and doctors carry a particularly high risk of viral infection.[888] Yet, contrary to the facts, Altman writes that, "it was the quick spread of SARS to health workers that was the first major clue that a new disease had emerged."[889]

Instead of triggering epidemic alarm, the WHO should actually have looked into the central question of why a 47-year-old doctor (Carlo Urbani) died as a result of a lung infection; something that is indeed unusual. But WHO officials suffer from virus tunnel vision, so neglected the fact that anyone who comes down with a lung infection typically has weakened immune and detoxification system. This leads to increased numbers of microbes—which consequently can end in an inflammation of the lower airways. And a whole range of substances can damage the immune system, particularly antiviral medications.

Articles on SARS in the *Lancet*[890] or the *NEJM*[891] show that it's common to administer all sorts of antiviral and antibiotic medications to SARS patients. So, Urbani was given the full arsenal of medications—the side effects of which can very likely be lethal.

We must also consider that lung infections have never registered as epidemics. If, for example, pneumonia cases accumulate, we should ask whether an unusually high number of immune-deficient people are involved—as was the case in Philadelphia in 1976, when veterans contracted pneumonia at a meeting of the American Legion, and some died.

The United States' highest virus officials, the Centers for Disease Control and Prevention (CDC), also got wind of this, and immediately sounded the alarm. A "monster killer" had caused the deaths of the ex-soldiers, the media cried out.[892] The legend of veteran's pneumonia caused by microbes was born.

The CDC as usual, was caught up in an infectious mania, and didn't even think it was necessary to set up laboratory experiments so that non-microbial causes could also be traced.[893] The discovery of a bacterium in a few victims shouldn't lead to the automatic assumption that the microbe is the primary or sole cause of the illness. Such a bacterium could very well be a secondary invader: a bacterium that multiplies on the foundation of a weakened body. We must also keep in mind that legionella bacteria are ubiquitous in the environment,[894] but large numbers of people (and animals) aren't getting sick because of them. There never was any danger of an epidemic.

Indeed, "epidemiologic analysis of epidemic and sporadic cases has identified a variety of risk factors for the development of Legionnaires' disease or for fatal infection," writes pathologist Washington Winn in the journal *Clinical Microbiology Reviews* after closely investigating the event. "Notable among these have been cigarette smoking, advanced age, chronic lung disease and immunosuppression [weakened immune system]. It is likely that a combination of risk factors produces the highest probability of infection."[895] Many patients, labeled as Legionnaires' disease victims, are already seriously ill (with cancer, diabetes, chronic bronchitis, kidney transplants, etc.) and take immunosuppressive medications.[896] [897]

And so the pneumonia that struck down veterans (legionnaires) at their 1976 gathering was a bacterial infection and the veterans were easy targets because they were immunologically weakened after partying day and night (with drugs, alcohol, nicotine, or sleep deprivation, all known to weaken the immune system). Even today, there are still "veteran's disease outbreaks," which amount to nothing more than a few pneumonia cases.

The rest of the "epidemic" victims are "test epidemic" cases that crop up only because healthy people are being tested serologically (by blood test), and this test also comes out „positive"—which in turn can have various causes (alcohol, drugs, malnutrition, etc.).

Antiviral Therapy: More Pain than Gain

A *bacterial* pneumonia may be easily determined from the white blood count, and sputum cultures. As a rule, a directed antibiotic treatment is successful (even though resistance to antibiotics can increasingly be observed). Now SARS is supposed to be a *viral* infection, so a strong immune system will typically allow the body to fight off the virus. Alternately, the weaker the immune system, the more pronounced the viral infection. But, what weapons does mainstream medicine primarily use to fight viral pneumonia or other diseases when a virus is alleged to be the cause? Ultimately, nothing but drugs whose side effects weaken the immune system.

A good example is shingles (herpes zoster), which affects one in three people in developed countries over their lifetimes. Mainstream medicine conjectures that dormant and then later "reactivated" herpes viruses in the body (or more precisely, chickenpox viruses) are to blame for shingles. Hence, for a fairly long time, it has been believed and postulated that antivirals, like bacteria-eliminating antibiotics, are an effective weapon against viruses.

One of the first antivirals, aciclovir (Zovirax), is said to fight herpes viruses and shingles. But clinical proof of this is, once again, missing. Not only do many shingles cases go away without treatment, for which reason people like to claim they react to being "spoken to" by wonder healers. Basically, the body's self-healing powers (immune system responses) are at work. Additionally, placebo-controlled studies for the approval of Zovirax—as with flu remedies (Relenza, Tamiflu, etc.)—provided no proof that antivirals significantly shortened the course of disease.

It is claimed that these medications can alleviate the disease symptoms affecting the nerves, but this is a very subjective sort of diagnosis and, since it is so difficult to objectify, the pharmaceutical industry simply makes assumptions that are ultimately tailored to generating profits. Yet, antiviral substances can trigger precisely the same symptoms that they profess to fight: from anemia , bone marrow damage, oversensitive skin, and breathing difficulties to defective kidney functions and liver damage (hepatitis). All of these adverse effects are noted on package inserts as well.[898]

Additionally, as a rule, these "antiviral" substances are nucleoside analogues or DNA terminators, meaning that they block the genetic material (DNA) and through this are supposed to impede virus replication. But this is not the only concept of antivirals that is tied to a hypothesis with many unproven and even contradictory factors. The basic requirement, then, for developing active antivirals is to first know the enemy—the virus—exactly, and then to know that it is a pathogenic enemy, working alone (without accomplices like chemical toxin, stress, etc.). But again, with the SARS virus, there are justified doubts that all of these factors have been adequately investigated.

SARS: Virus Enemy Not Found

As we've said before, the most reliable proof would involve of taking blood from a patient and isolating a virus by completely purifying it (separating it from all other cell components) and then imaging it with an electron microscope. Only true virus isolation allows for the development of reliable virus tests, since biochemical determination and identification of the genes and proteins typical of a virus require it to be available in a pure culture.

The presence of foreign particles, as well as the false determination of the particle would be fatal, for it distorts the results upon which, ultimately, the development of virus tests are based. The consequences then include misdiagnoses, unnecessary fear of death for thousands of patients, as well as the administration of side effect-laden antiviral medications, anti-fever medicines, etc.[899] But unfortunately, not one of the publications that have appeared to date, shows any proof of a genuine virus. Mainstream research has hardly managed to replicate what are termed coronaviruses (the so-called SARS virus is supposed to be one) "in conventional cell cultures," as can be gleaned from the German *Ärzte Zeitung*.[900] Also, according to orthodox virus theories, the suspected SARS virus should be present in every patient—and it should not be found in healthy individuals. But no studies confirm that this is the case.

On the contrary, in April 2003 at the first large global SARS conference in Toronto, it was reported that "very few" SARS patients tested „positive" for the coronavirus that has been introduced as the prime suspect right after SARS panic broke out, as reported in April 2003, at the first large global SARS conference in Toronto.[901] [902] Unfortunately, this information did not prompt orthodox medicine to ponder, even for a second, if the virus concept was really true. They're just too busy playing with their favorite toys: the molecular biological methods— above all with PCR—and, so, think that coronaviruses could be detected with them.[903]

As always, the medical establishment was confident that SARS was caused by a virus as well. On 15 May in *Nature*[904] and a month later in the *Lancet*, researchers in Rotterdam claimed to have delivered conclusive proof of a pathogenic SARS virus.[905] 436 patients, who fulfilled the case definition of SARS, were tested for the presence of a coronavirus. Then, the supposed coronavirus was injected into some macaque monkeys that responded not by becoming seriously ill, but by developing only light symptoms. Regardless, this satisfied the German *Tagesspiegel* enough to write that the "tests on monkeys at the national influenza center at Rotterdam's Erasmus University showed that the new coronavirus triggers SARS."[906]

The utility of sending patient samples for viral tests is, in fact, highly questionable. As the World Health Organization said via a press release on 22 October 2003 (months later), there was still no "gold standard" for detecting of the SARS virus. In other words, with regards to serological tests they could not be calibrated for a specific virus.[907]

Moreover, the presence of a coronavirus was said to be confirmed in only 329 of the 436 patients who fulfilled the case definitions for SARS, according to the *Lancet* study.[908] This means that more than 100 patients were misdiagnosed as having SARS, and were unnecessarily subjected to fear of death, restrictive quarantine measures and were given antiviral and antibiotic medications laden with side effects.[909]

A closer look at the monkey tests reveals another glaring weakness in these experiments. Researchers took a cellular culture which originally came from a SARS patient and further cultivated it with a complicated procedure, and administered it to four macaque monkeys through their throats, noses and under their eyelids.[910] The animals were examined daily for the appearance of disease. On the second, fourth and sixth days, the monkeys were anaesthetized with ketamine and ten milliliters of blood from were takenveins in the groin, and smears were obtained from the nose, mouth, throat and anus.

Three of the monkeys became lethargic after two or three days. On the fourth day, two developed temporary rashes. One monkey had breathing difficulties, while three were plagued by non-advancing alveolar damage to both pulmonary lobes. The lymph nodes near the trachea and the spleen were larger than normal. The other organs in these three macaques, as well as the airway and other organs from monkey number one appeared normal under microscopic examination.[911]

Attributing these symptoms to a specific virus, however, is impossible, since a gold standard (real detection and characterization of the virus) was missing. Apart from that, many different virus-sized particles were part of the cell culture, so without particle purification a distinction is impossible. Then there are the laboratory chemicals, at least traces of which still remain, and which could likewise have an effect.

Additionally, as already mentioned, the monkeys were anaesthetized with ketamine. Possible side effects of this medication in humans include increased blood pressure and heart rate, increased vascular resistance in the pulmonary circulation, pulmonary edema, heightened sensory perception and intracranial pressure, increased muscle tension, dehydration, redness of skin, dreams (of the unpleasant sort) and shock. During sedation or after waking up, side effects also include hallucinations, nausea, vomiting, dizziness, motor agitation and even respiratory arrest with too large a dose or too fast an administration.[912] These recognized human side effects can appear weaker, stronger, or altered in the monkeys, and are exactly the same symptoms observed in the monkeys (lethargy, rash, breathing difficulties, altered pulmonary tissue). But, incomprehensibly, the article doesn't broach whether these side effects could have been caused by ketamine. It is also amazing that researchers came to their final conclusions on the basis of only four test animals. Especially since the monkeys did not even continuously display the same symptoms, and the symptoms were far less typical than that of SARS (i.e. fever, shortness of breath and coughing). Only one animal had breathing difficulties at all (and SARS is, mind you, a pulmonary disease).

Furthermore, in these experiments, there was no control group of animals exposed to exactly the same (and possibly traumatic) conditions, including the physical containment and the treatments themselves, like being anaesthetized with ketamine. Moreover, the control animals should have received the same injections, only without the alleged virus. Only through such a control group could the researchers truly rule out that the symptoms that appeared in the monkeys could have been caused by something other than the claimed coronavirus.[913]

Apart from this, with antivirals, it is impossible to target specific viral genetic material (DNA). Rather, the use of antiviral substances is equivalent to a round of machine gun shots. Through this, the genetic material of healthy cells is always affected, meaning that their growth is constantly impeded. Finally, antivirals work like chemotherapy in the treatment of cancer patients, in that they are inescapably damaging to the immune system (immunosuppressive) or even carcinogenic (cancer-causing).

The reality is now that with virtually every little ache and pain, antivirals are too-often prescribed by doctors and requested by patients. And the money rolls in for pharmaceutical groups and doctors. But for the patients, this means that, in the long term at least, they will have to risk severe damage to their health (even including cancer).

Cortisone and Other Steroids: Questionable Effects

Steroids are another group of often-used and potentially problematic medications. Steroids, a family of drugs to which cortisone belongs, are extremely effective anti-inflammatories. With this, unpleasant symptoms like respiratory distress diminish, and doctor and patient are hopeful that the problem has been solved. At the same time, the patient's immune system is further weakened due to the anti-inflammatory effects of the medication, and the course of the disease, described as a "viral infection," can in certain circumstances become worse and even have lethal consequences.

The Kiel University Hospital had this unfavorable experience with steroids which were being used to treat so-called "viral liver inflammations." At first, laboratory values improved, but then, under cortisone therapy, severe shingles developed.

In May 2003, the *Lancet* reported that many SARS patients had been treated with high doses of cortisone and the antiviral (DNA terminator) ribavirin. But the case description, which is probably exemplary of most SARS cases, reads like a bad horror movie in which the characters make a serious of unfortunate choices.

The first unfortunate move was the decision to prescribe antibiotics that had no effect, because there was no bacterial infection. Thus a worsening in health occurred. The second unfortunate choice was to carry out an open lung biopsy. This means that a tissue sample was taken from the lungs for test purposes. But after the operation, the patient had to be put on a ventilator. This resulted in the third unfortunate decision: high doses of antivirals and cortisone were given intravenously. 20 days after arrival, the patient died. One can well imagine that the patient did not die despite, but rather as a result of the "therapy."

Admittedly, we could only scientifically draw such a conclusion if so-called placebo-controlled double-blind studies had been, or would be, carried out. These are tests where there are not one, but two groups of patients, from which one receives the preparation while the other gets an inactive pseudo-medication (placebo). At the same time, neither patient nor the doctors treating them knows which subject receives what (active substance or placebo), which is why they are termed "double blind." Only with such placebo studies can it be said that a medication is more effective than doing nothing — or causes more damage than an inert placebo, something that is not improbable, since many medications have severe side effects.

Adverse therapeutic outcomes can only be prevented through long-term placebo controlled studies. Otherwise, the doctor in charge never knows if the patient recovers, becomes ill, or even dies despite or due to the initiated measures (giving of pills, etc.).

And indeed, relevant studies, including ones carried out by the American drug approval authority FDA, argue that such placebo controls (contrary to usual practice) should always be carried out.

Without these placebo controls, it can by no means be ruled out that SARS patients who are mildly ill would recover without medications like ribavirin. At the same time, they could also become completely healthy again, *despite being* administered ribavirin, because their immune systems are still strong enough to withstand the effects of drugs with toxic and immunosuppressive effects. It is just as possible that SARS patients with already severely compromised immune systems are not aided at all by ribavirin, but that the disease's course is only accelerated.

A clear indication of how little sense it makes to administer antivirals, is depicted by the second case description in the *Lancet* study mentioned above. This paper points out that the symptoms gradually improved without ribavirin and steroid treatments.

The Therapeutic Dilemma of Our Time

We now come to the therapeutic dilemma of our time. It has become noticeably more difficult for doctors to engage in "therapeutic nihilism," that is, providing a severely ill patient with only life-support measures like supplemental oxygen and fluid replacement. Nowadays, in our completely overmedicated society, there is a knee-jerk reaction toward doling out drugs—from doctor and patient alike. Caution is rarely observed from either side.

Likewise, few doctors inform their patients about ways in which they can strengthen their immune systems themselves. For example, the influence of the intestinal flora [as the largest immune organ] upon health is very significant, as intestinal specialist Francisco Guarner says;[914] [915] it performs essential functions for the nutritional supply, the development of epithelial cells and the strength of immunity.[916] Numerous factors have an influence upon the intestinal flora's condition—primarily nutrition.[917]

Admittedly, doctors must also consider legal issues. They are seldom prosecuted if they have administered all sorts of medications but much more likely to be sued if they *didn't* administer anything. It's generally assumed that a patient may die *even though* he has been treated with medical substances (even when deadly side effects are known), but it is practically never assumed that the death is *due to* the medical treatment. As well-known British pharmacologist Andrew Herxheimer puts it, in reference to the poisoning of AIDS patients through antiviral medications like AZT: "Damage [caused by medical drugs] is usually underrepresented in media coverage."

Of SARS we can only to say that it is a "banal" pneumonia from which, if unfavorably treated, large numbers of people will die. Or as Ludwig Weissbecker, former chief of the department of internal medicine at the Kiel University Clinic, expressed: "Behind an unfortunate therapeutic outcome is often an unfortunate therapist."

Guangdong: The High-Tech Revolution's Dirty Secret

With SARS, like the other alleged epidemics, virus panic superimposed everything, even though other more reasonable explanations were right under our noses. It's interesting that the first patient to trigger SARS panic came from Guangdong province in China.[918] Here, it's important to emphasize that Guangdong province has 75 million inhabitants and thousands of farms, with humans and animals living extremely closely together.[919]

Yet *Die Zeit* spun a decidedly horrific tale when depicting living conditions in Guangdong province: "The environment from which the virus presumably[!] sprang is despicable: South China, a classic hotbed for deadly epidemics. Here, anything that has muscles and mucus membrane is eaten. Microbes easily jump from one species to another. This demands adaptation to new hosts. And this is how mutated viruses and new epidemics emerge."[920]

But this—as *Die Zeit* itself concedes—is pure speculation. The description also begs the question that if this were the case, how can it be that SARS first broke out in 2003, when the Chinese have lived closely together with their animals for thousands of years?

Through a microbe-fixated view, another piece of the puzzle was completely suppressed which was at least as characteristic for Guangdong province as the omnipresent chickens and other animals: Guangdong was China's largest industrial area, acting as a sort of global workshop with its textile, toy and microchip factories. This region is the hub for China's exponential global economic growth. It's a paradise for

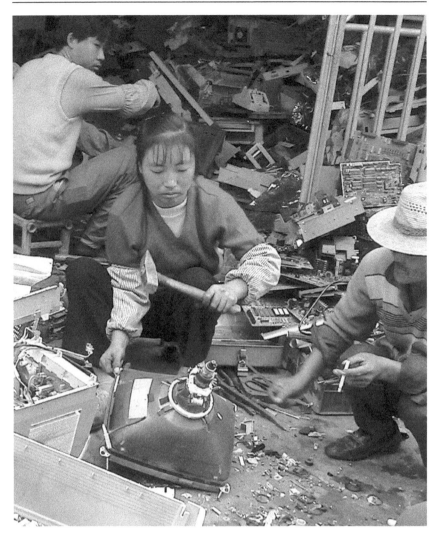

Guiyu (Guangdong), China: A woman is about to smash a cathode ray tube from a computer monitor in order to remove the copper laden yoke at the end of the funnel. The glass is laden with lead, but the most hazardous aspect of such an activity comes from the inhalation of the highly toxic inner phosphor dust coating. Monitor glass is later dumped in irrigation canals and along the river where it leaches lead into the groundwater. The groundwater in Guiyu is completely contaminated to the point that fresh water is trucked in constantly for drinking purposes. © Basel Action Network politicians, corporate investors and multinational corporations, but unfortunately the area has become extremely polluted. There was trash and garbage everywhere; above all high-tech waste.

Computers, mobile phones and the Internet are supposed to help poor countries achieve the kind of prosperity Western nations enjoy. But the age of information has caused many problems, including masses of electronic scrap and toxic waste. Up to 80 percent of electronic waste accumulated in the USA (10 million computers per year alone) is not disposed of in the land of boundless possibilities, but rather, through a series of dealers, the high-tech waste is sold to the best-paying customers on the international market.

At the end of this chain, as the study "Exporting Harm: The High-Tech Trashing of Asia" shows, are the poor in India, Pakistan and China—and above all, the people in Guangdong.

For $1.50 a day, locals disassemble computers, monitors and printers with their bare hands, endangering both their own health and the environment. "The export of E-trash is the high-tech revolution's dirty secret," says Jim Puckett of Basel Action Network, one of the study's co-authors.[921] "A short time ago, the import of high-tech junk was officially banned. But the waste makes it to China, be it because the regulatory authorities are simply overwhelmed or because corruption makes import possible."[922]

One of the places where the authors did their research was Guiyu in Guangdong, which developed from a rural spot into a booming centre of e-waste processing since the mid-1990s. There, workers empty toner cartridges from laser printers all day long without protective masks, breathing in fine carbon dust. Others, mostly women and girls, dip circuit boards into baths of liquid lead to separate and collect the soldering materials with which the memory chips and processors are attached to the plates.

Unprotected, they are exposed to toxic fumes. While the plastic plates are simply burned up, the chips and processors are put in acid baths, to extract their gold. Poisonous fumes are generated, and the unusable leftover acids are just dumped into the river. A lot of garbage is simply burned up or dumped onto rice fields, irrigation facilities or into waterways. The bodies of water and groundwater around Guiys have become so contaminated that drinking water has to be brought in daily from other cities.

Many heavy metals and other highly toxic substances are suspected to cause serious health problems, including cancer and neural damage. According to studies, "the high level of contamination [in Guangdong] caused by unsafe electronics disposal is a potentially serious threat to workers and to public health," said Arnold Schecter, a professor of environmental sciences at the University of Texas School of Public Health. "I think we're fooling ourselves. We think we're doing the right thing by recycling, but we're harming people in less developed countries."[923]

Chapter 7

H5N1: Avian Flu and Not a Glimmer of Proof

> *"There is no concrete proof that waterbirds at Qinghai that may have been*
> *infected with such a pathogenic strain and have survived, will migrate and*
> *be capable of transmitting the virus to other species of birds,*
> *animals or humans."*[924]
> Wetlands International, conservation organization

> *"As I look around, what I used to call 'human beings' have become more rare-*
> *ly. There was once a time—well, it's long ago—, when St. Augustine could say:*
> *'The heart speaks to the heart.' But now computer talks to computer. That we*
> *live in corrupt times needs no argument. Even the great doctors of our time,*
> *when I look at them through my lenses, seem to be quacks."*
> Erwin Chargaff
> Co-founder of biochemical research
> "The Heraclitean Fire" (1978)

The Media: Big Pharma's Megaphone

According to media reports in 2005, the world was threatened by a pandemic, triggered by a mutation of an avian flu virus with the mysterious and ominous-sounding name H5N1. In the weekly newspaper *Die Zeit* in late summer 2005, we shuddered to read the front-page headline: "Death on silent wings—the bird flu is approaching." And, as if the point was to create the title for the sequel to the Hollywood shocker *Outbreak*, in which actor Dustin Hoffman is on the hunt for a deadly virus: "H5N1 plays Blitzkrieg [lightning war]"; "impending attack of the killer ducks."[925] *Der Spiegel* quoted David Nabarro, named the UN chief coordinator in the battle against avian flu in September 2005: "A new flu pandemic can break out any moment—and it can kill up to 150 million people."[926] Reinhard Kurth, then director of Berlin's Robert Koch-Institute, didn't want to be outdone by Nabarro and, in an interview with the *Frankfurter Allgemeine Zeitung* he warned that, "an epidemic potentially threatens all six billion people."[927]

213

Sure, an inspection of media reporting on the subject shows one report or another that actually downplayed the virus panic. The Canadian news magazine *Macleans* (the country's equivalent to *Time* in the USA) printed an article headlined: "Forget SARS, West Nile, Ebola, and Avian Flu [H5N1]—The Real Epidemic Is Fear."[928] Marc Siegel, professor of medicine at New York University and author of the 2005 book *False Alarm: The Truth About the Epidemic of Fear*, presented his critique of the fear mongering climate in several media outlets simultaneously, including the *Ottawa Citizen*,[929] the Canadian capital's most significant daily newspaper, the *Los Angeles Times*,[930] and *USA Today*.[931]

In German-speaking regions, *Freitag*,[932] *Berliner Republik*,[933] and *Journalist*[934] were among the publications, that ventured to be critical; and the Swiss *Weltwoche* wrote: "Only when the last chicken has laughed itself to death will you see that horror reports are more contagious than BSE, SARS and H5N1."[935]

Sadly, the few levelheaded voices got completely lost in the tidal wave of H5N1 virus-manic reports. Under this apocalyptic cloud, there were few attempts to get to the facts, which should have happened from the beginning. Are the warnings churned out by newspapers, magazines and television stations and sold to a global public as the final conclusions of truth, backed up by scientific proof? Quite evidently not.

The scientists and their lobbyists seem more interested in acting as media celebrities. These mainstream virus experts do their rounds in newspapers and on television, creating a guise of legitimacy. The media repeats exactly what these so-called experts want to hear without asking for evidence. We discovered this after getting in touch with various publications asking the following questions:

1. Is an independent study available to you, which proves that the so-called H5N1 virus has been proven?
2. If there's proof of the virus' existence, is an independent study available to you, which proves that the H5N1 virus has pathogenic effects on animals?
3. Does sound evidence exist that rules out other factors (chemical toxins, foreign proteins, stress, etc.) as causes of the avian disease?
4. Is an independent scientific study available to you, which proves that H5N1 can jump to the human species and can trigger a pandemic with many millions of deaths?

Even opinion leaders like the *Spiegel, Frankfurter Allgemeine Zeitung* or the *Frankfurter Allgemeine Sonntagszeitung*, however, could not name a single study.[936] *Die Zeit* merely wrote: "All primary sources [studies] can easily be looked up using [the scientific databanks] DIMDI or Pubmed, and can then be ordered through [the document delivery service] Subito. Experts from the Robert Koch-Institute, for example, or the National Research Center for Viral Diseases in Riems [the Friedrich-Loeffler-Institute (FLI)] are open to questions from any journalist. And the relevant CDC and WHO publications are freely accessible."

In response, we told *Die Zeit* that the research methods they had mentioned were very familiar to us and we were only asking them kindly to name what we had requested: concrete studies. But there was no answer.[937] Many people will be bewildered by this information. Can the public really assume that the mainstream media (which pitches itself as a watchdog of political and economic powers-that-be) critically filters the statements of the medical industry and other interest groups—and do not simply function as megaphones, strengthening the industry's advertising messages?

The H5N1 hysteria made it clear that the media hangs on the words and opinions of the establishment, perhaps most especially regarding medical science. This was also shown by the paper "Bitter Pill," which appeared in, arguably, America's most significant media journal, the *Columbia Journalism Review (CJR)* in the summer of 2005. It describes in detail with numerous examples, how the medical industry uses the media to play out their modern marketing script: first by depicting scenarios of horror, creating the desire and demand for a remedy (typically in drug form)—and finally, the miracle substances come to the rescue, providing the pharmaceutical companies and their researchers high profits.

Not only do journalists naively trust the leading medical officials. "The news media too often seem more interested in hype and hope than in critically appraising new drugs on behalf of the public," as *CJR* writer Trudy Lieberman outlines. "[And] the problem has grown dramatically in recent years as direct-to-consumer advertising has increased, delivering ever-higher ad revenues to the nation's media."

In 1980, Big Pharma spent just $2 million in the USA on marketing and advertisements—but by 2004, this sum had swelled to several billions of dollars per year. And "instead of standing apart from the phenomenon and earning the public's trust," writes Lieberman, "the press too often is caught up in the same drug-industry marketing web that also en-snares doctors, academic researchers, even the FDA, leaving the public without a reliable watchdog."[938]

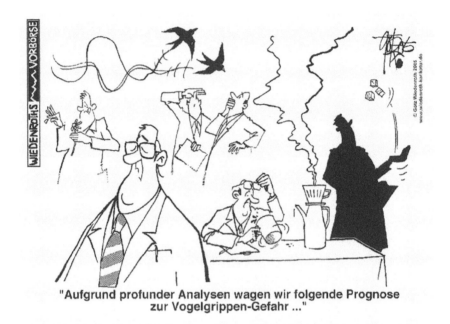

"Aufgrund profunder Analysen wagen wir folgende Prognose zur Vogelgrippen-Gefahr ..."

"On the basis of profound analyses, we venture to offer the following prognoses of avian flu danger ..."

H5N1: No Evidence of Virus Existence and Pathogenic Effect

Like the media, the German Federal Consumer Protection Ministry, government ministries of countries like the USA, Canada and France, and the World Health Organization firmly assume that H5N1 is a "highly contagious" virus. Or as Anthony Fauci (director of the powerful American National Institute of Allergy and Infectious Diseases and one of the eminent figures in American viral science who had already contributed decisively to the establishment of the HIV = AIDS dogma) put it: H5N1 is "a time bomb waiting to go off."[939] Later, in September 2006, the World Health Organization and the World Bank did a cost calculation, announcing that an avian flu pandemic could cost the world $2 trillion.[940]

These are words with explosive force, which begs the question: Can these authorities, upon whom the media relies in its H5N1 reports, back up their statements about an avian flu pandemic linked to such wide-reaching consequences with hard facts?

We sent the German National Consumer Protection Ministry (BMVEL) our four central questions, whereupon we received the following answer: "You are asking about very specific issues, which, at present, the Ministry—we ask for your understanding—cannot answer as quickly as would be necessary for your research." We wrote back that we had plenty of time, and would only like to know when we could expect an answer.

We also pointed out that the Ministry should actually have all the available evidence at hand. Otherwise, the Ministry could hardly be justified in making public statements expressing no doubt that H5N1 exists, is highly contagious, pathogenic (disease causing) and so on.[941] [942] Nor, without evidence at hand, should they have been spending millions of tax dollars on the battle against H5N1. But the Ministry could not name any studies and simply insisted: "Your requests for evidence of the pathogenicity and pandemic potential of the H5N1 virus and the studies that prove this can only be answered by the experts at the Robert Koch-Institute and the Friedrich-Loeffler-Institute."[943]

We then turned to the Friedrich-Loeffler-Institute (FLI), which, according to the Consumer Protection Ministry, was in possession of "pure H5N1 viral cultures."[944] As a response, the FLI sent four studies, published in the well-known American scientific journals *Proceedings of the National Academy of Sciences*,[945] *Science*,[946] *Journal of Virology*,[947] and *Emerging Infectious Diseases*.[948] But neither these papers, nor the paper by Subbarao et al (which appeared in *Science* in 1998)[949] cited in the *Emerging Infectious Diseases* paper claiming that H5N1 had been found in a human for the first time in 1997, yield actual proof of H5N1 existence (and these papers did not contain evidence for our other three questions either).

For avian flu, like the other alleged superviruses, biomedical research simply pulled its magic wand—the biochemical replication technique PCR (polymerase chain reac-

Chapter 7

tion)—out of its bag of tricks. Through PCR they claimed that the H5N1 virus' genetic material is replicated, and through this the virus had been detected. But in fact, PCR, as Terence Brown maintains in his standard work *Genomes*, cannot be used to detect viruses that have not been decoded ("sequenced") beforehand. And a complete decoding of H5N1's genetic material, which is necessary in order to know what exactly is being replicated using PCR, has never taken place. In any case, nobody could send us such a study (details on this topic can be read in: Engelbrecht, Torsten; Crowe, David, Avian Flu Virus H5N1: No Proof for Existence, Pathogenicity, or Pandemic Potential; Non-"H5N1" Causation Omitted, *Medical Hypotheses*, 4/2006; pp. 855-857).[950]

So, once again, there is evidently no electron micrograph of a pure and fully characterized H5N1 virus, either. There were pictures of alleged H5N1 viruses printed in media sources, but these were computer animations or completely normal cellular components that had been artificially produced in a test-tube (which is easily recognizable to any molecular biologist). The layperson can verify this by requesting a specialist peer reviewed publication in which H5N1 is illustrated and described in all the glory of its genetic information from the authorities in question, like the American CDC or the FLI. If anyone receives such a paper, please forward it on to us.[951]

Since H5N1 has never been seen, avian flu antibody tests—like SARS, hepatitis C, HIV and modern viral science in general—attempt to prove the existence of the deadly enemy in an indirect way. The claim is that an infected individual has very special antibodies directed against this particular H5N1 virus. But such highly specialized antibody tests could only be constructed if it were clear exactly what the tests reacted to when they came out „positive" or "negative." But here we've come full circle, for this would only be possible if tests were calibrated for an H5N1 virus, but there is no proof that such a thing exists.

Because of this, it is impossible to say that H5N1 can cause disease. Orthodox researchers say that the pathogenicity of viruses like H5N1 can be proven in the laboratory by "inoculating" it into fertilized eggs or animals that have already seen the light of day (the neon light of the test laboratory).[952] But, a look at the publications in which the experiments are described shows no proof of pathogenicity.

In the laboratory experiment which the FLI presented as evidence of H5N1's pathogenicity, large amounts of the test extract (which may have contained all sorts of cellular components and other potentially damaging material) was injected into ducks' windpipes, nasal cavities, eyes and throats for days. All the damage and destruction this extract caused was then passed off as the result of an H5N1 virus.[953] [954]

Such details do not interest the mainstream media. They keep playing their game of blown up horror stories and simultaneously credit scientists for their reports. In mid-January 2006, *Spiegel Online* jumped on the mega-story that H5N1 was said to have swooped in and killed three Turkish children; the headline read: "H5N1 virus adapts to humans." In the story they referred to WHO scientists who, after their analysis of the young victims, claimed to have discovered a genetic alteration in a virus that could become dangerous for humans.

However, it is not provable that this mutation had already adapted to humans, as the *Spiegel* admits in the body of the article: "It is still too early to estimate decisively whether the mutations are dangerous [for humans] as the WHO declared."[955] The WHO experiments were not published in any peer reviewed medical journals, so we inquired repeatedly to the WHO, requesting they send us papers on these experiments or simply tell us their titles so we could examine them for ourselves. But the World Health Organization did not respond.[956]

(Not Only) Factory Farming Makes Birds Sick

As with SARS, BSE, hepatitis C and HIV, it is necessary with H5N1 to move away from the fixation on viruses. For decades, we have been able to observe how animals in industrial poultry farming become sick: their combs turn blue, their egg production is reduced, or their feathers become dull.

The FLI, Germany's national institute of animal health and national avian flu reference laboratory, describes the symptoms that appear in birds in its information pamphlet "Classical avian influenza—a highly pathogenic form of avian influenza [highly contagious form of bird flu]": "Animals are apathetic, have dull, ruffled feather coats, and high fevers and reject feed and water. Many exhibit breathing difficulties, sneezing, and have discharge from eyes and beak. They develop watery-slimy, greenish diarrhea and sometimes exhibit disruptions to the central nervous system (abnormal posture of

219

the head). Water deposits (edemas) can appear on the head, wattle, comb and feet can turn purple through congestion or internal bleeding. Egg production is interrupted, and eggs that are produced have thin and deformed shells, or no hard shells at all (wind eggs). In chickens and turkeys, mortality rates are very high. Ducks and geese don't get sick as easily, and the disease does not always lead to death. Sometimes they suffer from an intestinal infection, which is outwardly almost unnoticeable, or else display central nervous disruptions."[957]

For years, a virus has been claimed as the sole cause of these disease phenomena, something which the FLI also takes for granted, writing in its information flyer on "Classical Avian Influenza": "How is avian influenza transmitted and spread? Diseased animals eliminate masses of the infectious agent with feces and mucous or fluid from the beak and eyes. Other animals become infected through direct contact—by breathing in or pecking at material containing the virus."[958]

By presenting something that has not been scientifically proven (no proof of virus existence, no proof of the transmittable or infectious mechanism) as irrefutable fact,[959] viral research commits a most basic error. It neglects its highest duty, namely, to investigate if factors other than microbes cause or at least are contributing causes of the disease in birds. In fact, these factors are characteristic of factory farming:

- Heavy psychological stress resulting from extremely close crowding in the cages and mass stabling with no natural sunlight
- Denatured industrial feed, including already spoiled feed
- Distortion of animal bodies' as a result of overbreeding for certain desired physical characteristics
- Preventive administration of all sorts of medications (antibiotics, vaccines, etc.) that may induce severe side-effects, even to chicks

You don't have to be a scientist to suspect that animals exposed to these unnatural conditions for a lifetime can become ill. A major offender, as studies show, is high-performance breeding, which pumps the animals up, while simultaneously deconditioning them in many physical areas, so that the livestock become ill almost independent of the farming system. This breeding is so extreme that many species would not be able to manage in more natural farming conditions.

Imagine trying to keep a high-performance cow with a super-sized udder that produces 8,000 liters of milk per year in a meadow without giving her concentrated feed? It wouldn't work at all. No less degenerate is the situation with poultry. "Eight-week-old chickens today are equipped with seven times the chest musculature as nine-week-old chickens 25 years ago," as John Robbins describes the gruesome reality of factory farming in his book "The Food Revolution."[960]

Numerous animals also suffer from skin diseases, chemical burns ("hock burns"), skeletal problems and paralysis. In the European Union alone, many tens of millions of hens in the mass pens are affected by lameness, which can be associated with severe pain caused by abnormal skeletal development and bone diseases[961] [962] (in many large facilities, half of the animals are affected by skeletal growth problems).[963] [964] These lame animals spend up to 86 percent of their time lying down, so that they sometimes cannot reach the drinking water container for days at a time.

Countless hens are also tormented by heart problems; many animals die of sudden cardiac arrest ("sudden death syndrome"). Experts estimate that in the EU, around 90 million chickens per year die as a result of heart defects, which can primarily be linked back to overbreeding—the heart simply cannot keep up with the extremely stimulated body growth.[965] Additionally, the air in the gigantic halls where the chickens are kept can be so full of dust and biting ammonia that the animals' eyes, throats or lungs begin to burn, resulting in diseases, collapsed lungs and a weakened immune system.[966] [967] [968]

Even assuming that a virus with pathogenic potential is somehow a culprit, it is science's duty to clarify the roles played by other possible disease-causing factors (like factory farming itself). And indeed, the FLI admits that the clinical pictures that the flu virus produces in the birds are similar to other clinical pictures.

Altogether, the FLI lists eight similar clinical pictures—so-called "differential diagnoses." But unfortunately, they only take these into consideration when they can't nab an influenza virus as the culprit.[969] Furthermore, the first seven spots on this eight-point list are diseases which mainstream medicine firmly assumes are caused by microbes (like so-called "pneumoviruses" or microbes believed to be the primary/single cause of "infectious bronchitis")—and only at the very end, in eighth place, are "poisonings" mentioned, with no further detailed explanation.[970]

Thus, before checking if the animals' symptoms have been caused by poisoning with medications, spoiled feed, chemicals like ammonia and so on, examiners first look to see if seven different infectious agents triggered disease. And if they think they have apprehended such a microorganism, they simply stop searching for other potential toxins. Poultry farm inspectors fall in step with this virus fixation. In 2003, when avian flu panic broke out in Holland, samples from diseased animals were sent in, but no samples of feed, water, litter or indoor air.[971] The study could hardly have been more single-mindedly directed at microbes.

The Friedrich-Loeffler-Institute did tell us that it had investigated if factors other than the alleged H5N1 virus could have led to the illnesses among Chinese wild birds that were believed to have triggered the 2005 avian flu and subsequently exterminated). But none of the studies we received from the FLI look at any causes beyond H5N1 – not even from the paper that is explicitly said to support the FLI's statements: "Role of domestic ducks in the propagation and biological evolution of highly pathogenic H5N1 influenza viruses in Asia," published in *Proceedings of the National Academy of Sciences*, 26 July 2005.

Obviously no further research was done after they thought they had discovered a virus with the assistance of indirect detection procedures (PCR and antibody tests). But, as already mentioned, these indirect "proof" procedures do not confirm the existence of a certain virus. And they certainly don't deliver evidence that this is a disease-causing virus.

Many experts like veterinarians and also small poultry breeders, meanwhile, continue calling attention to the fact that the so-called avian flu is by no means solely a phenomenon of factory farming, or that keeping laying hens in cages actually makes them less susceptible to disease than if they were kept in free range farms. But under closer observation, these clues do not add up.

The caged animals must battle substantial health problems and death rates. Even in the so-called enhanced cages, walking, running, fluttering and flying are just as impossible as in conventional cages, which are the size of a standard sheet of paper. "And a consequence of lack of movement is a reduced bone stability, osteoporosis, from which skeletal anomalies and painful broken bones can result," states Ute Knierim, professor of Applied

Farm Animal Ethology and Animal-Fair Husbandry in the Department of Ecological Agricultural Science at the University of Kassel.[972]

Here, disease is all too hastily equated with microbial or viral infection. But whether, for instance, free-range animals have also really become sick because of a virus or because of other factors must first be closely investigated in detail. In any case, when requests are made for concrete studies, no studies are named. The typical response is, "Oh, everybody knows that," or that the conclusion was made through personal experience.

Personal experience is certainly useful and here there is evidence to show that modern production methods make animals sick. We learn from our elders, who grew up on chicken farms in the 1920s and 1930s, a time when the birds could run around and peck away in a much more natural environment and were generally fed very natural food (corn, fresh vegetables, etc.). These birds never had a bluish comb discoloration or dull feathers. So, it's reasonable to conclude that the type of a farming is important, and perhaps even the deciding factor in the animals' health.

At first glance, modern free-range farming might sound like a good thing, but it is all too many times anything but— rather it also constitutes a sort of factory farming. Often, many thousand of chickens share a limited grass surface; up to ten chickens per square meter. Typically, "larger problems occur in larger flocks," according to Ute Knierim.[973] We must remember, though, that these conditions don't necessarily cause viruses. For example, an investigation by the Research Institute for Organic Farming (FiBL) shows that with the increase in flock sizes, feather picking, which compromises health, also increased. "Feather-picking is a serious problem that still has to be solved in order to establish whether it's fair to keep laying hens in larger flocks," says Helen Hirt, animal breeding and husbandry expert at the FiBL.

It's no coincidence that various livestock farming facilities have introduced an upper limit on flock sizes. Particularly as studies show that laying hens from large flocks use the important green space less than hens in small flocks. Why this is the case is not absolutely clear, but it has been observed that the green surface is unevenly used by the animals, which in turn leads to an overuse of the grass close to the coop, and in many cases to the turf's destruction and consequent overfertilization of the soil in this area. For animals constantly pecking at the ground, this can present a large problem.

223

According to Hirt, "the question of how turf can be kept intact is one of the most important for laying hens with pasture."

One possible way to make chickens spread out is to erect a shelter where the animals can take their dust baths. Our domestic chickens are descended from Bankiva chickens that lived in forests offering shade and places for retreat. "And the need to be in an environment offering covered areas continues with our domestic chickens," says Hirt. Indeed, investigations show that chickens do spread out better over the green surface when sand-bath shelters are made available to them.[974]

These short explanations clearly show that poultry breeding appropriate to each species that encourages robust health is a difficult undertaking. But the primary goals of many livestock owners are not just maximizing profits but also maintaining the animals' health. Unfortunately, all too often, they do not have sufficient professional knowledge to guarantee that their birds stay healthy. Just like in human medicine, the animals are hastily and frivolously administered highly toxic medications, and are fed all sorts of things, from artificial industrial feed to human favorites like popcorn or chocolate—things to which the animals are certainly not genetically adapted. All of this is really worth bearing in mind, as is the practice of regularly giving young chicks numerous vaccines.

"Besides general know-how, the smaller rural structures, in which owners take care of the animals themselves and thus may have better training and more interest in the animals' well-being, probably also play a part in the realization of considerably better results," summarizes Knierim. "But individual factors, like access to a cold scratching shed and the origin of the hens, evidently have strong influence upon the success of an alternative way of keeping laying hens."[975]

Moreover, studies have shown that an artificially triggered laying interruption has benefits. This usually occurs through substantial light reduction and feed restriction. At first, it can put considerable strain on the animals. But at the end of the laying pause it was shown that both the strength of the eggshells and the quality of the proteins had significantly improved. The weight of the eggs had also sharply increased and markedly less feather damage was observed in the animals at the end of the laying pause.[976]

"Chickens—like all animals used in agriculture—are natural beings," reminds Hans-Ulrich Huber from the Swiss animal protection organization STS. "For this reason, they should not spend their lives exclusively in coops, but should also experience sun, earth, plants, air and light. This corresponds to their inherent needs and boosts their health! For wherever the sun doesn't reach, comes the vet."[977]

Guesswork on Rügen

The H5N1 scare, which affected Germany via the island of Rügen in the Baltic Sea, was also no more than an artificially produced test epidemic. Dead birds were searched for, found, and collected by the German armed forces and tested by so-called epidemic experts. That the occasional bird had s „positive" test was no reason to panic, since nobody can precisely say what causes a „positive" or „negative" reaction to the tests. In any case, that it is an evil H5N1 virus is, as outlined, anything but proven.

Another striking fact these scientists chose to overlook is that only a fraction of dead birds discovered reacted „positively" to the H5N1 tests. At this point, health officials should have asked what had caused the death of all the H5N1 „negative" birds. And did more birds die that year than the previous year? Or did they search more for dead birds? These are self-evident questions that the scientists, the politicians and the media chose not to ask. A rare exception appeared in the German *Tageszeitung,* which quoted ornithologist Wolfgang Fiedler of the Max-Planck-Institute: "Despite bird flu, avian mortality rates on Rügen have not to date been higher than in other years."

An even more difficult question to answer is why the assembled experts chose not to carry out proper research. They certainly didn't look for the source of the (purported) avian flu infection on Rügen. "How on earth could Rügen's swans become infected with the dangerous H5N1 virus?" asked *Der Spiegel,* referring to reports from the Associated Press and the German Press Agency (Deutsche Presse-Agentur, dpa). "Researchers have a mystery before them. For the birds had wintered in Germany—and as a result didn't come from the [alleged!] epidemic areas."[978] The bird population on Rügen, as ornithologists reported, is basically isolated in winter, something which clearly speaks against the possibility that the swans somewhere became infected with an H5N1 virus.

But scientific and political powers ignore every doubt, pass over every inconsistency and simply stick to this: H5N1 is the deadly enemy. They're not interested in proof—speculation is enough. And so the allegations continue to pose as truths: that H5N1 came out of the Far East, where, since late 2003, it is said to have caused several outbreaks of avian influenza in various Southeast Asian countries, including Korea, Indonesia, Vietnam, Japan, Thailand, Cambodia, China (including Hong Kong), Laos and Malaysia—and by mid-2005, more than 100 million animals had died.[979] Mind you, even according to official statements, only a fraction of the deaths are accounted for by H5N1. By far the largest proportion of the bird deaths were a result of the mass-exterminations prompted by the virus-panicked authorities.

The prevailing practice is as follows: a chicken (or another bird) is singled out because it lays fewer eggs or gets a blue comb; it's then sent to virus hunters and tests „positive" for H5N1; and an epidemic of panic breaks out among humans! Consequently, all chickens in close proximity are gassed to death. And ultimately, statistics show that these 100 million chickens were killed by the avian flu virus H5N1, further fanning the flames of panic.

The Dutch Bird Flu Panic, 2003: Caught in Virus Tunnel Vision

It would be a mistake to assume that these bird gassings are the product of some cruel Third World practice. In early 2003, Dutch officials on the border of the German state of North Rhine-Westfalia (NRW) reported that "health problems" with a "very high" death rate had been observed on six poultry farms.

This immediately triggered epidemic hysteria. The next day (a Saturday), no-go zones within a radius of 10 kilometers of the affected farms were erected and poultry shows were prohibited. Additionally, the Netherlands banned exports of poultry and eggs. On the same day, the government of NRW issued an import and export ban on poultry products coming from their EU neighbor. Dozens of operations that had delivered chickens or feed from the Netherlands in the days before were put under official observation. Immediately, the search for a virus began using indirect test procedures—and look at that! The very next day, there was an announcement that a highly pathogenic virus of the type H7N7 had been found.

"Over the following four months, 26 million chickens in the Netherlands, around 2.5 million in Belgium, and approximately 100,000 in NRW were gassed with carbon dioxide, poisoned by lethal injection, electrocuted or manually slaughtered," according to Hans Tolzin, editor of the German vaccination publication *Impf-Report*, who did extensive analysis of the event.[980]

Yet the media jumped on the virus bandwagon. German *Stern* magazine falsely reported, "approximately 30 million animals perished from the bird flu in the Netherlands."[981] And the weekly newspaper *Die Zeit* said that, "The impending attack of the killer ducks could destroy the existence of German chicken breeders. A bird flu like in 2003 is imminent. Then, millions of chickens lost their lives in the Netherlands and in the town of Viersen on the lower Rhine"[982]—which likewise suggests that a virus had wiped out the birds. But these media claims are ridiculous because a claimed H7N7 virus was only found in single animals (or more precisely, a claimed H7N7 virus was said to be identified in individual animals). In the end, 30 million birds died from another all-too-human strain of virus mania.

Zeit and *Stern* rode the waves of public virus panic—in this case, giant killer waves. The killings ultimately swelled to such a size that the capacity of extermination and cremation facilities was no longer sufficient. A state of emergency was imposed on Dutch communities, and they were barricaded off by the military. When a few diseased chickens were found on a farm, the farm's complete chicken stock was "preventively" exterminated, along with the stocks of surrounding farms. The economic damage in the Netherlands alone cost more than €100 million.

But the existence—or even the dangerousness—of this so-called H7N7 virus was likewise never proven. And while there was, once again, reason enough to look for other causes (the effects of factory farming on the animals' health, for example), the authorities declared H7N7 the enemy—and eureka!—another epidemic was born. "The epidemic was announced on 23 February 2003, and since then, I have collected and evaluated all accessible press releases and official reports," says Tolzin. "But there was only a single report with researchable details, from which it emerged that other causes besides the avian influenza had been taken into consideration. But even this report, which was penned by the Dutch Agriculture Minister Veerman on 3 March, was never mentioned again."[983]

Everyone was clucking about a virus in the Canadian province of British Columbia, when, in November 2005, a single duck was allegedly detected as having the avian flu virus H7N3–using modern indirect molecular biological "proof" procedures. It was was officially reported that the animal only had a "mild form" of this virus type, which produces no or only "mild disease" symptoms. That is to say, the duck was not sick.[984]

According to Canadian authorities, it was "not the virus circulating in Asia [H5N1]. There is no new threat to human health."[985] However, as a "preventive" measure the authorities not only killed the single duck, they immediately slaughtered a further 56,000 healthy duck and geese. Yet international statutes certainly did not require such drastic measures like killing entire flocks of birds if, as was presumed in this case, only a "low pathogenic" virus is in the game.

"There's paranoia, there's politics and there are perceptions that come into play here that cause people to do things for other reasons than what you would call true science," says David Halvorson, an avian flu expert at the University of Minnesota. "I tend to look at it from the scientific perspective that [the killings are] a waste of animals' lives."[986]

Rat Poisons Carry off Birds

The haste, with which authorities and media hit the virus panic button by exclusively suspecting a virus instead of considering a wide spectrum of possible causes from the beginning, is also shown by the incident of the geese deaths in the German province of Rhineland-Palatinate in October 2005. A boy had found the dead greylag geese and informed the police. "The dead geese were floating in the pond," described a police spokesman in Koblenz. "And some animals perished from severe cramps before the eyes of the action force."

In response, the dead birds were collected in cases by firemen wearing special protective suits, and brought into the state investigations office, which immediately prompted the media to stir up the H5N1 panic. "Avian flu suspicion: mysterious deaths of geese near Koblenz and Göttingen have strengthened fears of an avian flu outbreak in Germany," reported the news channel N24.[987] In turn, this prompted Jürgen Trittin, then German Minister of the Environment, to announce that he would initiate resolute counter measures, in case the dangerous H5N1 virus was detected in these birds.

It turned out that the birds had been poisoned, as the regional inspection office reported. Its president, Stefan Bent, said that a rat poison had been detected in the stomachs of twelve of the 22 cadavers. The toxin phosphide had clearly caused the deaths of the wild geese. And even if the presence of the rodent poison phosphide had only been proven in twelve stomachs, Bent said it could be assumed that all the animals died from it. The toxin caused abnormal alterations in the inner organs of the animals, like round hemorrhages on gastric mucous membrane and increased fluid in the lungs.[988]

Rodent poison, mind you, is not only used in Germany. In a comprehensive 2003 report, the Japanese Agriculture Ministry tried to trace the progressive routes of flu virus outbreaks in birds in factory farms: "Poison bait type rodent poison was used during the summer and was applied continually [against mice and other wild animals] replenished when required."[989]

On How to Avoid Seeing What Is Right under Our Noses

These incidents show how important it is to look at the full picture when researching possible causes. Such a broad-spectrum viewpoint would also have been most advisable in the case of the many thousands of wild birds found dead near China's largest salt-water lake, the Qinghai Hu, between May and July 2005. It reignited global panic over avian flu, because epidemic hunters, politicians and the media immediately, and with rock-solid conviction, put their bets on an H5N1 outbreak.

Once again, many other causes come into question. Pollution, for instance, presents a huge problem in China, as in most developing countries, not least because of the chemical industry, one of the country's fastest-growing economic industries.

In the first half of 2005, quantity of production rose by 27 percent compared to the previous year. Additionally, many new chemical factories had sprung up shortly before. These facilities also produce products for developed countries, in which dangerous chemical factories are not welcome, as Greenpeace expert Kevin May explains. Factories are often built on rivers, since water is needed for the production process. "And of course, this is dangerous for inhabitants who drink the water," says May. Even without major accidents, factories in China present a danger to peoples' health and the health of the environment—including wild animals.

70 percent of all Chinese rivers were polluted at that time, because the industry directed its waste into the waterways, according to official statements.[990] There is also "no concrete proof that waterbirds at Qinghai that may have been infected with such a pathogenic strain and have survived, will migrate and be capable of transmitting the virus to other species of birds, animals or humans," according to Wetlands International, a global nature protection organization linked with many institutions.[991] One of its partners is the UN Environmental Program (UNEP), a group that deployed an expert task force composed of representatives from nine different organizations in late 2005, as it was held to be urgently necessary to get to the bottom of the avian flu hype. The knowledge concerning central aspects of the birds' deaths, it was said—including the question of how the virus is transmitted from wild birds to domestic animals—could by no means be considered certain.

The UNEP warned of growing hysteria. Additionally, they criticized the "one-eyed approach in the media which grossly oversimplifies the causes and the methods needed to counter-act in the interests of human and animal health." The media, so it was said, should provide more balanced reports "focusing on the facts." Simultaneously, "the Task Force calls for much greater emphasis by governments and local authorities on combating the role of factory farming," writes William Karesh, member of the task force and director of the Wildlife Conservation Society's Field Veterinary Program.[992]

Most striking is that even the medically very orthodox WHO[993] admits, "the role of migratory birds in the spread of highly pathogenic avian influenza is not fully understood. Wild waterfowl are considered the natural reservoir of all influenza A viruses. They have probably carried influenza viruses, with no apparent harm, for centuries."[994] But, if even from mainstream science's perspective, wild birds rarely or never become ill or die from avian flu viruses, this must have prompted even more curiosity to research other non-viral causes. Why would the wild animals get sick or even die from viruses at the beginning of the 21st century when they have lived in peaceful coexistence for millennia?

More than 150 Dead People—What Really Caused Their Deaths?

According to official statements, H5N1 caused the deaths of 153 people from the end of 2003 until November 2006 (most of them in Asia; see diagram).[995] But if we study the reports on the deceased closely, there is no evidence for the theory that H5N1 was the killer. At the same time, the reports allow completely different possibilities appear as plausible explanations. For example, that some of the victims were suffering from cold symptoms of an unknown source and then simply had the bad luck to fall into the hands of medical professionals who turned out to be H5N1 hunters.

Immediately, doctors prescribed prodigious amounts of medications in order to wipe out an imaginary virus—but in truth, it was never shown that these medications could combat the alleged virus. On the contrary, it is a fact that the medications are highly toxic, for which reason it is completely possible that the doctors only helped snuff out the weakened patients' lives.

The Friedrich-Loeffler-Institute sent us a paper that claims to show that H5N1 has pathogenic effects in humans (Uiprasertkul et al: "H5N1 Replication Sites in Humans" published in the journal *Emerging Infectious Diseases* in July 2005). The report features just one six-year-old boy who was diagnosed with a progressive pneumonia (a superimposed aspergillus fungal infection was later diagnosed). The young boy was treated with antimicrobial medications that can seriously damage the immune system, as well as with the antiviral medication Tamiflu (oseltamivir), that has even been connected with fatalities (more on Tamiflu below). The boy's fate? "The patients died during the late phase of the disease after intensive treatment with antiviral drugs."

Methylprednisolone had also been prescribed to the boy a few days before he died, 17 days after initial diagnosis. The steroid is known to weaken the immune system and should not be used in the presence of a severe bacterial, viral or fungal infection (as was the case with the boy).[996] Additionally, the report admits that, "The multiorgan dysfunction observed in human H5N1 disease, despite the apparent confinement of infection to the lungs, has remained an enigma." That is to say, what is termed H5N1 could not be detected in various diseased organs at all, which researchers simply shrugged off as an "enigma" instead of calling it what it clearly was and is: evidence that the established H5N1 theories make no sense.

In the 1998 *Science* paper by Subbarao et al,[997] (also cited in the article in *Emerging Infectious Diseases*), they described a previously healthy three-year old boy, who presented with symptoms of pharyngitis on 9 May 1997. Doctors responded by giving him Aspirin and

Affected areas with confirmed human cases of H5N1 avian influen

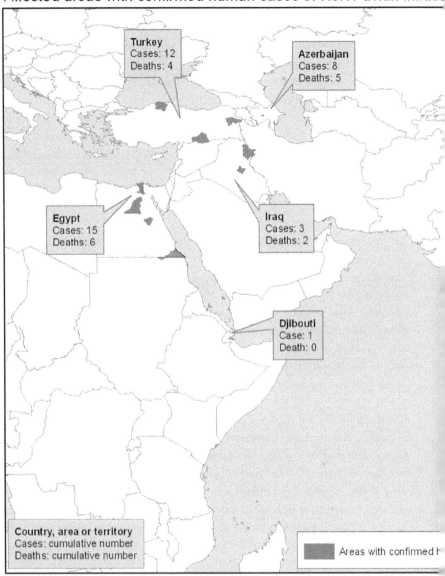

Turkey
Cases: 12
Deaths: 4

Azerbaijan
Cases: 8
Deaths: 5

Egypt
Cases: 15
Deaths: 6

Iraq
Cases: 3
Deaths: 2

Djibouti
Case: 1
Death: 0

Country, area or territory
Cases: cumulative number
Deaths: cumulative number

Areas with confirmed h

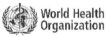 World Health Organization

The World Health Organization (WHO) estimated that by May 16, 2006, the alleged virus H5N1 had infected approximately 200 people and killed 100. But there is no proof of this.

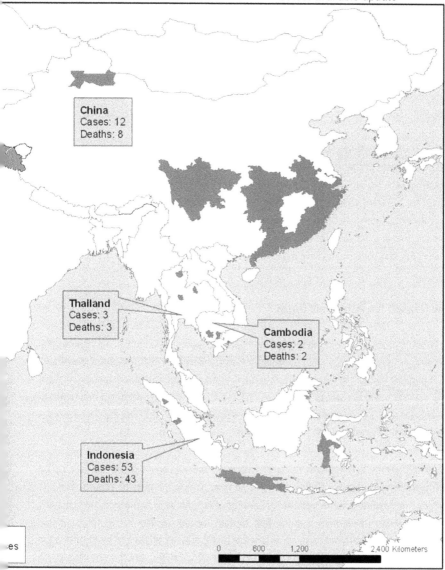

China
Cases: 12
Deaths: 8

Thailand
Cases: 3
Deaths: 3

Cambodia
Cases: 2
Deaths: 2

Indonesia
Cases: 53
Deaths: 43

es

0   600   1,200   2,400 Kilometers

on of any opinion whatsoever   Data Source: WHO / Map Production: Public Health Mapping and GIS
or area or of its authorities,   Communicable Diseases (CDS) World Health Organization
mate border lines for which there may not yet be full agreement.

Instead, much speaks for the possibility that other causes like the administration of highly toxic medications led to the patients' deaths. © www.who.org

antibiotics. Six days later, his symptoms deteriorated and he was admitted to hospital to be treated with "broad antibiotic coverage." Subsequently, the child developed Reye's syndrome which is a severe disease associated with nausea, personality changes, organ damage and coma—and in many cases ends in death.[998] [999] Just like the other boy, he died on 21 May. The H5N1 virus was cited as his cause of death, but here as well, evidence of H5N1 was not provided. The authorities didn't even confirm if the boy had ever been in contact with birds.

Apart from this, studies suggest that Aspirin can trigger the Reye's syndrome (that was also diagnosed in the boy).[1000] In fact, around ninety percent of cases in children are associated with aspirin use.[1001] The National Reye's Syndrome Foundation even explicitly says: "Do not give your child Aspirin."[1002] But even this information did not prompt the study's authors to investigate the role Aspirin or other substances might have played in the three-year-old's demise. They spared no trouble, on the other hand, back in 1997 to warn of a "rapid and explosive spread of a pandemic virus."[1003]

No Reason for Pandemic Panic

H5N1 fear mongers continued to predict impending horror for Germany. "A pandemic will come over us in several waves," confidently asserted Bernhard Ruf, director of the Leipzig Competence Centre for Highly Contagious Diseases and top warrior against avian flu at the WHO.[1004] "And we would be lucky to survive the year 2015 without a pandemic. In Germany alone, up to 40 million will become infected and 150,000 will die. The economy will collapse. The world will be paralyzed."[1005]

But there are no justifications for such warnings if H5N1 cannot be isolated as a pure virus, and thus cannot scientifically be proven to exist. And if there's no proof that H5N1 can be highly contagious in animals, by jumping from wild birds to domestic animals and mutating into an infectious mini-monster. And if it cannot be shown that this so-called H5N1 can also jump to humans, cause disease as a deadly avian flu virus and then come into contact with human influenza virus, exchange genes and as evil "parent viruses," (as they're called) give birth to an even more horrible "daughter virus."

And furthermore, if other factors like factory farming, pesticides, rodent poisons, stress and natural death are overlooked as potential contributing factors.

The FLI even admitted this to us: "Concerning your inquiry about the pandemic properties of H5N1, it can only be said that there are currently no scientific methods with forecasting effects which could evaluate the possibility of an influenza virus triggering a new pandemic."[1006] And in late October 2005, the *British Medical Journal* stated that, "the lack of sustained human-to-human transmission suggests that this H5N1 avian virus does not currently have the capacity to cause a human pandemic."[1007]

Here it's worth noting the comments of Julie Gerbering, the then director of the Centers for Disease Control in Atlanta. In mid-April 2006, at a conference on avian flu pandemic in Tacoma, Washington, with 1200 experts from all over the country in the audience, she said, "There is no evidence [H5N1] will be the next pandemic." Further, "[there is] no evidence it is evolving in a direction that is becoming more transmissible to people," and there is "no reason to think it ever will" pass easily between people. These statements are in complete contrast to the continued panic reports by CDC officials. After the conference, *The News*

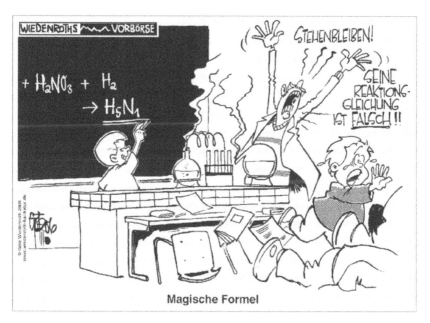

Magische Formel

Teacher: „Stop! His reaction equation is wrong!!" Magic Formula

Tribune reported that, "given those facts, bird flu, like SARS, swine flu and other once widely publicized health threats, might never become a significant human illness."[1008]

It is scandalous that as a result of unfounded pandemic warnings, more than 200 million birds had been killed by April 2006. Additionally, as a UNO report continued, costs total-ing $20 billion had been incurred by the affected countries by this time and a million farmers had already slid into poverty.[1009] In Germany, the government ordered that poul-try be kept indoors which even led to suicide among some breeders. As the Westfalian newspaper *Westfalen-Blatt* reported "the breeders did not see any way out." Indeed, at the very least, ordering small poultry breeders to keep their birds inside is tantamount to banning them from their profession.[1010]

Tamiflu: From Shelf-Warmer to Big Seller—to Death Bringer?

There was no foundation for demands for antiviral medications. Nevertheless, media like *Die Zeit* insisted it was "high time that Germany buys vaccines and enough medicine."[1011] The dangers of such hasty demands for a quick-fix becomes clear by tracking the rise of Tamiflu, a flu remedy that became a hot-seller only after the virus mania machine cranked up. "Tamiflu, conceived as a remedy for common flu, did not sell well because it was too expensive and had too little effect," according to a rare industry critique by the Swiss news magazine *Rundschau* on 19 October 2005. "The pharmaceutical groups promised a lot, but in practice it was shown that doctors could hardly prescribe the medicine to anyone."

So, the virus hunters and their media sidekicks released terrifying pictures of infection experts in white spacesuits and remote factory farms with piles of dead birds. These images were beamed around the globe, accompanied by sensationalized tales of people who had already allegedly become infected with or died from the horrible H5N1 virus. In 2004, the WHO office in Manila promptly recommended oseltamivir (Tamiflu) for "endan-gered individuals." The substance was produced by the Swiss pharmaceutical giant Roche, under the brand name Tamiflu.

Roche took advantage of the moment and quickly issued a press release saying, "Tamiflu may be effective against avian flu." But the media didn't seem to take notice of the phrase "may be" and crafted their headlines to tout a miracle remedy for avian flu. For Roche, this was the best kind of advertising: free and with an incredible effect. Some pharmacies soon sold out of the medication. "In the media and television, they always say that Tamiflu works against the avian flu virus," said a pharmacist from Istanbul in an interview with the *Rundschau*. "Now, they all come and want Tamiflu."[1012]

Reuters news agency reported on 20 July 2005, that the "global flu precautions had granted [Tamiflu manufacturer] Roche a leap in profits." Worldwide, "Tamiflu sales increased by 363 percent to 580 million franks [€380 million] in the first half of 2005, in comparison to the same period in the previous year."[1013]

Ultimately, in 2005, Roche increased its Tamiflu profits by 370 percent to around €1 billion"[1014] — primarily thanks to massive government purchases (financed by tax dollars). As the *Zeit* relates, the German province of North Rhine-Westfalia "announced that they would put €30 million worth of medications into storage."[1015] In the first nine months of 2006, worldwide Tamiflu sales rose to $1.3 billion, Roche reported, an increase of 88 percent over the year prior.[1016] To keep up with demand, Roche factories in Europe, North America and Japan worked full throttle. By the end of 2006, capacity has doubled once again, to an annual production of 300 million packages of Tamiflu.[1017]

But what scientific basis is there for this Tamiflu hype? Franz Humer, Chairman of Roche's Board of Directors, assures that Tamiflu "is a very important product for our patients, above all in case of an influenza pandemic." But this statement doesn't hold up, since Tamiflu has never been tested as a remedy for avian flu in humans, as even stated by a press release from Roche. In this, it says that there is no clinical data on the effectiveness of Tamiflu against H5N1.

This is also why Robert Dietz at the World Health Organization in Manila, which jump-started Tamiflu's sales-explosion with its promotion of the flu remedy, could not avoid admitting to the Swiss news program *Rundschau*: "We had no specific medical foundation for our decision to recommend Tamiflu as a remedy for avian flu."[1018] In fact, in early December 2005, the Vietnamese doctor Nguyen Tuong Van, director of the Intensive Care unit at Hanoi's Institute for Clinical Research into Tropical Diseases (who had followed WHO guidelines for patient treatment), came to the conclusion that "Tamiflu is useless; [for this reason,] we place no importance on using this drug on our patients."[1019] And just prior to this statement, appeared the first reports on deaths connected to the intake of Tamiflu.

First came a report from Japan. The pharmaceutical company Chugai, a Roche subsidiary, had notified the Health Ministry that after Tamiflu intake, two boys aged 14 and 17 became disoriented, showed abnormal behavior and ultimately died (one was thought to have jumped from his apartment; the other had thrown himself in front of a truck).[1020] Only a few days later, news made the rounds that the influenza medication was connected to the deaths of twelve children in Japan. And the American Food and Drug Administration (FDA) called it "unsettling" that "after Tamiflu intake, children in 32 cases had had hallucinations or shown abnormal behavior."[1021]

Of course, these cases are not restricted to Japan. For example, near the end of 2006, Canadian officials at Health Canada warned of hallucinations among Tamiflu users. As of November 11, there had been seven cases of psychiatric side effects linked to Tamiflu in Canada and 84 reports of side effects occurring in Canadians taking the medication, including 10 deaths.[1022]

But the media doesn't push reports of Tamiflu's side effects nearly as much as the earlier completely unfounded declarations that Tamiflu was the best protection from avian flu (H5N1). This is certainly due to the fact that, in connection with the reported fatalities, the medical establishment immediately warned people not to panic just because a few people had died after taking Tamiflu – and in the typical manner, the media followed the medical establishment's placations. The FDA stressed that they wanted to investigate why people had died, but they implied that it was extremely difficult to establish the exact causes.

As early as the 1990s, Tamiflu was found to cause inflammation in the brain (encephalitis). But the medical establishment twisted these findings by saying that neural symptoms were also often triggered by influenza infections, so they said that it was difficult to tell whether Tamiflu could be responsible for the neurological complications.[1023] This was made even more difficult because many victims had been taking not just Tamiflu, but also other medications.[1024] Basically, the issue could only be clarified if controlled studies (one group/patient receives the active substance, the other a placebo) were available. But, they weren't available.[1025]

Why was this medication never tested through the necessary clinical trials before being released to the public? The information provokes disbelief, particularly since the medical establishment and the politicians actively participate in virus mania, they celebrate medications like Tamiflu and only calls for caution and restraint when news of medication-related deaths start to circulate. At which point, they rush to the side of the pharmaceutical companies whose bottom lines might be negatively affected.

Should the Tamiflu safety data become so bad that it has to be taken off the market, it could turn into a financial disaster for Roche. But, until clarity prevails, there is no reason to buy or take Tamiflu, neither prophylactically nor as a remedy for flu symptoms. Tamiflu is connected with numerous side effects, including vomiting, diarrhea, bronchitis, abdominal pain, headaches, dizziness, hallucinations and hepatitis.[1026] [1027]

This was confirmed by a comprehensive study evaluation of the Cochrane Collaboration on Tamiflu published in 2014. Result: Tamiflu is not suitable to prevent the spread of flu or to reduce the occurrence of dangerous complications. The media acknowledged this with headlines such as "The Great Tamiflu Disaster".

And three years earlier, a paper appeared that concluded: "Taking Tamiflu can lead to a sudden deterioration in health and subsequent death."[1028]

A patient who had taken Tamiflu for just two days reports: "I couldn't sleep for three days and I hallucinated. My family was very worried about me. I will never take this horrible medicine again and would not advise anyone to. I completely lost my personality, I felt as if I was a different person. It was four weeks before I started feeling myself again."[1029]

Tamiflu Studies and the Problem of Independence

There must also be studies that show that Tamiflu works against the flu, right? Of course, such studies would be worthless without placebo controls, along with a guarantee that the scientists involved were free from conflicts of interest. Has the media ever taken the trouble to double check if the Tamiflu trials were sound? We do know one thing for certain: fraud is well established in biomedicine, and conflicts of interest are widespread. Making it absolutely imperative that we sort fact from fiction.

It doesn't take much scientific research to find out if the pharmaceutical company Roche has financed Tamiflu (oseltamivir) studies. You only need to google, for example, "Roche funded pubmed oseltamivir"– and many hits come up.[1030] Let's click on just *one* paper: for instance: Effectiveness of neuraminidase inhibitors in treatment and prevention of influenza A and B: systematic review and meta-analyses of randomized controlled trials, published in the *British Medical Journal* in 2003. It includes the following information:

"Competing interests: KGN [Karl G. Nicholson, one of the study's authors] has received travel sponsorship and honorariums from GlaxoSmithKline, the manufacturer of zanamivir, and Roche, which makes oseltamivir, for consultancy and speaking at international respiratory and infectious diseases symposiums. His research group has received research funding from GlaxoSmithKline and Roche to participate in multicenter trials of neuraminidase inhibitors."[1031]

Unfortunately, such conflicts of interest are common practice, something which the public is rarely made aware of. But as the British Parliament observed in a comprehensive investigation in 2005, three-quarters of clinical studies that appear in the leading scientific journals, *The Lancet, The New England Journal of Medicine* (*NEJM*) and *The Journal of the American Medical Association* (*JAMA*), are funded by pharmaceutical companies.[1032] And if the industry is paying, they will use all sorts of tricks to attain the desired results,[1033] by omitting the critical questions or negative results and exclusively publishing positive results.[1034]

Nonetheless, the *NEJM* explicitly modified its policy for writers in 2002, so that review articles and editorials could also be written by experts who receive fees of up to $10,000 a year from pharmaceutical companies. The fees can also come from companies whose products are plugged by the author in his or her *NEJM* articles. This presents a classic conflict of interest. What was the key reason for the alterations to their writers' policy? The *NEJM* said that they were simply no longer in a position to find enough experts without any financial connections to the pharmaceutical industry.[1035]

For an allegedly independent scientific journal, this explanation seems ludicrous, but it depicts the stark reality of modern medical science. Arnold Relman, Harvard professor and former Editor in Chief of the *NEJM* says that, "The medical profession is being bought by the pharmaceutical industry, not only in terms of the practice, but also in terms of teaching and research."[1036]

Precisely these financial interconnections threaten to undercut the independence of medical research. The issue only recently reached top circles in the USA after it was revealed that hundreds of scientists employed by the National Institutes of Health had received millions of dollars in commissions and big stock packages from the pharmaceutical industry. The story was researched by the *Los Angeles Times* and triggered a broad discussion on the independence of NIH researchers.

US Congress members accused NIH leaders and their predecessors with supporting the "option of corruption" among its employees. In response, Elias Zerhouni, the health authority's director, announced the introduction of new rules which banned higher NIH managers from signing paid consulting contracts, and prohibited all NIH employees from holding stocks and stock options. But it turned out that many thousand NIH employees were exempt from the obligation to disclose their acquisitions. Through this loophole they could continue to be paid in secret by pharmaceutical companies without fear of punishment.[1037] [1038]

Donald Rumsfeld Makes Giant Profits

With Tamiflu specifically, doctors and other experts have begun to ask critical questions regarding the US government's vehement commitment to the purchase of stockpiles of the Roche medication. Death by avian flu, according to President George W. Bush, threatens two million Americans.[1039] This statement, based on nothing more than wild speculation, seemed to justify the massive purchase of 20 million bottles of Tamiflu at $100 each. For a total cost of $2 billion.[1040]

Particularly alarming is the fact that, at taxpayers' expense, enormous sums are spent on a medication whose efficacy against avian flu has never been proven and will never be proven either. For, even assuming that H5N1 does exist and causes disease in humans, nobody can predict what the mutated form of the H5N1 virus, which is supposed to first trigger the pandemic, will look like. This means that no medication, not even Tamiflu, can be conceived against such an alleged mutant virus.

And this is exactly why the UK government's decision to order 14.6 million doses of oseltamivir for use in the event of a flu epidemic has been questioned even by orthodox experts. Among them Joe Collier, professor of medicines policy at St George's Hospital Medical School, London, and former editor of the *Drug and Therapeutics Bulletin* who has been quoted in the *British Medical Journal* with the words: "I would like to know what evidence there is that Tamiflu actually alters mortality. And if it doesn't then what are we doing?"

On the other side of the Atlantic Canada's federal health minister, Ujjal Dosanjh, told listeners during an interview on a Canadian Broadcasting Corporation radio program (*The Current*, 27 October 2005) that oseltamivir did not prevent infection with the flu virus.[1041]

This is why many were upset that Donald Rumsfeld, a once-leading member of the George W. Bush administration, was making a tidy sum of cash thanks to massive state Tamiflu purchases. As a once-leading member of the Bush administration, he makes a tidy sum of cash from massive state Tamiflu purchases. From 1997 until 2001, before taking office, Rumsfeld chaired the Board of Directors of the American biotechnology corporation Gilead. And after 2001, according to his own statements, Rumsfeld continued to hold huge share packages in Gilead valued at $5-25 million.[1042] Gilead had originally developed Tamiflu, and in 1997, the Nasdaq-listed corporation sold an exclusive license to Roche for the production of Tamiflu, though Gilead kept the substance's patent.

Gilead has since cashed in license fees from Roche (as is reported, between 10 percent and 19 percent of net price, or 10 percent of profits).[1043] [1044] In the three (hot) autumn months of 2005, Tamiflu licensing brought in $12 million for Gilead; up from $1.7 million in the third quarter of 2004.[1045] Simultaneously, Gilead market values climbed from $37 to $47 within just a few months, something that made Rumsfeld—one of the richest men in the Bush cabinet—at least $1 million richer.

Rumsfeld wasn't the only political heavyweight in the USA, who was said to have very close connections to Gilead. George P. Shultz, US Secretary of State from 1982 to 1989, was on Gilead's Board of Directors. In 2005, Shultz sold stocks of the Californian biotech company at a value of more than $7 million. Another member of Gilead's board was the wife of former California governor Pete Wilson. "I don't know of any biotech company that's so politically well-connected [as Gilead]," Andrew McDonald, of the analyst firm Think Equity Partners, told *Fortune*.[1046]

A *Saar-Echo* article, published under the title "Bush Makes Panic and Rumsfeld Profit," hits the nail on the head:

"Bush and his vice-president, 'Dick' Cheney, the 'human embodiment of the combination of oil and military interests' had developed the pattern of this capitalistic escapade for the good of the American billionaire's oligarchy in connection with the Iraq War, when they explained their invasion of the oil-rich Middle Eastern country with the shameless lie that Iraq was in possession of weapons of mass destruction. After the defeat of Saddam Hussein, one of the main profiteers from the Iraq invasion was the American company Halliburton, whose core business is trade and conveyance of crude oil.

The CEO of Halliburton, until his leap to the seat of the American vice-president, was Richard Cheney, who in turn is a close friend of Tamiflu profiteer Donald Rumsfeld. Together, they founded the neoconservative think tank 'Project for the New American Century' in 1997. Since they have held office, the billion-dollar side projects of these and other US politicians have run like clockwork."[1047] [1048]

Although massive accusations of fraud are levied against Halliburton, because, for example, the group charges exorbitant prices for many services (for the cleaning of just 7 kilograms of laundry, more than $100 was charged), the US Army placed a new order in 2005 to support the troops in Iraq. The price tag: $5 billion.[1049] [1050] In 2004 and 2003, the oil and gas subcontractor based in Texas, George W. Bush's home state, had already pocketed $10 billion.[1051] [1052]

In his farewell speech in 1961, outgoing president Dwight D. Eisenhower warned of the increasing entanglement of military and industry, and of the growing influence of this "military-industrial complex" on American politics. This enlightened warning was repeated in the award-winning documentary *Why We Fight*, a focus on today's billion-dollar war machine. 40 years later, history seems to be proving Eisenhower right.[1053]

One of the many parallels between the military-industrial complex and the medical-industrial complex is huge funding by tax dollars. In 2005, the Bush administration announced that they were introducing a $7.1 billion program to protect the USA from a possible avian flu epidemic. Just a few weeks before, Bush had been heavily criticized around crisis management in New Orleans after Hurricane Katrina. Ironic as it may seem, the government saw an excellent opportunity to polish up Bush's battered public image in the announcement of an (incredibly expensive taxpayer funded) avian flu package.

According to George W. Bush, they wanted to buy enough vaccine against the avian virus to protect 20 million Americans. For this, they would attempt to get the US Congress to approve US$1.2 billion. Additionally, they hoped to get approval of nearly US$3 billion for the development of new flu vaccines, as well as US$1 billion for the storage of antiviral medications. And a further US$600 million was allocated for local authorities, so that they could create emergency plans for containment of an epidemic.[1054]

Bush also demanded that Congress ease liability regulations for vaccine manufacturers. Only this way, it was said, could production capacity grow, since pharmaceutical firms refused to manufacture vaccines without protection from liability lawsuits. This plan was part of a legal initiative—the "Biodefense and Pandemic Vaccine and Drug Development Act of 2005"—which had the goal to allow no more lawsuits, even if vaccinations or medications are administered by force.[1055]

"A drug company stockholder's dream and a consumer's worst nightmare," according to the National Vaccine Information Center.[1056]

Not to be swayed by scientific interest groups, Bush countered back with, "No country can afford to ignore the threat of avian flu." He did admit that nobody knew if the H5N1 flu virus could lead to a deadly human epidemic, but he warned that history dictates we must once again anticipate a terrible large epidemic.[1057]

Bush was referring to the so-called Spanish flu of 1918, to which many millions of people fell victim. This "Spanish flu" was so named because the Spanish media were the only ones to report about the virus while most other nations decreed an information ban on the pandemic, allegedly in order to avoid fear among World War I troops. But is it really a suitable virus model for any sort of pandemic predictions nowadays?

"Spanish Flu" 1918: Result of the First World War, Not of a Virus!

Virus Hypothesis of *Nature* and *Science* without Foundation

"Within a few months, the Spanish flu achieved what all the epidemics in history have not managed," wrote *Spiegel Online*. "In 1918, the pandemic killed between 20 and 50 million people, more than any other disease before. In the USA alone, there were 550,000 deaths. Infected patients suffered from high fever and their lungs became inflamed. Within a few days, victims drowned in their own fluids."[1058]

It sounds dramatic—and it was dramatic. But it's much too hasty to assume that a virus triggered mass mortality. There are certainly no facts to support such a theory. These mass deaths occurred at the end of the First World War (July 1914 to November 1918), at a time when countless people were undernourished and under incredible stress after four years of war.

Additionally, the medications and vaccines applied in masses at that time contained highly toxic substances like heavy metals, arsenic, formaldehyde and chloroform, all of which could very likely trigger severe flu symptoms. Numerous chemicals intended for military use also moved unregulated into the public sector (agriculture, medicine).[1059]

In 1997, a paper by Jeffery Taubenberger's research team appeared in *Science*, claiming to have isolated an influenza virus (H1N1) from a victim of the 1918 pandemic.[1060] "But before one can be certain that a pandemic virus had in fact been detected, some important questions must be asked," writes Canadian biologist David Crowe, who analyzed the paper.

The researchers had taken genetic material from the preserved lung tissue of a victim—a soldier, who died in 1918. Lung diseases were extremely typical of the "Spanish flu," but it is a big leap to conclude that the many other million victims also died from the same cause. And particularly "the same virus" as Crowe points out. "We simply do not know if the majority of victims died for exactly the same reason. We also do not know if a virus can be held responsible for all mortalities, because viruses, as they'd now be described, were unknown at this time."

So even if one does accept that an influenza virus was present in the soldier's lungs, this hardly means that this virus was the killer.

Taubenberger's group admits that the soldier was an atypical case, since most of the so-called influenza victims ("influenza" suggests a viral cause) actually died from bacterial lung inflammation (for example, tuberculosis). These bacteria, it is conjectured, ultimately gained the upper hand and supplanted the viruses. But this speculation doesn't necessarily make any sense.

The genetic analysis of pulmonary tissue form the single soldier was based on the assumption that certain genetic sequences (RNA sequences) are characteristic of all flu viruses. That is, it is theorized that there are certain proteins in flu virus shells, the RNA sequences of which were ultimately claimed to have been discovered using PCR. These proteins are hemagglutinins (this is where the "H" in H1N1 or H5N1 comes from: "H1" and "H5" stand for certain hemagglutinin types) and neuraminidases (the "N"). But in biochemistry, many different substances are termed hemagglutinins, not just proteins that cause red blood cells to clot together.

Nevertheless, it is said that proof of a virus can be exhibited by mixing red blood cells in the laboratory with samples, in which the alleged virus is said to be found. This was done by taking tissue samples from organs in which the virus is presumed to lurk (in this case from a lung) and placing them (*in vitro*) into a petri dish filled with red blood cells. Then if clots form, the theory goes that a hemagglutinins from a flu virus must have been the cause of the coagulation.

But a complete virus had never been isolated from this sample. This method is also weak since it cannot differentiate between the RNA of an external virus and human RNA. "This cannot be *normal* human RNA, otherwise everyone would react 'positively' to the method," says Crowe. "But it would certainly be possible that the RNA 'collected' by the PCR does not come from a virus protein, but is rather produced by the body itself, for instance in connection with a disease process."

The enzyme neuraminidase, for instance, which is held to be specific to a flu virus, is actually produced naturally by the body and performs significant metabolic functions. If there is a deficiency of this enzyme — because of an innate metabolism disorder, for example — it is known as Mucolipidosis I[1061] or Sialidosis which causes serious dysfunctions such as impaired vision, disorders of the nervous system , skeletal abnormalities, myasthenia (muscle weakness), seizures, disturbances of equilibrium, or cerebral development disorders. Anyone who takes flu remedies and neuraminidase inhibitors like Tamiflu should keep this in mind. We can then conclude that Taubenberger et al, have not verifiably shown that a flu virus was present in the soldier. Their experiment cannot prove that this soldier died from a flu virus, let alone that the other umpteen million victims lost their lives because of a specific virus.

The same is true of the papers published in the scientific journals *Nature* and *Science*[1062] in October 2005. The media reports spun the information into a global sensation with news that "US researchers revive old killer virus" and "American scientists have recon-structed the extremely dangerous Spanish flu pathogen in a military laboratory."[1063] But even if headlines suggest this, the fact is that a virus with complete genetic material (ge-nome) had never been discovered. Lung tissue samples were simply taken from several corpses from that time, including an Inuit woman buried in Alaska's permafrost layer in 1918. Then, the scientists conducted practically the same procedure as in 1997. Research-ers had not proven that the genetic material they found really belongs to a pathogenic "old killer virus." With many samples, the tests even came out "negative." The whole thing, then, is pure speculation.

Mysterious Epidemiolgy Debunks the Virus Dogma

According to traditional epidemiological precepts, an infectious disease begins in one place and spreads out from there in certain directions, depending on the envi-ronmental conditions, in certain directions. Such a development didn't occur with the "Spanish flu."

In 1918, there were two different disease waves: an initial milder one in spring and then a much more severe wave, which claimed many lives, in late summer and autumn. Here, experts can't even agree whether the disease was introduced to the United States from Europe, or the other way around.

According to one source, the epidemic began in February 1918 in the Spanish town of San Sebastian, close to the French border on the Atlantic coast.[1064] But another source names the same outbreak date, but a completely different place thousands of kilome-ters away from San Sebastian, on the other side of the Atlantic: New York City. That these outbreaks happened at the same time cannot be explained by either ship route or migrating bird patterns.

Then in March 1918, there were reports of cases in two army camps in Kansas, hundreds of kilometers away from New York. In April, the "Spanish flu" appeared in Paris for the first time, in May in Madrid, until it reached its peak in Spain at the end of May. In June, cases first began accumulating in war-torn Germany, but simultaneously in China, Japan, England and Norway as well. On 1 July, Leipzig had its first case. And over the course of that month, approximately half a million Germans were affected.

The second serious wave began almost at the same time in Boston's Harbor, on the Indian subcontinent, in Southeast Asia, in the Caribbean and Central America. In September, various army camps in the western USA along with the states of Massachusetts, Pennsylvania and Philadelphia were affected. In October Brazil was hit, and in November Alaska.

But even if we factor in the fastest ships of the time, railway routes and migrating birds, there's no sound epidemiological basis to conclude a virus-caused influenza. Unless one assumes that the virus mutated into a deadly infectious agent on all continents simultaneously—which is probably less likely than winning the lottery ten times in a row.[1065]

Failed Infection Attempts

In order to be able to better assess the puzzling mass disease, an attempt to simulate infection was undertaken with volunteers in Boston in November 1918. This comprised of 62 healthy sailors charged with delinquency and sent to prison. They had been promised a pardon under the condition that they take part in an experiment. 39 of them had not had influenza, so the theory was that they would be particularly susceptible to infection and illness.[1066] But the results proved nothing of the sort, as American scientific journalist Gina Kolata describes in her book "Influenza":

"Navy doctors collected the mucus from men who were desperately ill from the flu, gathering thick viscous secretions from their noses and throats. They sprayed mucus from flu patients into the noses and throats of some men and dropped it into other men's eyes. In one attempt, they swabbed mucus from the back of the nose of a man with the flu and then directly swabbed one patient's nasal septum and rubbed it directly onto the nasal septum of one of the volunteers.

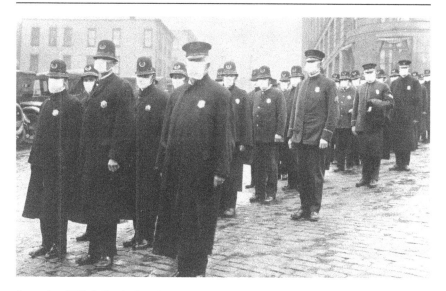

December 1918: Police in Seattle with protective masks from the Red Cross, thought to protect against flu viruses. © National Archives at College Park, MD

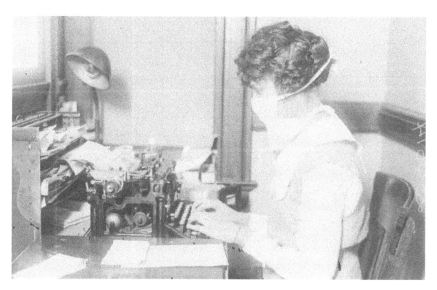

New York City, 16 October 1918: Even typists wore protective masks against the alleged flu viruses. © National Archives at College Park, MD

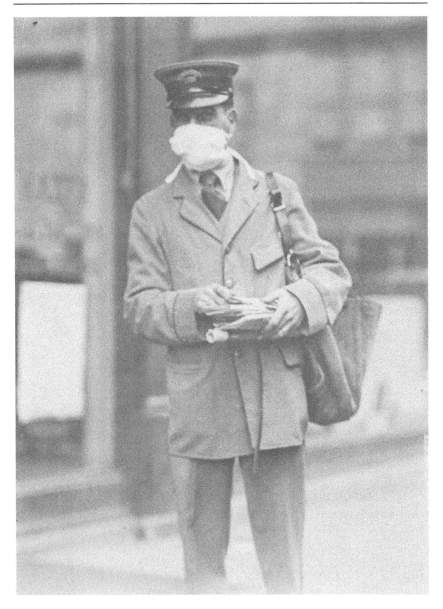

16 October 1918: A New York postman with a mask to protect from influenza viruses.
© *National Archives at College Park, MD*

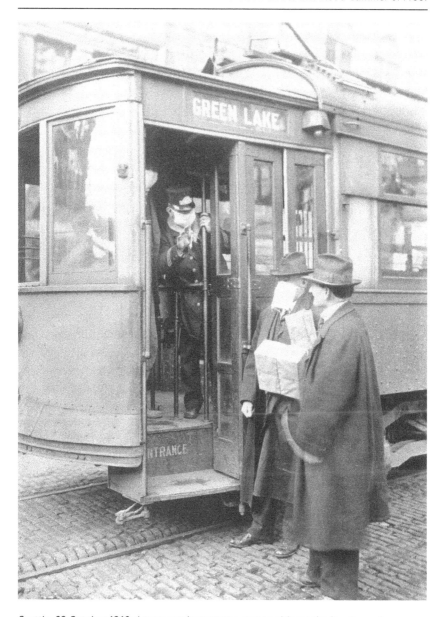

Seattle, 29 October 1918: A tram conductor turns away a citizen who is not wearing a protective mask. © *National Archives at College Park, MD*

Trying to simulate what happens naturally when people are exposed to flu victims, the doctors took ten of the volunteers onto the hospital ward where men were dying of the disease. The sick men lay huddled on their narrow beds, burning with fever, drifting in and out of sleep in a delirium. The ten healthy men were given their instructions: each was to walk up to the bed of a sick man and draw near him, lean into his face, breathe in his fetid breath, and chat with him for five minutes. To be sure that the healthy man had had a full exposure to the sick man's disease, the sick man was to exhale deeply while the healthy man drew the sick man's breath directly into his own lungs. Finally, the flu victim coughed five times in the volunteer's face.

Each healthy volunteer repeated these actions with ten different flu patients. Each flu patient had been seriously ill for no more than three days—a period when the virus or whatever it was that was causing the flu should still be around in his mucus, in his nose, in his lungs.

But not a single healthy man got sick."[1067]

A comparable experiment, carried out under much stricter conditions, took place in San Francisco, with 50 imprisoned sailors. But, once again, the results did not correspond with what the doctors had expected: "Scientists were stunned. If these healthy volunteers did not get infected with influenza despite doctors' best efforts to make them ill, then what was causing this disease? How, exactly, did people get the flu?"[1069]

Overmedication, Massive Vaccinations and War Turmoil as Key Factors
A look at history books and statistics shows that epidemics always develop where human immune systems have been weakened, primarily because of lack of food and clean water. This was also the case with the pandemic of 1918. A panoply of causes, which naturally could also have worked in combination, comes into consideration:[1070 1071 1072 1073 1074]

- Psychological stress, evoked by fears of war.

- Over-treatment with chemical preparations, which can seriously compromise the immune system, including painkillers like Aspirin and chloroform. Chloroform was used as a preservative in medications and is metabloized in the liver into phos-

ΛXIOS   Sections   About Axios   Sign up

Special report: War, fever and baseball in 1918

Λ   Kendall Baker, Jeff Tracy

f   🐦   in   ✉

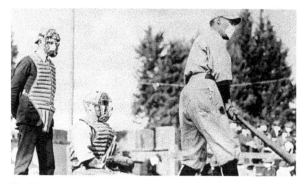

A baseball player wearing a mask in 1918. Photo: George Rinhart/Corbis via Getty Images

On April 6, 2020, the news website Axios *published an article that opened with a photo showing baseball players wearing protective masks during the 1918 so-called Spanish flu epidemic. While many mainstream media outlets claimed that records from back then "fatally remind us of the corona crisis" in 2020 (*Süddeutsche Zeitung*),[1068] Axios was a bit more sophisticated and wrote:*

"In some respects, the coronavirus and Spanish flu aren't all that comparable. After all, the war provided a vastly different backdrop, little was known about viruses at the time (imagine having no idea what you were suffering from) and medicine was far less advanced. In 1918, the basic treatments that were offered were enemas, whiskey and bloodletting. Hospitals as we know them today were quite different. There were no intensive care doctors [and] no antibiotics to treat any secondary infection. So it was a very different time and a very different way of practicing medicine,' [said] Dr. Jeremy Brown, National Institutes of Health, per CBS." Source: Screenshot from axios.com

253

gene[1075] — an agent used as poison gas in the First World War. In the late 19th century, manufacturers of medicinal products also increasingly began selling products that contained highly toxic substances like morphine, codeine, quinine and strychnine as medicines; as at that time there were no regulations for such manufacturers. From 1898, the German inventor of Aspirin, Bayer, sold heroin, for example, as an allegedly non-addictive morphine substitute, and also as a cough remedy in many different forms, ranging from syrup—in noble-looking flacons –to plugs, powders, liquids, and tampons soaked in it for gynecological treatments.[1076]

- Damage to airway organs resulting from "preventive" measures, like rubbing the throat with antiseptic preparations or inhaling antibacterial substances. Many of the substances used at that time also contained the toxic metal silver and have since been prohibited (for example, Formalin/formaldehyde has strong corrosive and irritating effects on the skin, eyes, and airway, and can cause kidney, liver and lung damage; a carcinogenic potential is also attributed to it).[1077]

- No effective antibiotics: many people were afflicted by bacterial and fungal infections; however, the first really effective means of killing bacteria and fungi was penicillin, which was discovered much later, in 1928 and became a medication during the Second World War.

- Vaccines often contained toxic heavy metals and were produced out of poorly filtered mucus or other fluids from infected patients.

A frequently observed disease symptom of the so-called "Spanish flu" was bleeding inside the lungs (typical of tuberculosis patients, for example)—a phenomenon that was also described as a result of smallpox vaccinations.[1078] In fact, numerous sou rces report that mass vaccinations (up to 24 vaccinations per person) decisively contributed to the pandemic. American author Eleanora McBean relates her own experiences:

"All the doctors and people who were living at the time of the 1918 Spanish Influenza epidemic say it was the most terrible disease the world has ever had. Strong men, hale and hearty, one day would be dead the next. The disease had the characteristics of the Black Death added to typhus, diphtheria, pneumonia, smallpox, paralysis and all the diseases the people had been vaccinated with immediately following World War 1. Practically the entire

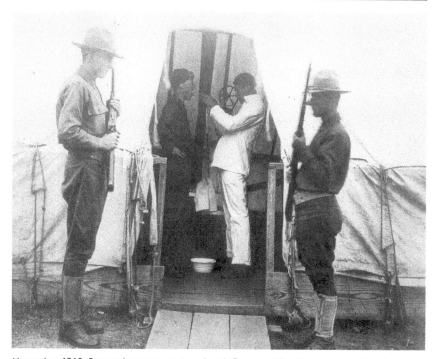

November 1918: Preventive treatment against influenza with a throat spray; American Red Cross, Love Field, Texas. © *With permission of the National Museum of Health and Medicine, Armed Forces Institute of Pathology, Washington, D.C., Reeve33986*

population had been injected/ 'seeded' with a dozen or more diseases—or toxic serums. When all those doctor-made diseases started breaking out all at once it was tragic.

That pandemic dragged on for two years, kept alive with the addition of more poison drugs administered by the doctors who tried to suppress the symptoms. As far as I could find out, the flu hit only the vaccinated. Those who had refused the shots escaped the flu.
My family had refused all the vaccinations so we remained well all the time. We knew from the health teachings of Graham, Trail, Tilden and others, that people cannot contaminate the body with poisons without causing disease.

When the flu was at its peak, all the stores were closed as well as the schools, businesses—even the hospital, as the doctors and nurses had been vaccinated too and were down

LOG IN   SUBSCRIBE

Déjà vu? Public gathering places were ordered closed in 1918 during deadly Spanish flu crisis

Written By: Pioneer Staff Report | Mar 20th 2020 - 11am.

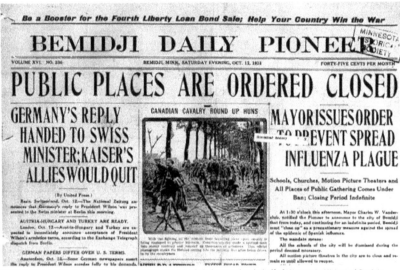

The front page of the Bemidji Daily Pioneer on Oct. 12, 1918. Prepared on behalf of Minnesota Historical Society.

On 20 March 2020, the US newspaper The Bemidji Pioneer *published an article about the COVID-19 lockdown, picturing it with a 1918 cover story from its own publication. In the 2020 article it says: "Gov. Tim Walz closed Minnesota's restaurants and bars to dine-in and drink-in customers this week. A similar thing happened a century ago, when a headline in the Oct. 12, 1918 edition of the* Bemidji Daily Pioneer *blared this message in all capital letters: PUBLIC PLACES ARE ORDERED CLOSED." Unfortunately, the newspaper did not tell its readers that the parallel drawn here is completely wrong. Because back then, the roughly 675,000 Americans, who were said to have been victims of the so-called Spanish flu, did not die of a virus, but of the turmoil of war, i.e. malnutrition, psychological stress, treatment with chemical poisons or highly toxic vaccines (why COVID-19 is not a viral disease, see chapter 12). Source: Screenshot from* bemidjipioneer.com with the flu. No one was on the streets. It was like a ghost town. We seemed to be the only family [that] didn't get the flu; so my parents went from house to house doing what they could to look after the sick, as it was impossible to get a doctor then. If it were possible for germs, bacteria, virus, or bacilli to cause disease, they had plenty of opportunity to attack my parents when they were spending many hours a day in the sick rooms. But they didn't get the flu and they didn't bring any germs home to attack us children and cause anything. None of our family had the flu — not even a sniffle — and it was in the winter with deep snow on the ground.

When I see people cringe when someone near them sneezes or coughs, I wonder how long it will take them to find out that they can't catch it — whatever it is. The only way they can get a disease is to develop it themselves by wrong eating, drinking, smoking or doing some other things which cause internal poisoning and lowered vitality. All diseases are preventable and most of them are curable with the right methods, not known to medical doctors, and not all drugless doctors know them either.

It has been said that the 1918 flu epidemic killed 20 million people throughout the world. But, actually, the doctors killed them with their crude and deadly treatments and drugs. This is a harsh accusation but it is nevertheless true, judging by the success of the drugless doctors in comparison with that of the medical doctors.

While the medical men and medical hospitals were losing 33 percent of their flu cases, the non-medical hospitals such as Battle Creek, Kellogg and MacFadden's Health-Restorium were getting almost 100 percent healings with their water cure, baths, enemas, etc., fasting and certain other simple healing methods, followed by carefully worked out diets of natural foods. One health doctor didn't lose a patient in eight years.

"If the medical doctors had been as advanced as the drugless doctors, there would not have been those 20 million deaths from the medical flu treatment. There was seven times more disease among the vaccinated soldiers than among the unvaccinated civilians, and the diseases were those they had been vaccinated against. One soldier who had returned from overseas in 1912 told me that the army hospitals were filled with cases of *infantile paralysis* [polio] and he wondered why grown men should have an infant disease. Now, we know that paralysis is a common after-effect of vaccine poisoning. Those at home didn't get the paralysis until after the world-wide vaccination campaign in 1918."[1079]

Author Anne Riley Hale alludes to all of the above factors in her 1935 book *Medical Voodoo*: "As every one knows, the world has never witnessed such an orgy of vaccination and inoculation of every description as was inflicted by army-camp doctors upon the soldiers of the [First] World War." Hale also observed that the "amazing disease and death toll among them occurred among 'the picked men of the nation'– supposedly the most robust, resistant class of all, who presumably brought to the service each a good pair of lungs, since they must have passed a rigid physical examination by competent medical men."[1080] And yet, precisely these supermen with super-lungs were the ones who were dropping like flies from pulmonary tuberculosis.

In this context, a report in the *Idaho Observer* (July 2003) is also worth noting. It mentions a contemporary vaccination trial by one Dr. Rosenow, published in the *Mayo Collected Papers* of the world-renowned Mayo Clinic. According to this paper, the vaccinated guinea

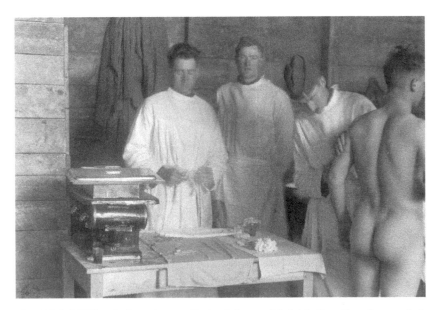

„Spanish flu" 1918: entrainment camp, Genicart, France; Administration of vaccines against flu and lung infections. © With permission of the National Museum of Health and Medicine, Armed Forces Institute of Pathology, Washington, D.C., Reeve015663

pigs primarily suffered from severe lung damage—a typical symptom of tuberculosis and other diseases related to the "Spanish flu."[1081]

Doctors Respond to the Catastrophe with Overwhelming Silence

Meanwhile, medical historians are amazed that doctors and the media have remained silent about the catastrophes that resulted from Spanish flu. As Kolata writes in her book, Victor Vaughan, at that time, America's top military doctor, dealt with the mega-catastrophe in just one paragraph of his 464 page long memoirs. And yet, Vaughan must have recollected everything very well, as his book appeared in 1926, not long after the war's end (and he probably would never forget the horrific events). "If anyone might be expected to write about the epidemic it was Vaughan," writes Kolata. Like Vaughn, other army doctors remained steadfastly silent.[1082]

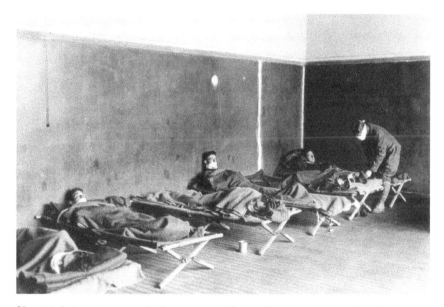

"Spanish flu": interior view of influenza ward, US Army Field Hospital No. 29, Hollerich, Luxembourg, 1918. Look at the men's faces: they're covered to try and check the alleged airborne spread of the disease. © With permission of the National Museum of Health and Medicine, Armed Forces Institute of Pathology, Washington, D.C., Reeve015663

The pandemic, one of the worse to ever afflict the earth, was simply virtually erased from newspapers, magazines, books and society's collective memory, says Kolata.[1083] This could be psychologically explained in two ways. The catastrophe presented a very personal catastrophe for physicians, because, although they were basically given all the money and material resources in their world to fight the alleged flu, they were unsuccessful in preventing the disaster. In a brutally clear way, doctors and pharmacologists were shown the limits of their power. It is clear that mainstream medicine prefers not to dwell on such a total defeat, let alone expand upon it in memoirs or newspapers.

Perhaps the occasional scientist, doctor or politician began to mull over the lost campaign against an imaginary virus and entertained the thought that the mass administration of highly toxic vaccines and medications could have been at least partially responsible for the pandemic. Clues for this were by all means visible. But who likes to take responsible for the deaths of millions of people—even unintentionally—and admit failure to fulfill the duty to investigate all factors that come into question?

Chapter 8

Cervical Cancer and Other Vaccines: Policy vs. Evidence

"There has been a great concentration of research on the viruses which can produce cancer, but there is no convincing evidence that any human tumour is virus-induced. Considering the extreme rarity of cancer in wild animals I can see no way by which an ability to induce cancer could favour the survival of a virus species. Neither can I see anything in human biology which could have power to evolve human cancer viruses; except by deliberate human effort directed to such an end. I believe we can forget about the possibility of any of the common forms of cancer being of virus origin."[1084]

Sir Frank Macfarlane Burnet
Nobel laureate for Medicine

"[Looking not only at vaccine research one must conclude that] our public health policies are not even remotely evidence-based. Rather, our public health policies are faith-based decrees by government 'authorities'– no better than voodoo medicine."[1085]

Vera Sharav
Alliance for Human Research Protection (AHRP)

Flu Vaccines: Do They Make Sense?

Louis Pasteur, Robert Koch and their heirs have inoculated us with a monocausal theory of disease. The picture is alluring and comforting because it completely shifts the blame away from ourselves to microbes, and suggests that if we simply throw enough money at pharmaceutical research— presto!— we're safe from all sorts of diseases, including the flu. But we're still waiting for side effect-free miracle pills that will liberate us from flu symptoms.

Mainstream medicine holds that flu medications and vaccines have worked wonders. But a glance at the history books and statistics reveals, as mentioned, that these so-called epidemics only developed when people's immune systems had been weakened, starting with lack of food or clean water and compounded by chemical toxins like medications, warfare agents and pesticides. The diseases, held to be caused primarily by viruses, had long begun their retreat when vaccine campaigns were finally introduced (as with diphtheria; see diagram 9). For example, population statistics in the USA show that the death rates in senior citizens were quite stable from 1980 onwards, although the vaccination rate had climbed steeply from 1980 to 2001 (from 15 to 65 percent) — and parallel to this, the number of flu victims had also climbed.[1086] [1087]

Diagram 9   Diphtheria cases in Germany (1920-1995)

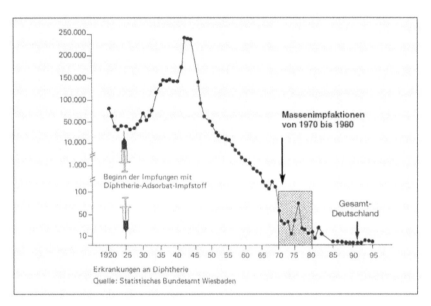

Source: Buchwald, Gerhard, Impfen – Das Geschäft mit der Angst, Knaur, 1994, p. 81

In 2018, the Cochrane Database of Systematic Reviews also staggeringly commented on the lack of evidence for flu vaccination in older people. They concluded, "The available evidence relating to complications is of poor quality, insufficient, or old and provides no clear guidance for public health regarding the safety, efficacy, or effectiveness of influenza vaccines for people aged 65 years or older. Society should invest in research on a new generation of influenza vaccines for the elderly"[1088]

Greed, Negligence and Deception
in the Vaccine Industry
By Robert F. Kennedy Jr.

"In early May 2019, the magazine *Politico* published an article written by three of my relatives, criticizing my advocacy for safe vaccines.[1089] After numerous requests, the magazine
has refused to publish my response. Here is my answer:

Three of my Kennedy relatives recently published an article criticizing my advocacy for
safe vaccines. Our contentious family dispute highlights the fierce national donnybrook
over vaccinations that has divided communities and raised doubts about the Democratic Party's commitment to some of its defining values: abhorrence of censorship,
wariness toward excessive corporate power, support for free speech, religious freedom,
and personal sovereignty over our bodies, and the rights of citizens (codified in the
Nuremberg Code and other treaties to which we are signatories) to decline unwanted
government-mandated medical interventions. The debate has also raised questions
about the independence of our press and its role as a champion of free speech, and First
Amendment rights as a bulwark against overreaching by government and corporations.

I love my family and sympathize with their anxieties when I call out government officials
for corruption. The Kennedys have a long, close, and continuing relationship with public
health agencies so it is understandably difficult for us to believe that powerful regulators
would lie about vaccines. "All issues are simple," the saw goes, "until you study them."

CDC, FDA, WHO: Under Big Pharma's Spell and Dishonest for a Long Time
I've arrived at my skepticism after 15 years spent researching and litigating this issue. I
have watched financial conflicts and institutional self-interest transform key sectors of
our public health bureaucracies into appendages of the very pharmaceutical companies
that Congress charged them to regulate.

Multiple investigations by Congress and the United States Department of Health
& Human Services (HHS) Inspector General have consistently found that an overwhelming majority of the FDA officials directly charged with licensing vaccines, and
the CDC officials who effectively mandate them for children, have personal financial

entanglements with vaccine manufacturers. These public servants are often share-holders in, grant recipients from, and paid consultants to vaccine manufacturers, and, occasionally, patent holders of the very vaccines they vote to approve. Those conflicts motivate them to recommend ever more vaccines with minimal support from evidence-based science.

The pharmaceutical industry also enforces policy discipline through agency budgets. FDA receives 45 percent of its annual budget from industry. The World Health Organization (WHO) gets roughly half its budget from private sources, including Pharma and its allied foundations. And CDC, frankly, is a vaccine company; it owns 56 vaccine patents and buys and distributes $4.6 billion in vaccines annually through the Vaccines for Children program, which is over 40 percent of its total budget.

Further, Pharma directly funds, populates and controls dozens of CDC programs through the CDC foundation. A *British Medical Journal* editorial excoriates CDC's sweetheart relationship with pharma quotes UCLA Professor of Medicine Jerome R. Hoffman 'most of us were shocked to learn the CDC takes funding from industry … It is outrageous that industry is apparently allowed to punish the CDC if the agency conducts research that has potential to cut into profits.'

HHS partners with vaccine makers to develop, approve, recommend, and pass mandates for new products and then shares profits from vaccine sales. HHS employees can personally collect up to $150,000 annually in royalties for products they work on. For example, key HHS officials collect money on every sale of Merck's controversial HPV vaccine Gardasil, which also yields tens of millions annually for the agency in patent royalties. Furthermore, under the 1986 Act that created the National Vaccine Injury Compensation Program, HHS is the defendant in Vaccine Court and is legally obligated to defend against any claim that a vaccine causes injury. Despite high hurdles for recovery, HHS pays out hundreds of millions of dollars annually (over $4 billion total) to Americans injured by vaccines. Hence, if HHS publishes any study acknowledging that a vaccine causes a harm, claimants can use that study against HHS in Vaccine Court. In June 2009, a high-level HHS official, Tom Insel, killed a $16 million-dollar budget item to study the relationship between vaccines and autism by the Interagency Autism Coordinating Committee. Insel argued that petitioners would use these studies against HHS in vaccine court.

Such conflicts are a formula for 'agency capture' on steroids. 'Instead of a regulator and a regulated industry, we now have a partnership,' says Dr. Michael Carome, a former HHS employee who is now the director of the advocacy group Public Citizen. Carome says that these financial entanglements have tilted HHS 'away from a public health perspective to an industry-friendly perspective.'

In 1986, Congress—awash in Pharma money (the pharmaceutical industry is number one for both political contributions and lobbying spending over the past 20 years) enacted a law granting vaccine makers blanket immunity from liability for injuries caused by vaccines. If vaccines were as safe as my family members claim, would we need to give pharmaceutical companies immunity for the injuries they cause? The subsequent gold rush by pharmaceutical companies boosted the number of recommended inoculations from twelve shots of five vaccines in 1986 to 54 shots of 13 vaccines today. A billion-dollar sideline grew into the $50 billion vaccine industry behemoth.

Since vaccines are liability-free—and effectively compulsory to a captive market of 76 million children—there is meager market incentive for companies to make them safe. The public must rely on the moral scruples of Merck, GlaxoSmithKline, Sanofi, and Pfizer. But these companies have a long history of operating recklessly and dishonestly, even with products that they must market to the public and for which they can be sued for injuries. The four companies that make virtually all of the recommended vaccines are all convicted felons. Collectively they have paid over $35 billion since 2009 for defrauding regulators, lying to and bribing government officials and physicians, falsifying science, and leaving a trail of injuries and deaths from products they knew to be dangerous and sold under pretense of safety and efficacy.

Doesn't it require a kind of cognitive dissonance to believe that vaccines are untainted by the greed, negligence, and corruption that bedevil every other pharmaceutical product?

No Safety Testing, Missing Placebo Trials
Such concerns only deepen when one considers that, besides freedom from liability, vaccine makers enjoy another little-known lucrative loophole; vaccines are the only pharmaceutical or medical products that do not need to be rigorously safety tested. To win an FDA license, companies must safety test virtually every other drug for years in randomized comparisons

against an inert placebo. Yet, not a single vaccine currently on the CDC's childhood schedule was tested against an inert placebo before licensing. Without placebo testing, regulators have no capacity to assess a medicine's risks. During a January 2018 deposition, Dr. Stanley Plotkin, the world's most influential vaccinologist, acknowledged that researches who try to ascertain vaccine safety without a placebo are in "La La land."

According to Dr. Drummond Rennie, Deputy Editor of the *Journal of the American Medical Association*, 'It is the marketing department, not the science, that is driving the research.' It seems plain wrong to me that Democratic-controlled legislatures across the country are frantically passing coercive mandates for pharmaceutical products for which no one knows the risks.

Furthermore, safety testing, which typically requires five or more years for other medical products, often lasts only a few days with vaccines — not nearly long enough to spot cancers or chronic conditions like autoimmune disease (e.g., juvenile diabetes, rheumatoid arthritis, multiple sclerosis), allergic illnesses (e.g., food allergies, allergic rhinitis, eczema, asthma), or neurological and neurodevelopmental injuries (e.g., ADD, ADHD, narcolepsy, epilepsy, seizure disorders, and autism). Manufacturers' inserts accompanying every vial of mandated vaccines include warnings about these and over 400 other injuries including many serious immune, neurological, and chronic illnesses for which FDA suspects that vaccines may be the cause. Federal law requires that the package insert for each vaccine include 'only those adverse events for which there is some basis to believe that there is a causal relationship between the drug and the occurrence of the adverse event.'

Many of these illnesses became epidemic in American children after 1986, coterminous with the exploding vaccine schedule. For American kids born in 1986, only 12.8 percent had chronic diseases. That number has grown to 54 percent among the vaccine generation (those born after 1986) in lockstep with the expanding schedule. Evidence including HHS's own surveillance reports, manufacturers' inserts, and peer-reviewed studies link all of these injuries to vaccines. However, the associations are not definitive because CDC has failed to conduct the necessary randomized studies to prove or disprove causation.

HHS has directed the Institute of Medicine (IOM, now the National Academy of Medicine) to oversee the CDC's vaccine safety science. IOM has repeatedly rebuked the agency for failing to study whether vaccines are causing these epidemics. In my experience, vaccine proponents rarely cite specific peer-reviewed studies to support their assertions that all vaccines are safe, relying instead on appeals to authority; CDC, FDA, WHO, or the AAP. My relatives, for example, argue that vaccines are safe because WHO, HHS, CDC, and FDA say so. But HHS designated the IOM as the ultimate arbiter of vaccine safety. And IOM says that the existing scientific literature does not support these claims. Despite requests by the IOM, CDC has steadfastly refused to perform safety studies.

In total, three IOM reports (1991, 1994, and 2011/2012) investigated 231 adverse events associated with vaccines. For 34 conditions, IOM found that the evidence supported a causal connection between the vaccine and the adverse event. But for 184 adverse events, fully 80 percent of the conditions reviewed, the IOM found that HHS's evidence was inadequate to accept or reject vaccine causation. How can our public health officials claim safety when there is no follow-up research on reported adverse events?

Autism and Vaccines

Let's drill down on bedrock dogma that science has thoroughly debunked any links between autism and vaccines. That assumption is so engrained that media ridicules anyone who questions this orthodoxy as a dangerous heretic. But, look for a moment, at the facts. In 1986, Congress specifically ordered CDC to determine if pertussis-containing vaccines (DTP, later DTaP) were causing autism. Then, as today, many parents with autistic children were claiming that vaccines were a cause of their child's autism and DTP/DTaP vaccines were/are a popular suspect.

On its website, CDC declares that, "Vaccines don't cause autism," citing IOM's comprehensive 2011/2012 literature review of vaccination safety science. However, the IOM study and the follow-up HHS study in 2014 both say that CDC has never performed a study to support CDC's claim that DTaP does not cause autism. The same is true for Hep B, Hib, PCV 13, and IPV. The only vaccine actually studied with regard to autism is MMR, and a senior CDC scientist claims the CDC did find an increased rate of autism after MMR in the only MMR/autism study ever conducted by the CDC with American children. Moreover, HHS's primary autism expert recently provided an affidavit to the DOJ explaining that vaccines can cause autism in some children.

Autism has grown from about 1 in 2,500 prior to 1986 to one in 36 among vaccine generation children today. Why are we content with the CDC's claim that the exponential explosion of autism is a mystery? CDC spares no expense systematically tracking the source of 800 measles cases. But when asked about the cataclysmic epidemic of upwards of 68,000 new autism cases annually, CDC shrugs. Why are we not demanding answers? 'CDC is paralyzed right now when it comes to anything to do with autism,' explains former senior vaccine safety scientist Dr. William Thompson, who is still a CDC employee. Thompson told Congressman Bill Posey under oath that CDC bigwigs ordered him to destroy data that showed a link between autism and vaccines and to publish a fraudulent study dismissing the link. Today, he is remorseful, 'When I see a family with a child with autism, I feel great shame because I have been part of the problem.'

We Are Killing Children
HHS has also ignored its statutory obligations to study vaccine injuries and improve vaccine safety. In 1986, Congress—recognizing that drug companies no longer had any incentive to make vaccines safe—ordered HHS to study vaccine injuries, work to improve vaccine safety, and report to Congress on its progress every two years. A year ago, I brought a lawsuit that forced HHS to admit that in 36 years it had never performed any of those critical studies.

Post-licensure vaccine safety surveillance is also in shambles. The CDC's Vaccine Adverse Event Reporting System (VAERS), to which doctors and patients may voluntarily report adverse vaccine events, received 58,381 reports in 2018, including 412 deaths, 1,237 permanent disabilities, and 4,217 hospitalizations. An HHS-funded review of VAERS concluded that 'fewer than 1 percent of vaccine adverse events are reported' to VAERS. This suggests that there are a hundredfold more adverse vaccine events than are reported. The CDC has nonetheless refused to mandate or automate VAERS reporting.

On March 9, 2019, Dr. Peter Aaby issued a scathing rebuke to the world's public health agencies for continuing to allow pharmaceutical companies to sell vaccines without proper safety testing. Dr. Aaby, who has authored over 300 peer-reviewed studies, is one of world's foremost authorities on WHO's African vaccine program and the winner of Denmark's highest honor for health care research. Dr. Aaby was one of five co-authors of a 2017 study of the diphtheria tetanus, and pertussis (DTP) vaccine, the most widely used vaccine on earth, which found that children who received DTP had ten times the risk of dying compared to DTP-unvaccinated children.

For thirty years, doctors, including Aaby, never noticed the danger because vaccinated children were succumbing to illnesses and infections apparently unrelated to the vaccine. It turns out that while the vaccine protected children from diphtheria, tetanus, and pertussis, it so badly weakened their immune systems that they were dying in droves from unrelated infections. The researchers concluded: 'The DTP vaccine may kill more children from other causes than it saves from diphtheria, tetanus and pertussis.' In March, an alarmed Aaby plead for a policy change, 'Most of you think we know what our vaccines are doing. But we don't .... We are killing children.'

The world's most aggressive vaccine schedule has not given our country the world's healthiest children. We now rank 35th in overall health outcomes—just behind Costa Rica, making the U.S., by most measures, including infant mortality, the sickest in the developed world. In addition to those 400 chronic diseases and injuries that FDA suspects may be vaccine related, the vaccine generation suffers unprecedented levels of anxiety and depression and behavioral disorders running the gamut from aggression to anorexia. Peer-reviewed animal and human studies have linked all these symptoms to vaccines. The present generation is the first in a century to lose I.Q., having suffered an extraordinary drop of seven points. Researchers concluded that some environmental cause is the trigger. In the U.S., SAT and, more recently, bar exam scores are plummeting.

Could these declines be the outcome of injecting virtually every child with multiple doses of two of the world's most potent neurotoxins—mercury and aluminum—in bolus doses beginning on the day of birth? Shouldn't we be doing the research to reject this hypothesis? The logical approach to doing so would be to compare health outcomes between vaccinated and unvaccinated children. For years, public health officials, including the IOM, have urged CDC to conduct such studies.

In 2013, the IOM found that, 'No studies have compared the differences in health outcomes ... between entirely unimmunized populations of children and fully immunized children .... Furthermore, studies designed to examine the long-term effects of the cumulative number of vaccines or other aspects of the immunization schedule have not been conducted.' In a 2008 interview, former NIH Director Bernadette Healy explained that HHS

269

refuses to perform safety studies out of fear that they will expose dangers, 'that would scare the public away' from vaccines. Healy continued, 'First of all, I think the public is smarter than that ... I don't think you should ever turn your back on any scientific hypothesis because you're afraid of what it might show.'

Media Malpractice

The suppression of critical safety science documented by the IOM would not be possible without a mass epidemic of media malpractice. Mainstream and social media outlets which collectively received $9.6 billion in revenues from pharmaceutical companies in 2016 have convinced themselves they are protecting public health by aggressively censoring criticism of these coercively mandated, zero liability, and untested pharmaceutical products. But, the absence of press scrutiny leaves industry no incentive to improve vaccine safety. Muzzling discussions of government corruption and deficient safety science and abolishing vaccine injuries by fiat is not a strategy that will solve the growing chronic disease epidemic.

The children who comprise this badly injured generation are now aging out of schools that needed to build quiet rooms and autism wings, install wobble chairs, hire security guards and hike special ed spending to 25 percent to accommodate them. They are landing on the social safety net which they threaten to sink. As Democratic lawmakers vote to mandate more vaccines and call for censorship of safety concerns, Democratic Presidential candidates argue about how to fix America's straining health care system. If we don't address the chronic disease epidemic, such proposals are like rearranging the deck chairs on the Titanic. The good news for Pharma is that many of these children have lifelong dependencies on blockbuster products like Adderall, Epi-Pens, asthma inhalers, and diabetes, arthritis, and anti-seizure meds made by the same companies that made the vaccines.

My belief that all or some of these injuries might be vaccine related has been the catalyst that wrenched so much of my focus away from the environmental and energy work that I love, and prompted me to become an advocate for vaccine safety. I have sacrificed friendships, income, credibility, and family relationships in an often-lonely campaign to force these companies to perform the tests that will definitively answer these questions.
People will vaccinate when they have confidence in regulators and industry. When public confidence fails, coercion and censorship became the final options. Silencing critics and

deploying police powers to force untested medicines upon an unwilling public is not an optimal strategy in a democracy.

My uncle and my father argued that in a free and open society, the response to difficult questions should never be to shut down debate. What we need is science, not censorship. I am not anti-vax. I am pro-safety and pro-science. I want robust, transparent safety studies and independent regulators. These do not seem like the kind of radical demands that should divide our party or our families. As Americans and Kennedys, we ought to be able to have a civil, science-based debate about these legitimate concerns."

Fraud, Waste, Bribery — Corruption in the Health Service

Even if the perfect vaccine did exist, effective and without any side effects, it would still be a far cry from a "magic bullet." People tend to overlook the fact that flu vaccines are manufactured before those viruses (virus stems) they are supposed to work against even exist.

Even mainstream studies have shown that during flu "peak season," only 10 percent of infections that form in the upper airway can be traced back to influenza viruses.[1090] The statistic sounds reassuring and would make for great news if it weren't for the epidemic hunters from the CDC, RKI or WHO, who speak every year about another 10,000 flu deaths and urgently warn that only vaccinated people are protected from influenza. On close examination of the data upon which their warnings are based, the question crops up: "Are US flu death figures more PR than science?"

This is precisely the title of a study published in late 2005 in the *British Medical Journal*. Author Peter Doshi, of Harvard University (in 2006, Doshi switched to the Massachusetts Institute of Technology, MIT), provides a resoundingly decisive answer: "US data on influenza deaths are a mess."[1091] Doshi's main criticism is that the CDC works under the assumption that 36,000 Americans die from viral flu each year — but they still owe us proof that an influenza virus really kills these people. Doshi's conclusion: The CDC's communication strategy is equivalent to "marketing of fear."

Several astute observers critiqued the government's promotional campaign urging the public to vaccinate against the flu by challenging the 36,000 annual death count the CDC attributes to the flu. Especially worth mentioning is the meta-analysis of the published flu vaccine reports by Tom Jefferson of the Cochrane Center, replicated in the *British Medical Journal*[1092] as well as a column in *Red Flags* by Edward Yazbak, a pediatrician.[1093] The findings of these 2006 articles are sobering: a major gap exists between evidence and public health policy.

The summary points of the *BMJ*'s meta-analysis are clearly alarming:

1. Because non-randomized studies predominate, systematic reviews of large data sets from several decades (meta-analyses) provide the best information on vaccine performance.
2. Evidence from systematic reviews shows that inactivated vaccines have little or no effect on the effects measured.
3. Most studies are of poor methodological quality and the impact of confounders is high.
4. Little comparative evidence exists on the safety of these vaccines.

The lead author Tom Jefferson concludes: "The optimistic and confident tone of some predictions of viral circulation and of the impact of inactivated vaccines, which are at odds with the evidence, is striking. The reasons are probably complex and may involve a messy blend of truth conflicts and conflicts of interest making it difficult to separate factual disputes from value disputes or a manifestation of optimism bias, that is to say an unwarranted belief in the efficacy of interventions."

In fact, the bottom line is that the CDC has not provided data to back up its claim about the number of deaths it attributes to the flu. The CDC appears to be acting on behalf of flu vaccine manufacturers, even as the evidence shows the vaccine to be worthless at best—or to be fatal at worst. A Vaccine Adverse Events Reporting System (VAERS) search performed on 10 October 2005 yielded three reports in the past two years of children younger than 23 months of age who died shortly after receiving a dose of influenza vaccine. No other vaccines were administered at the same time and all three children had underlying diseases.

"We can only conclude that we are in the era of post-evidence-based medicine," states Vera Sharav from the Alliance for Human Research Protection in New York. "Our public health policies are not even remotely evidence-based. Rather, our public health policies are faith-based decrees by government 'authorities'—no better than voodoo medicine."[1094] Underlying this collapse of Western medicine is the collusion between science and business. Our public health policies are currently shaped by corporate interests.

The CDC's German counterpart, the Robert Koch-Institute plays similar games with the statistics. They allege that in the winter of 2004-2005, 15,000 to 20,000 people died from viral flu in the country.[1095] But there is no proof to back up these statements. Rather, examining the data of Germany's Federal Statistical Office (Statistisches Bundesamt), just nine people died of influenza viruses in 2004 (2003: 25; 2002: 10; 2001: 9). The picture painted by hospital statistics is just as undramatic: 12 deaths[1096]—a mere speck in comparison to the RKI's claim of 20,000 mortalities.

Ask RKI to explain this extreme discrepancy and the institute answers that "official statistic on 'influenza deaths' underestimate the true influence [of flu viruses], because very many [influenza] deaths are 'hidden' in other diseases." For this reason, according to RKI, "even the Statisches Bundesamt's data hardly reflects the true number of influenza deaths."[1097]

But where's the study showing concrete evidence that a virus was really at play, or was the single or primary cause in the cases where the RKI suspects a "hidden" flu virus? The RKI had no answer to this, even after repeated inquiries (see: Can We Trust Blindly The Figures of CDC, RKI, etc.?, Rapid Responses to Peter Doshi's article in the *British Medical Journal* "Are US flu death figures more PR than science?", *British Medical Journal* (Website), December2005/January 2006).

Neither did we receive studies from Berlin's virus hunters to prove that 1) the flu virus declared a killer has been completely detected (purification and electron micrographs); 2) the virus, insofar as it does exist, has lethal properties; 3) all other factors (nutrition, toxins, etc.) can be ruled out as primary or major causes of the so-called "flu victim's" death.[1098]

The RKI says it arrived at the 15,000 to 20,000 flu deaths by applying an "internationally recognized" and "peer reviewed" calculative method. But whether a calculation makes sense cannot be determined by the fact that it is "recognized" and has been verified by other researchers, but only by being verified by independent technical experts. We wanted to do this, but so far it has not been possible.

In December 2005, the RKI did agree to send us their detailed calculations by the end of January 2006 at the latest; we have yet to receive them.[1099] Yet the RKI should actually have the requested calculation at hand.

The RKI also claims "it is often the case," that influenza death figures are estimated values.[1100] [1101] And in this regard as well, they agreed to send us the documents that support this by the end of January 2006. But unfortunately, we have not yet received a single document from the RKI. One thing is certain: contrary to what the RKI told us, in its database of significant papers and statistics, the RKI does not explicitly say that only estimated values are available. This is true on their website, for instance, where influenza mortality figures are listed,[1102] and in a press release from late 2004.[1103]

The RKI identifies the influenza work-group (Arbeitsgemeinschaft Influenza, AGI) as the source of their influenza data. The AGI was founded by the pharmaceutical industry in 1991, and receives financial support from four vaccine manufacturers.[1104] So, if the RKI relies on an organization funded by the pharmaceutical industry, how can the institute make sure that published data is absolutely sound?[1105]

It would be wise to ask the same question of the German vaccine committee STIKO (Ständige Impfkommission), a part of the RKI system. STIKO Chair, medical professor Heinz-J. Schmitt, is also on the Board of Directors of Stiftung Präventative Pädiatrie (Foundation for Preventive Pediatrics),[1106] a children's health foundation which in turn works closely with and is funded by pharmaceutical companies like GlaxoSmithKline and Chiron-Behring.[1107] Schmitt additionally functions as consultant to the GlaxoSmithKline project "Gesundes Kind" ("Healthy Child"), which plugs protective vaccinations.[1108]

To be able to evaluate whether RKI can still act independently of the pharmaceutical industry, we requested that the institute disclose all the ways their scientists are remunerated (lecture fees, research grants, etc.). By their scientists, we mean the ones working for the RKI or for other institutions directly subordinate or integrated into the RKI.[1109]

But to date, we have not received a response to any of these questions.

In any case, it is certain that several STIKO members cultivate close relationships with Big Pharma or are active for pharmaceutical companies, including the major ones

Table 3   Members of the Ständige Impfkommission (STIKO), which belongs to the Robert Koch-Institute, and their connections to the pharmaceutical industry (excerpts), as of 2008

Dr. Robert Dobbelaer Head, Biological Standardization Scientific Institute of Public Health (SIPH, Brussels)	According to the World health Organization, he is himself a manufacturer of polio vaccines
Prof. Dr. Ulrich Heininger Department of Pediatric Infectious Disease and Vaccinology University Children's Hospital Basel (UKBB, Universität-Kinderspital bei der Basel	Maintains the website http://www.rund-ums-baby/de/impfen, and is a member of the German Society for Pediatric Infectious Disease (DGPI) scientific advisory council. Sponsors of this society are: - Aventis Pasteur MSD Ltd. Leimen - Aventis Pharma Germany Ltd. - Bristol-Myers-Squibb, Munich - GlaxoSmithKline Ltd. & Co. limited partnership - Infectopharm, Heppenheim - MSD Sharp & Dohme Ltd., Haar - Wyeth Pharma Ltd., Münster
Prof. Dr. Wolfgang Jilg Institute of Medical Microbiology and Hygiene at the University of Regensburg	Chair of the German Society of Virology's (GfV) Immunization committee (the GfV is a non-profit organization presently with around 900 members, which aims to promote virology in all fields through increasing and exchangibg knowledge from virologic research, primarily in the German-speaking area). The GfV's treasurer is Dr. Michael Bröker of Chiron-Behring (Chiron Vaccines, Chiron Behring Ltd. & Co. limited partnership, Emil-von-Behring-Str. 76, 35041 Marburg)
Prof. Dr. Rüdiger von Kries Department of Children and Adolescent Epidemiology Institute of Social Pediatrics and Youth Medicine, Ludwig Maximilian's Universität, Munich	Kries is in the scientific advisory council of the German Society for Pediatric Infectiology (DGPI, sponsors as above)
Prof. Dr, Thomas Mertens Clinic, University of Ulm Virology Department Institute of Microbiology and Immunology, Ulm	Member of the German Society of Virology (on the GfV, see above, Prof. Dr. Wolfgang Jilg)
Prof. Dr. Heinz-J. Schmitt Pediatric Infectiology Children's Clinic of the Johannes Gutenberg University, Mainz Schmitt is chair of STIKO	President of the Stiftung Präventive Pädiatrie, a German pediatric foundation which co-operates with the following partners/companies: - GlaxoSmithKline - Chiron Behring Consultant to the GlaxoSmithKline project "Gesundes Kind" (healthy child)
Prof. Dr. Fred Zepp University Children's Clinic, Mainz	Directs the department of Pediatric Immunology and Vaccine Development, which co-operates with the pharmaceutical industry; Zepp is also Chair of Stiftung Präventive Pädiatrie's advisory council (as above)

For current information about the STIKO members, see www.rki.de

like GlaxoSmithKline (see table 3). It is also telling that the RKI, as *Focus* magazine reported in a rare critical article on epidemic authorities, were confronted with the revelation of a corruption case in early 2006, which cast a very negative light on the highly esteemed institution.

Social researcher Friedrich T. [full surname not mentioned], who had worked as a top official at the RKI, was sentenced by the district court Berlin-Tiergarten to six months in prison and a fine of €3,000. In late 1998, T. had internally proposed awarding the contract for a reputedly extremely important AIDS study ("RKI Sentinel") to a private polling institute by the name of Images. And indeed Images' bid for the study worth 396,000 German marks (approximately $200,000) was accepted. Two months later, an Images employee turned over 10,000 marks in cash to T.

The presiding judge saw the elements of corruption here, as she explicitly declared this a "not unserious case." During the trial, the judge had declared that there were evidently a few alarming "interconnections" at the RKI. She was "convinced" that more was known at the institute "than came out in the trial." The final verdict also stated that "the court cannot resist the impression that here on a large scale, the RKI has been used as a good source of money."

The company Images functioned namely only as a dummy firm for the identically staffed and located Intersofia GmbH (Ltd.), whose founder and sole shareholder is none other than RKI official T. Two Intersofia employees had founded Images expressly for the purpose of landing the AIDS study contract, since T. couldn't directly hand the contract to his own company Intersofia. T. penned not only the "service description" for the RKI Sentinel but also Images' offer. On 3 November 1998, T. proposed the dummy company as contractual partner, but Images was not founded until 15 November, and five days later, the then RKI director Reinhard Kurth personally signed the contract.

Focus is completely correct in writing that T.'s corruption case had turned into a worst-case scenario for Reinhard Kurth as well. Kurth had evidently also lied to the public. The RKI's press office and even the RKI president declared to know nothing of any possible conflicts of interests for T. at the time the contract was awarded. But this claim is impossible. In her verdict, the judge cited the testimony of a certain Wolfgang Kurtz, who was Director of Central Administration at the RKI during the time in question (first half of November). According to

Kurtz, the epidemic authority's "Research Council," which was responsible for awarding the contract, were fully aware that T. was doing the AIDS study "with his old mates."

Additionally, the researcher's financial sleights of hand had been a constant gossip topic at the institute for years. By the end of 2000, top management had detailed information on the Intersofia/Images scam. An employee of T.'s private company had filed a disciplinary complaint against her boss with the RKI, revealing details about the scheme. A whole year later, Kurth declared that internal clarification of the accusations was proving to be "difficult and time-consuming."

But in T.'s trial, the district attorneys simplified this allegedly complex issue. The accused had seen the RKI simply as a sort of "self-service shop." Perhaps he thought he was invulnerable. Not only did T. have good contacts at the top of the Federal Health Ministry, he also collaborated very closely with his superior, no less than Bärbel-Maria Kurth, RKI department head, and the president's wife.

T. also took care of a particularly awkward assignment for his boss. Mrs. Kurth had tried to safeguard GDR scientist Michael Radoschewski's career for many years, after it had gone into a tailspin post-reunification. Because of his former Stasi (East German secret police) activity, he could not get a steady job in unified Germany's health administration. Mrs. Kurth, herself a former GDR student, helped with labor contracts, and ultimately accommodated him in the firm Images, T.'s dummy company. Radoschewski even worked on the AIDS study. In this way, the RKI continued paying his salary indirectly.

The AIDS study, financed to the tune of approximately $200,000 worth of tax dollars, was incidentally not published. T. and his Images troupe had sunk the project.

Images' former Managing Director, Liane S. appeared as a witness in the trial. The judge dismissed her attempts at exoneration, calling them "lies." But why would Mrs. S. have said anything bad about T. and his insider dealings? S. now works at the RKI—in Mrs. Kurth's department.[1110]

As has repeatedly been portrayed in this book, there is certainly no reason to assume that such conflicts of interest and corrupt activities are the exception, and to suppose that, on the whole, everything is just fine. Transparency International's "Corruption

Annual Report 2006" is worth another mention. The report was presented to the public in May of the same year, and unequivocally says that waste, fraud and corruption have eaten into the local public health service and annual damages are at least €24 billion.

This rarely publicly addressed mismanagement is very difficult to fix because the industry in question is run by powerful corporations and its allies—including decrepit government organizations that lack transparency and federal oversight. Transparency International clearly awards chief responsibility for this mess to the pharmaceutical industry, which forges studies, influences authorities, suppresses risks and undermines alternative health and self-help groups.

40 percent of medical studies from 2005 were demonstrably faked or manipulated by sponsors.

Politics has yielded to health lobbyists for too long, says the watchdog organization. Health service bodies governed by public law at the Federal State level have been left to their own devices for too long. It is time to look for a means of compulsory accountability for everything. This includes, above all, the highest level of transparency for contributors and taxpayers.

Often though, nothing happens, because doctors, scientific researchers and pharmaceutical lobbyists have strong connections to politics. Corruption fighters also demand a "radical professionalization" among the health care system players, especially the insurance companies, the panel doctor's associations and government institutions in order to make their decision-making processes more transparent. There must also be a stronger enforcement of the law, in order to ban bad doctors from the profession.

Transparency International also recommended requiring disclosure of financing and relationships to sponsors, as well as the registration of all clinical trials. To avoid deadly mistakes, the health care field should not be allowed to purchase medical experts for their pharmaceutical studies and consequent marketing. Additionally, there needs to be legal regulations for health insurance companies to maintain accountability and public safety. The establishment of specialized district attorneys would also be sensible.

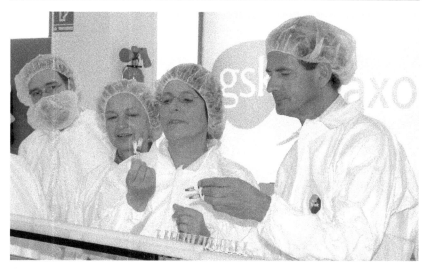

Governments and pharmaceutical industry work hand in hand: On 24 March 2006, pharmaceutical manufacturer GlaxoSmithKline (GSK) informed German Health Minister Ulla Schmidt about their latest development of a vaccine against a flu epidemic. With GSK director Thomas Werner, she visited the GSK factory in Dresden. And the German government made no less than €20 million available to fund the development of a "broadband vaccine" against avian flu infections. With this, they would be in the position to vaccinate the population before the virus mutates, as Schmidt announced.[1111] And if it were up to GlaxoSmithKline, vaccination of the public would not wait until a pandemic breaks out[1112] But that is the pinnacle of absurdity, because if vaccinations were to make any sense in the first place, the genetic structure of whatever (virus) is being vaccinated against would have to first be known. But as mentioned, this is not the case (not only for H5N1)[1113] Source: Screenshot from www.presseportal.de/pm/39763/802530

But "structural corruption" cannot be tackled simply with new laws, reforms and better law enforcement, according to the anti-corruption organization. A culture has to be generated that outlaws fraud in medicine. "It is immoral and indecent to make money from a system that is putting an increasing strain on people with low incomes, and allow increasing gaps in a comprehensive complete medical care, through faulty calculations."[1114]

It would be extremely helpful if the media—the State's (self-declared) "Fourth Estate"—would turn itself again to its true task and consistently try to bring the "structural corruption" in the health service to light, instead of playing henchman to Big Pharma.

HPV Vaccination against Cervical Cancer: Not Proven Safe and Effective

Today, jubilation is expressed by both orthodox science and the mass media about the recently developed vaccine against the human papillomavirus (HPV) assumed to cause cervical cancer. The HPV vaccine is being marketed heavily, especially for use in girls 9-15 years of age. In the literature, we read that the vaccination has been proven to be the most efficient and logistically feasible preventive intervention against cervical cancer. And the vaccine makers "promise an almost 100 percent protection," according to a lead story in the *Frankfurter Allgemeine Zeitung* written by the head science editor himself, headlined: "Vaccinating Against Cancer – In the Drugstore a Dream Comes True."

According to one of Germany's most important daily newspapers, "we now see the start of a new epoch. Heading the march into a new golden age is pharmaceutical company Sanofi Pasteur MSD, with a new vaccine called Gardasil. The announcements by the manufacturer could be dismissed as typical pharmaceutical industry pursuit of giant markets, profits, power and prestige.

Yet, *en masse*, physicians and scientists have joined the chorus, which speaks to a paradigm shift. All are gushing about the potential to abruptly stanch one of the worst villains for women with only three harmless injections. The results of the [vaccine's] approval studies are so convincing that by now there is no limit to euphoria."[1115]

Again, the news sounds more than good. But, before we uncork the champagne, should we really believe the promises of this pharmaceutical giant, brush aside all the conflicts of interests today's biomedical science and forget all the previous empty promises made by even the most prestigious researchers?

In order to clarify this, we approached one of the relevant institutions from which all these predictions, assertions, and claims stem from: The German Cancer Research Centre (Deutsches Krebsforschungszentrum, DKFZ). What we asked for was:[1116]

1. A solid study proving the existence of a human papillomavirus, in short HPV (including a description of the purification and isolation of the particle as well as the characterization of the full genome and the mantle, plus an image done by electron microscopy).
2. A solid study proving beyond doubt that HPV causes cervical cancer.
3. A solid study showing that non-viral factors such as nutrition or chemical toxins alone or in combination can be excluded as possible (primary) causes for cervical cancer.
4. A solid study demonstrating conclusively that the vaccinations entering the market are safe and effective.

Indeed, in response we received a "wonderful literature list," as the DKFZ declared,[1117] of which there were several studies addressing items 1, 2, and 4. Unfortunately, missing from the list was a study proving item 3, that non-viral factors such as nutrition, pesticides, stress, etc. alone or in combination can be excluded as possible (primary) causes for cervical cancer. Interestingly, even the medical establishment itself identified non-viral factors such as smoking or the use of oral contraceptives which are "viewed as relevant co-factors" in the development of cervical cancer.[1118] And there is no proof that these factors could not act as primary factors.

In this context it is also worth mentioning that in the search for the causes of cervical cancer it has been disregarded that up to 80 percent of all women at least temporarily shall contract this so-called papillomavirus during their life, but in 80 percent of these women the virus just disappears after a while. That is to say in only 20 percent of the cases the doctors identify (with their test methods) a persistent infection that according to orthodox researchers carries the risk of causing cervical cancer.

As a matter of fact, according to Lutz Gissmann from the DKFZ in Heidelberg far less than 1 percent of these "infected" women come down with cervical cancer. "We just don't know why most women are able to cope with the virus," Gissmann concedes.[1119] That means—assuming we believe the methods of virus detection are valid—in most cases of cervical cancer there is a „positive" HPV test, but in only a tiny minority of cases is cervical cancer found.

There must be other factors responsible for the development of cervical cancer. Obviously, there is no proof that these non-viral factors cannot play the major or primary role. And so it is not really surprising to hear from one of the leading established cervical cancer researcher,

Matthias Dürst from the University of Jena, that "the infection with the papillomavirus alone still does not cause cancer."[1120] The tumor is said not to develop until there are genetic changes on the chromosomes causing this abnormal growth. But here we have the same problem: there is not a single study proving that a (papilloma)virus initiates these genetic changes or chromosomal alterations.

But let's step backwards again and ask: Can we really believe the methods of virus detection? As mentioned before, the DKFZ sent us a "wonderful literature list" in which there were two studies both conducted by zur Hausen et al. that they claim serve as proofs for the "first isolation of specific HPV from cervical cancer tissue."[1121] [1122] "But a closer look reveals that actually there is no such kind of proof," says Canadian biologist David Crowe.

For example, the first of these two papers published in 1983 in the journal *Proceedings of the National Academy of Sciences*: A Papillomavirus DNA from a Cervical Carcinoma and Its Prevalence in Cancer Biopsy Samples from Different Geographic Regions, lacks the following critical issues:

1. It is not clear where the cloned DNA of the presumed virus comes from. Without knowing the origin of the DNA it is impossible to prove that a virus was there.
2. A large number of cervical tumors were screened without success, increasing the possibility that the discovery of one tumor with this DNA is just a coincidence. The cancer establishment is always talking about the "high correlation" between HPV-prevalence in women and cervical cancer. But it should be noted that particles called HPV are quite common, so to say that HPV is usually found in people with cervical cancer might not mean much.
3. The authors use the term "nonstringent" conditions which probably means that hybridization occurred with less than a perfect match. (Hybridization is a technique that measures the degree of genetic similarity between DNA sequences; it can be used to determine the genetic similarity between two organisms.) That is to say, the two DNA strands they were using were not identical. "Of course, they will just say that viruses mutate rapidly," Crowe points out. "But this is pure speculation."
4. They extracted DNA and hybridized it with "known" HPV samples—but they got less than a 0.1 percent match. Because of this they declared that it was a newly identified type of Humanpapillomavirus (HPV 16), as opposed to declaring that they had pulled out DNA that had nothing to do with HPV at all.

5. Because of the presence of this new "HPV 16" DNA in 11 out of 18 cervical cancer biopsy specimens, the authors concluded, "It reveals a remarkable specificity of HPV 16 infections for malignant tissue." Yet they haven't proved that this is a virus at all!

We approached the DKFZ twice with our points of criticism asking for clarification.[1123] But we didn't gat any response.

That rises the important question: Why should a woman undergo a PAP smear or an HPV test supposed to detect papillomavirus-DNA (not even for the detection of the virus itself!) if (1) there is no scientific proof of this virus and (2) even the cancer establishment admits that the papillomavirus does not cause cancer on its own?

Apart from this, critics of the cancer orthodoxy emphasize that the PAP smear test developed in 1928 by the Greek medical doctor George Papanicolaou is practically meaningless. The test just rests on the evaluation of cell changes found in smears taken from the uterine orifices that are said to cause cancer. But this is pure theory, and the test just classifies too many women as being at risk of getting cervical cancer.

Established cancer scientists such as Dürst don't agree and counter that in 99.6 percent of cases a negative PAP smear test result would accurately suggest that a woman does not have a precancerous lesion (tissue alteration that is associated with a higher risk of becoming a malignant degeneration) or cervical cancer.[1124]

Sounds very good, but this magnificent promise can only be qualified by taking a look at the statistics. In Germany, for example, every year around 7,000 women fall ill from cervical cancer, that is to say 0.017 percent of the 40 million women living in Germany. This means, 99.983 percent of these women do not develop cervical cancer. In other words, cervical cancer is a very rare disease, and it is very easy to achieve a 99.6 percent safety margin, not from the PAP smear test, but from the incidence statistic alone.

Furthermore, the PAP smear test has a high error rate. For example, often sick cells are misdiagnosed because simple inflammation can be confused with mutated cells. In one examination at the University of Hanover, the screening-tests yielded 86 suspected cases, but posterior control tests could confirm only 46 of the suspected cancer diagnoses. This is an error rate of almost 50 percent. Karl Ulrich Petry, gynecologist and one of the leading researchers of the study, stated: "Cervical cancer screening sometimes is like trying to nail 'jello" onto the wall. The collected data is not really reliable."[1125]

Nevertheless, in the USA alone, every year around 200,000 women have their uterus re-moved, many of them to prevent cervical cancer. But in fact only 14,000 American women come down with cervical cancer each year. That is to say, tens of thousand of women in the United States are being operated on—or shall we say: misled—unnecessarily or at least hastily. The reason is that the PAP smear test is not searching for early forms of cervical cancer cells, but for pre-forms of cancer which very often resolve by themselves or stay innocuous.

In 2003 the *British Medical Journal* published a study about the outcomes of screening to prevent cervical cancer. And the results were not encouraging: around 1,000 women need to be screened for 35 years to prevent one death; 150 of these women will receive a stress-causing test result, and 50 women will go through cancer treatment with all its highly toxic side effects. "For each death prevented many women have to be screened and many are treated who would not have developed a problem," writes Angela Raffle, the leading author of the trial.[1126]

In other words: There is just no scientific proof for the effectiveness of the screening tests,[1127] and their collateral side effects (stress, operation, medication) are more than worrying.

The same holds true for HPV tests, introduced in Europe some years ago. They are con-sidered and promoted as providing much more reliable and exact cancer check-ups. But the lack of an HP-virus proof alone makes these tests worthless. In addition to this these tests entail the significant risk of classifying even more women, who will most likely nev-er get a cervical tumor during their life, as "in danger" of getting cervical cancer—leading to even more needless operations and medications.

In this context let's not forget the fact that only around 0.1 percent of the women said to be infected with HPV fall ill with cervical cancer—so in consideration of this extremely low "frequency" it remains an enigma how established cancer authorities can speak at all of a high correlation between cancer and HPV.

Nobel laureate for Medicine Sir Frank Macfarlane Burnet warned us against jumping to any conclusions about a potential link between cancer and viruses back in 1971, in the book "Genes, Dreams and Realities":

"In the last dozen years there has been a great concentration of research on the viruses which can produce cancer or leukaemia of mice, hamsters, and chickens. There is no doubt at all about the genuinely malignant character of the tumours which are produced but so far there is no convincing evidence that any human tumour is virus-induced. One must be definite that despite ten years' intensive study the virus theory has established itself as nothing further than speculation. There may be almost a majority of younger cancer research men who think it likely that eventually cancer will be shown to be due to the action of 'slow viruses' which in the great majority of people persist without any visible effect. To me this is an unjustifiable and unscientific act of faith based on a failure to understand the significance of the work on viruses of laboratory animals.

My great objection to the hypothesis that any human cancer is a direct result of virus infection is my inability to conceive of a selective process in nature that could be equivalent to the laboratory procedure. Considering the extreme rarity of cancer in wild animals I can see no way by which an ability to induce cancer could favour the survival of a virus species. Neither can I see anything in human biology which could have power to evolve human cancer viruses; except by deliberate human effort directed to such an end. I believe we can forget about the possibility of any of the common forms of cancer being of virus origin."[1128]

HPV Vaccine: A Possible Disaster for the Next Generation

If we visualize the facts about HPV—no proof for virus detection; no proof for HPV's pathogenicity or for HPV being the primary, let alone single cause of cervical cancer; non-HPV causation omitted; only 0.1 percent of the so-called HPV-infected women coming down with cervical cancer—one must conclude that the vaccinations entering the market cannot be safe and effective.

All the worse that the US drug approval agency FDA appears to have learned nothing from recent catastrophic disasters due to the agency's approval of unsafe drugs—such as Merck's anti-inflammatory drug, Vioxx. The FDA hastily approved Merck's HPV vaccine "Gardasil" which is designed to prevent cervical cancer and genital warts in sexually active women. However, the vaccine has not been proven safe and effective in clinical trials, either. The trials are being criticized for using a placebo containing aluminum adjuvant (whose adverse reaction profile makes the vaccine appear safer than it is), rather than using a non-reactive saline solution placebo.

Here's how: the vaccine triggered adverse event reports in 90 percent of the test subjects within 15 days—hardly an indication of safety. However, the controversial placebo formula triggered 85 percent adverse event reports. How does the FDA know what long-term adverse effects the vaccine might produce?[1129] Even more so as Gardasil comes along with heavy side effects ranging from reddening and swelling around the injection site, fever, hives, arthritis,[1130] and even death.[1131]

It seems as if the medical establishment learned nothing from the disastrous DES (diethylstilbestrol) effects on the daughters of women who took the hormone during pregnancy triggering cancer and genital deformities.[1132] This is a particular concern because the HPV vaccine is being promoted for use in girls between 9 and 15 years of age. But the vaccine has never been tested for girls in this age group who are in a most sensitive phase of their development.

Vaccinating these girls and young women has to be called negligent. Not least because not even the minimum protecting antibody concentration is known, nor the duration of the protection of the vaccination nor the necessity of booster inoculations.[1133]

Sure, the DKFZ and other established cancer institutions never tire of saying that the vaccine's protective effect is 4 to 5 years,[1134] but this is nothing more than pure and unfounded speculation that benefits the marketing of a medical substance that is promising very high profits for the pharmaceutical giants making it.

National Vaccine Information Center president, Barbara Loe Fisher, says "Merck's pre and post-licensure marketing strategy has positioned mass use of this vaccine by pre-teens as a morality play in order to avoid talking about the flawed science they used to get it licensed. This is not just about teenagers having sex, it is also about whether Gardasil has been proven safe and effective for little girls."[1135]

Let's not forget that the idea of immune therapy for cancer is 100 years old. Paul Ehrlich already postulated that one can use immunity to fight against cancer. In the April 2005 issue of *Nature Medicine* a trial vaccine is described that for the first time ever is supposed to be able to extend the life expectancy of patients with prostate cancer.[1136] But Erhlich's trial and all other attempts to make a virus-disease out of whatever type of cancer was, are and always will be hopeless ventures.

The reason is as simple as it is evident: "The cancer cell does not contain new genetic material—but the immune system still only recognizes foreign material," as cancer researcher Peter Duesberg points out. "If mutated genes could activate the immune system, then we all would be long dead, because the immune system would kill cells daily en masse. In actuality, ordinary gene mutations are channeled through the body under the 'radar screen' of the immune system. The topic is often revived, but always it turns out to be a false alarm."[1137]

If HPV were the cause of cervical cancer, then it must be transferred also from the female partner to the male partner. But even if we assume that the HPV tests indeed measure HPV, it is still fact that HPV is practically not detectable in men, nor does it induce health problems in males. "This speaks strongly against an infectious cause of cervical cancer," says Vienna-based gynecologist Christian Fiala. "Furthermore, a PAP smear test being conducted badly in many cases results in a resection of uterine orifice tissue exactly where the tissue degenerations are. After the tissue is cut out, further degenerations are rarely observed. But if all this is caused by an infection, it couldn't be treated surgically."[1138]

When the science becomes politicized—whether from the conservative right or from the liberal left—we cannot trust anything that's being said. Absent scientific evidence demonstrating the safety of the HPV vaccine, there is no guarantee that this will not prove to be a disaster for the next generation.

"We can only conclude that we are in the era of post-evidence-based medicine," states Vera Sharav from the Alliance for Human Research Protection in New York. "Our public health policies are not even remotely evidence-based. Rather, our public health policies are faith-based decrees by government 'authorities'—no better than voodoo medicine."[1139]

Chapter 9

The Big Swine Flu Hoax

„The boards of health have been taken in by a campaign of the pharmaceutical companies that simply wanted to earn money with the supposed threat.“[1140]
Wolf-Dieter Ludwig, Medical professor and chairman of the drug commission of the German medical profession

„Early on the official sources declared that pregnant women were at a special risk as compared to the seasonal flu. As we shall see later, this was a grand lie. The Minister of Fear, the Centers for Disease Control and Prevention, was working overtime peddling doom and gloom, knowing that frightened people do not make rational decisions. Nothing sells vaccines like panic.“[1141]
Russell Blaylock, US neurosurgeon

„What experience and history teach us is that people and governments have never learned from history and never acted on lessons they should have learned from the past.“[1142]
Georg Wilhelm Friedrich Hegel, philosopher (1770-1831)

The Facts About Swine Flu

The topic of swine flu is complex. In order to make it easier to understand the details, here are the essentials in compact form about the great panic that spread through the world in the summer of 2009:[1143]

1. The so-called swine flu is a "normal" flu

Even according to official sources, the so-called swine flu was more harmless than normal virus flu that we experience every year. Severe cases usually only occured in regions where hunger and misery reign or in people already suffer from pre-existing conditions.

2. Arbitrary diagnoses

The diagnosis of the "swine flu" was based solely on laboratory tests that do not detect viruses, but rather certain protein and gene molecules, which are found in droves in every human being. That these molecules belong to viruses that cause illness was a—not proven—claim of the US epidemic authority CDC. With the help of these questionable laboratory tests, people with cold symptoms are arbitrarily labelled as swine flu death candidates and healthy people as "virus carriers."

3. Where one tests a lot, one also finds a lot

The epidemic hysteria was basically unavoidable, as it is the direct result of a "laboratory test epidemic" that is rampant worldwide: there is more testing going on than ever before.

4. "Letters of Indulgence" for the clueless people

The virologists behave like high priests who lead a campaign against imaginary demons and sell ineffective letters of indulgence in the form of Tamiflu and vaccines to the clueless people for a lavish fee (billions of taxpayers' money). Research results that do not serve the purpose of virus scaremongering are generally ignored, because that would harm careers, research funds and Nobel prizes—and of course the almost unbelievable turnovers of their financial backers.

5. (Alleged) pandemics are even more lucrative today than wars

The impact of the real beneficiaries of the pandemic panic-mongering—the pharmaceutical companies—on the world's leading US health authorities is grave. The manufacturers of antiviral drugs, vaccines and laboratory tests can expect additional global sales of tens of billions of euros. So the benefitting major shareholders can live quite well with a little pseudo-science and panic mongering—and without a conscience ...

6. Vaccines: Effectiveness not proven

The approval studies of the vaccines were designed from the outset in such a way that they do not require any statements to be made about actual protective effectiveness (i.e. no statement that vaccinated people have better health outcomes than unvaccinated people). Thus, the German admission board, the Paul-Ehrlich-Institute (PEI) acted like a marketing branch of the manufacturers.

7. Warning for pregnant women: Miscarriages are to be expected

The pandemic vaccines stimulate antibody formation as well as the so-called "cellular immunity". This can have fatal consequences for the pregnancy, because "cellular immunity" is normally shut down by the maternal immune system during pregnancy in order to shield the unborn life.

8. Secrecy without end

At the beginning of May 2009, the WHO leadership decided on camera, that a wave of influenza with a "severe course" was no longer necessary to declare the highest pandemic level. In other words, the overwhelming majority of patients suffered only mild symptoms and the number of deaths was low worldwide—hence, there was no sign of a real pandemic, yet the highest pandemic level had been declared. A contradiction in terms. But the reason for this becomes clear when you consider that this trick created the legal precedent for the use of pandemic sample vaccines. No one knows exactly which substances are contained in these vaccines and in what quantities.

Virus Proof Is Also Lacking in Swine Flu

It is hard to believe, but for decades one virus panic after another has run rampant through the world—from HIV/AIDS to hepatitis C and SARS to avian flu (H5N1)—and the global community has been taken in by the virus hunters again and again. In 2009, the so-called swine flu virus was turned into a monster threatening humanity. Once again, the mainstream media that dictated the public debate largely parroted whatever the corrupted medical authorities told them.

Although the evidence on swine flu was extremely thin, the greed of the pharmaceutical companies for profit was enormous. Reason enough, therefore, to become sceptical from the bottom up.

The very first question that should have been asked in the case of swine flu was: Is the detection of the swine flu virus plausible and scientifically validated? If the journalists had addressed this question, they would have quickly realized that considerable doubts are justified as to whether this actually happened (just like with HIV and also with the so-called bird flu virus H5N1).

It is true that the German Federal Government's information flyers titled "What you need to know about the new flu ('swine flu')" and "Vaccination against the new flu ('swine flu')" show photos in which an "electron microscope image of the new influenza virus A (H1N1)" is supposed to be depicted. However, the photo showing particles that are purported to represent swine flu viruses does not name a source and even the Robert Koch Institute (RKI) was not able to find out who took the photo and in which scientific publication it appeared.

In this respect, the claim of the RKI that the photographs depict an "evil" swine flu virus[1144] is scientifically extremely questionable, not to say groundless.

So what are these particles if they are not externally invading and disease-causing influenza viruses? In 2007, for example, *the Biochemical Journal* described how these particles are artificially produced:[1145] it simply involves the killing of chicken embryos or cell cultures. In effect, these cells are killed in order to extract proteins that cause red blood cells to clump together. These proteins, called hemagglutinins, are then claimed to come from viruses without any further scientific proof.

In addition, all human and animal cells contain enzymes, including neuraminidases whose functions have yet to be fully elucidated. They have important intra and extra-cellular signalling roles and are proposed to have a major role in immune function. They are linked to regulation of cholesterol metabolism, and have been implicated in diseases such as diabetes and cancer.

These enzymes are produced and released in greater quantities when cells are destroyed (e.g. by means of adjuvants in vaccines or other stress factors such as pesticides or heavy metals). But neuraminidase activity is frequently passed off as the result of fictitious viruses that allegedly use these enzymes to multiply.

These hemagglutinins and neuraminidases are used to give the viruses their names. The "H" always stands for hemagglutinin, the "N" for neuraminidase, whereby, for example, the "H1" of H1N1 or the "H5" of H5N1 always stands for a particular type of hemagglutinin. But once again: It has not been scientifically proven and seems unlikely that these hemagglutinins and neuraminidases can be assigned specifically to viruses that cause disease.

Nevertheless, detection of these particles are asserted as proof of an evil virus. It is then proclaimed to be absolutely necessary to block the neuraminidase enzymes to prevent the virus from spreading in the body. To do this, people are offered drugs such as Tamiflu (which was infamously connected to the bird flu panic) or Relenza. However, neuramin-idase inhibitors can have serious complications including anaphylaxis, toxic epidermal necrolysis (with potential sepsis and multi-organ failure) and even death. The dead are then referred to as victims of the alleged virus ...

Big Business Swine Flu:
How the US „Pandemic Agency" Fooled the World

That this could go so far was mainly due to the omnipotence of the American Centers for Disease Control and Prevention, or CDC for short. The agency had already been threat-ened to become superfluous twice in its history: after World War II and again at the end of the 1970s.

But both times it managed to pull itself up by its own bootstraps. By the end of the 1970s, the agency was able to overcome the crisis through its promotion of HIV/AIDS on the world stage. Now, it seems to be able to do whatever it wants—its word is always consid-ered to be the word of God, without enough critical questioning by any other institution.

The World Health Organization (WHO) apparently also trusts the holy word of the CDC. At the end of April 2009, the WHO made its first statement and, quite surprisingly, an-nounced that the CDC had completely decoded the genome of the swine flu virus. Such a statement is precarious not least because it goes against scientific etiquette to publish such momentous statements without it first being published in a renowned journal. Only through such a "peer reviewed" publication would other scientists, journalists, institutes, etc. have had the opportunity to verify the statement that the swine flu virus had been fully proven in its entirety.

It should be noted that in other scientific fields, careful examination and confirmation by other institutes is a common procedure. For example, the official recognition of the new element "Coopernicium" discovered in 1996 at an institute in Darmstadt took a whole 13 years.[1146] Scientific confirmation of newly discovered viruses, however, is obviously not considered necessary by the WHO, ostensibly the highest health authority on our planet. The word of the CDC is enough.

The American CDC seems to enjoy the complete privilege of fools—and even the WHO is dancing to its piping. Yet the CDC in reality is anything but a trustworthy source, as has been pointed out several times in this book. And the swine flu panic-mongering was an eloquent testimony to the fact that one should by no means blindly trust what the CDC says if one wants to get to the facts.

For example, on the 18th of October 2009, in one of the rare at least somewhat critical media reports on swine flu, the American television show *60 Minutes* led the CDC to say that the swine flu vaccine was similar to other flu vaccines and therefore "safe." But such a statement is outrageous because the swine flu vaccine was only tested for a few weeks— which is definitely too short to conclude that the vaccine was "safe."

In addition, CDC officials warned elsewhere that the swine flu virus is so dangerous precisely because it is so different from other influenza viruses. To be immune from an impending deadly pandemic, the CDC said it was imperative that the world had to be vaccinated. But if the swine flu virus is so different from other influenza viruses, then the swine flu vaccine must also be different from other vaccines. So please, dear CDC: Is the swine flu virus very similar to other flu viruses or not? You can't have it both ways.

But that is not all: another central statement from the CDC is scientifically simply not tenable, if not a lie. In the fall of 2009, the CDC announced on its website that the flu was becoming increasingly widespread and that "so far most flu viruses are of the H1N1 type (sometimes also called swine flu virus)."[1147] But this statement is not true even if one does not want to give up the belief that a pathogenic so-called swine flu virus actually exists.

Indeed, the American TV station *CBS News* researched the story for months and then reported in another rare critical media report on swine flu that H1N1 was in reality not nearly as widespread as institutions like the CDC claim. "If you've been diagnosed 'probable' or 'presumed' 2009 H1N1 or 'swine flu' in recent months, you may be surprised to know this: odds are you didn't have H1N1 flu," reported *CBS News* journalist Sharyl Attkisson. "In fact, you probably didn't have flu at all."[1148]

Additionally, *CBS News* found out that in July 2009, the CDC advised states to stop testing for H1N1. They also stopped counting patients who tested „positive" for H1N1 from that date. The reason for the DCD's new instructions was, according to *CBS News*, that the authorities felt it was a waste of resources to continue testing for H1N1 and counting the cases, allegedly because it was already proven that swine flu was an epidemic.

But this was an outright lie, because in fact the predicted major epidemic (pandemic) did not break out even many months later. The death rate of those counted as swine flu victims by the authorities rose from just 1,274 to 3,406 cases in the USA between August and October 2009. In Europe, the number of people officially dying of swine flu even rose from just 53 to only 207 cases. And on a global scale, the number of cases only rose from 1,462 to 4,735 between August and October 2009. This meant that by October 2009, less than 0.2 percent of those affected had died worldwide.

In Germany, only two deaths were reported by that time and it should be noted that these two people were suffering from serious underlying diseases. This means that in Germany, as well, far fewer people had died than predicted (because with assumed mortality rates of 0.1 to 0.6 percent of the suspected cases, not only two, but between 23 and 138 people should have died).[1149]

Even if every single death is a tragic fate in itself, with such a low number of cases, it is certainly not possible to speak of an epidemic, let alone a pandemic.[1150]

In any case, once the CDC had instructed testing for H1N1 to stop, the consequence was that the diagnosis of swine flu could and was made completely arbitrarily. Virtually every person who came into a doctor's office with flu-like symptoms was now assumed to have swine flu. This opened the door to manipulation.

Conflicts of Interest and Greed for Profit
Also Dominate Swine Flu Research

In this book, we have already documented how frequently conflicts of interest in the medical industry exist. Nevertheless, we would like to briefly go into this subject again, because it is of central importance, especially for the swine flu insanity.

The term "insanity" may sound forceful to some people, but when you bring to mind that the people who manufacture and distribute the vaccines are ultimately the same people who test the vaccines for safety and efficacy, then one can only speak of insanity.

For example, Paul A. Offit, chief physician at the Children's Hospital of Philadelphia, is said to have earned at least $29 million when the hospital sold its license for the rotavirus vaccine Rotateq of Merck for $182 million. Furthermore Offit sat on an advisory committee of the U.S. Food and Drug Administration (in the Advisory Committee on Immunization Practices ACIP) to help build a market for Rotateq[1151] (regarding Paul A. Offit, see also chapter 8).

In August 1999, the U.S. government reviewed its vaccine policy. The review revealed that many of the same people who were active in committees discussing vaccine approval and recommendation, also had financial ties to pharmaceutical companies that produced vaccines. In fact, the law requires that such conflicts of interest be disclosed and that people with such close ties to the vaccine industry are not allowed to participate in such discussions and decisions.

It also came to light that three out of five members of the FDA panel that approved the rotavirus vaccine in 1997 were financially linked to the companies that produced different versions of the vaccine. Just one year after approval, the rotavirus vaccine was withdrawn from the market after it had been found to have caused serious side effects.[1152]

The independence of the regulatory authorities in other countries was just as pitiful. In Germany, for example, at the Permanent Vaccination Commission STIKO, which is affiliated to the Robert Koch-Institute, "the existing mechanisms to ensure their independence are obviously not sufficient", as Angela Spelsberg, physician, epidemiologist and at the time board member of the anti-corruption organization Transparency International, wrote in the German journal *Blätter für deutsche und internationale Politik* at the end of 2009.

This applies in particular to the conflicts of interest of STIKO members. "In order to change this, the minutes of the meetings and the decisions taken, but above all their reasons, must be published as a matter of principle," said Spelsberg.

Since August 2008 the members of STIKO have been disclosing their potential conflicts of interest on the STIKO website after years of pressure from Transparency International Germany. "The information from March 2009 shows that the majority of the 16 members have more or less intensive contacts with the most important vaccine manufacturers." as Spelsberg noted. "Individual members also conduct vaccination studies or work in close cooperation with vaccine manufacturers."

It can also be read there that some of the STIKO members are committed to the "Forum Impfen" (vaccination forum), which in turn enjoys financial support from the company Sanofi-Pasteur-MSD, among others. "The website of the 'Forum Impfen' unfortunately gives no indication of the financial amount of this support", complained Spelsberg.[1153]

At the end of 2009, it also came forth that Walter Haas, coordinator of the influenza expert group at the state-run Robert Koch-Institute (RKI), was a scientific advisor to the European Scientific Working Group on Influenza (ESWI). ESWI is an association financed exclusively by the pharmaceutical industry. A total of ten pharmaceutical companies supported the ESWI. Among them were GlaxoSmithKline, manufacturer of the German swine flu vaccine Pandemrix, and the Swiss Roche Group, which produces the antiviral drug Tamiflu.

The ESWI website also featured a promotional film by Tamiflu producer Roche. An ESWI spokesperson told the news magazine *Der Spiegel* that they were proud to have won a "top-class institution" such as the RKI and Walter Haas as a free consultant. Angela Spelsberg, on the other hand, complained that the RKI was operating in a grey area, both ethically and legally: "It is unacceptable that an office holder who is supposed to serve the welfare of the population alone is so closely connected to a lobbying association."[1154]

Professor of medicine Reinhard Kurth, who headed the RKI from 1996 to 2008 and immediately afterward was appointed chairman of the Schering Foundation's board, also casts a dark shadow on the RKI. At first glance, Kurth's move to the Ernst Schering Foundation may look at least slightly better than, for example, the move of Kurth's former colleague Heinz-J. Schmitt.

After his retirement as chairman of STIKO in 2007, Schmitt switched to Novartis, one of the world's largest vaccine companies, to take on a leading position in the vaccine field. But

Kurth's move to the Ernst Schering Foundation is piquant when one considers that this foundation, which promotes young scientists, is also likely to favor the welfare of the pharmaceutical company Schering and its investors—rather than the welfare of the general public.

This is also supported by the fact that the Schering pharmaceutical group has been part of the Bayer Group since the end of 2006. And the latter acts remarkably unscrupulously on the world market when it comes to its own interests.[1155]

Incidentally, a look at the history of the RKI is not very refreshing. Not only was Robert Koch himself involved in science fraud (see beginning of chapter 2), but according to a comprehensive investigative report published in 2008, the RKI was heavily involved in the National Socialist policies of violence. It had a central position in the state health administration and was also part of the Reich Health Office between 1935 and 1942. Further, just three months after the National Socialists seized power in January 1933, there were a wave of redundancies at the RKI, during which the entire central structure of the institute had been replaced. Later, the director of the RKI and almost all department heads were in the NSDAP (National Socialist German Workers' Party).

It's particularly sad for contemporary researchers to also see the lack of moral courage of their predecessors. No evidence of protest was found in the files, nor was it only a few individual scientists who had crossed moral boundaries. These themes were still present in the 1991 commemorative publication on the 100th anniversary of the founding of the institute, but at least the RKI conceded that revision was required. Indeed, it is said that these problems were much worse at the RKI compared to many other institutions. According to historians, among other things, physicians had a disproportionately high affinity to National Socialism than other professional groups.[1156]

Whoever looks back onto such a dark history should be inspired to do everything possible today to advocate the truth. From a scientific point of view, however, this cannot be said in regard to the behavior of the RKI with regard to topics such as the so-called swine flu.

In the case of the swine flu, the approval of the vaccine was ultimately granted by the European approval authority EMEA, whose work was extremely critically observed by Transparency International Germany. It is highly problematic that the EMEA reports to the Directorate-General for Economic Affairs of the European Commission and not to the Directorate-General for Health and Consumer Protection. It is equally alarming that almost two thirds of its work is financed by the pharmaceutical industry—and that the review of the approval documents by external scientists is only possible after the vaccine has been approved.

There was also a blatant conflict of interest case in the UK. As early as the 1st of May 2009, Professor Sir Roy Anderson declared: "Now we have a swine flu pandemic." When Anderson told this outright lie (at no time did a swine flu pandemic even come close to occurring), there never was a , he was not only a British government advisor, rector of Imperial College London and member of the British Scientific Advisory Council for Emergencies (SAGE), which developed the pandemic plan for Britain—Anderson was also a highly paid board member of the vaccine manufacturer GlaxoSmithKline.[1157]

The swine flu hysteria brought the British pharmaceutical company a gigantic shower of money—mainly thanks to the active support of the state authorities. The German government alone ordered 50 million doses of the swine flu vaccine Pandemrix from GlaxoSmith-Kline in Dresden. Value of the deal: €700 million. Worldwide, the pharmaceutical giant sold as many as 440 million doses within a short time and thus gained billions in turnover.[1158]

Shortly after the announcement of the (never occurred) "swine flu pandemic," the value of Glaxo shares rose by an impressive 10 percent, while quarterly profits swelled to €2.4 billion in the third quarter of 2009. A further €2.3 billion profit was expected in the fourth quarter, when the "swine flu vaccine" was delivered.[1159]

Despite the size of the contract that the German government awarded to GlaxoSmith-Kline, the associated terms and conditions were not made publicly available. This ob-scured the conflicts of interest of those who negotiated the deal.[1160]

The obvious assumption that the authorities were "bought" by the pharmaceutical com-pany is further substantiated by the fact that "the federal states jointly and severally dispensed GlaxoSmithKline from claims for damages," as reported by the pharma critical journal *arzneitelegramm*.[1161] [1162]

Such a far-reaching concession cannot be plausibly explained as legitimate. In fact, it has all the appearances of the government being a puppet of the pharmaceutical industry while putting on an act for the public. (Something that was to repeat in 2020 on a grand scale with COVID-19.)

The price of €18 per double vaccine plus twice €5 (for each vaccination) for a total of €28 was much higher than the price of the usual flu vaccination, which was about €14 based on the selling price from the manufacturer. "Withal the large-scale order is extremely cost-saving for the supplier," as Angela Spelsberg remarks. Not least because the state purchase guarantee eliminates the otherwise usual costs for sales promotion.

The new alleged "pandemics" can thus be described as a safe business model for the manu-facturers—and it seems to become more and more lucrative. The other development pipe-lines of the corporations are threateningly empty, new blockbuster drugs are hardly in sight and patents for medications, with which huge profits were once made have expired thus allowing cheap imitation preparations (generics) onto the market. vaccines are no longer a niche business and now represent a kind of savior for threatened balance sheets.

No wonder that more and more pharmaceutical companies are seeking their salvation in the vaccine market. At the beginning of 2009, the US pharmaceutical company Pfizer absorbed the vaccine producer Wyeth. A few months later, three other pharmaceutical giants—Abbott Laboratories, Johnson & Johnson and Merck—announced their intention to buy shares or rights in vaccine manufacturers. By the end of 2009, analysts predicted an annual growth rate of 18 percent for the vaccine industry, compared to 4.4 percent for the pharmaceutical industry as a whole.[1163]

The times in which it was not possible to earn more than "a few tired marks" with a vacci-nation are apparently finally over. Proof of this can also be seen with the cervical cancer vaccination, which should be viewed just as critically as the swine flu vaccination[1164]— and it similarly devours vast amounts of taxpayers' money. In Germany, a single vaccina-tion initially cost more than a whopping €150.[1165] It makes one wonder if what actually threatens humanity is unscrupulous profit seeking through rinse-and-repeat panic-mon-gering "epidemics" in the style of HIV/AIDS, BSE, SARS, bird flu and swine flu (on cervical cancer, see chapter 8).

"This could happen again every year unless stop-rules are introduced as soon as possi-ble to give the all-clear for suspected but harmless pandemics—and unless public decision-making processes are controlled and contractual agreements between vaccine manufacturers and the government are disclosed", said Spelsberg. "Health resources of such a magnitude, which are urgently needed elsewhere, must not simply be distributed behind closed doors in the future. Non-transparency and potential conflicts of interest undermine the credibility of the responsible recommending and regulatory authorities. Furthermore, in the current case, they are feeding the suspicion that the H1N1 flu wave, as a swine flu pandemic, was deliberately used by the pharmaceutical industry for marketing purposes. A thorough investigation of the events by an investigation committee is therefore urgently indicated."[1166]

Unfortunately, however, no such investigation was carried out. Perhaps then it was not surprising that in 2020, with the worldwide "lockdown" and Corona/COVID-19 panic campaign in full swing, Spelsberg's fears played out on a gigantic scale (on corona, see chapter 12).

What happened instead of a complete reappraisal of the scandalous events? The authorities came up with the most abstruse proposals, which can only be explained by the fact that the people responsible were totally blinded or acting with the absolute will to deceive.

For example, children in the pre-schools and primary schools in Le Guilvinec in French Brittany were in all seriousness no longer allowed to greet each other with the traditional kiss. This was an actual decree issued by the mayor. Shaking hands was also forbidden. Instead, the little ones should rise "like Native Americans" to greet.

According to islacanaria.net, doctors in Madrid, the capital of neighbouring Spain, have put up a banner with advice like "No kissing, no handshakes—just say hola!" And in Germany they also thought about a ban on kissing. For example, Minister Karl-Josef Laumann, then Minister of Health in the state of North Rhine-Westphalia, sent a written declaration to all school principals at the begining of school in late summer 2009. This stated: "Since the new flu is highly contagious, welcoming rituals such as shaking hands, hugs or kisses should be avoided."[1167]

Even the carnival revellers were supposed to start the carnival on the 11th of November at 11.11 a.m. according to the motto "Bützen* ja—Knutschen nicht!" ("Bützen yes, but

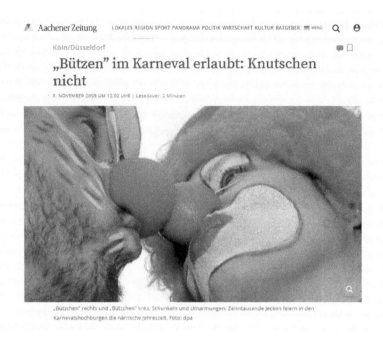

During the "swine flu" panic-mongering there were foreshadowings of what was to come, with the contact bans that were issued in 2020 in connection with Corona/COVID-19. At the end of 2009, various media outlets ran headlines such as „Bützen' allowed in carnival: smooching not" („bützen" means to kiss with a pointed mouth). At the time, Düsseldorf carnival revellers mischievously replied that the fear of bad weather was greater than that of swine flu. Source: Screenshot from aachener-zeitung.de

not smoochingl!"; "bützen" means to kiss with a pointed mouth, see screenshot from aachener-zeitung.de).

"Nobody has to skip carnival. But whoever goes out to celebrate must know that he can come very close to swine flu — especially if he behaves accordingly", warned Klaus-Peter Brenner from the Cologne health authority in all seriousness . "For example, if I kiss all the people there, I open the door to the virus." And the director of the Institute of Virology at the University Hospital of Cologne, Herbert Pfister, added in all seriousness that one "would actually be well advised to avoid such mass events [like carnival] in these times." At least at risk groups such as chronically ill people or pregnant women should not throw themselves into the thick of the hustle and bustle, he advised.[1168] Obviously, virus research and what doctors, officials and journalists often unilaterally present to the public without debate has degenerated into foolishness, if not downright malevolence.

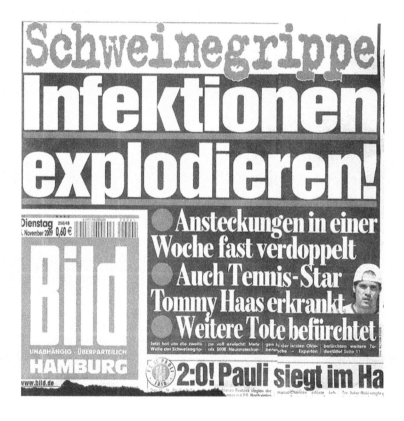

On 3rd November 2009, Germany's leading tabloid newspaper Bild *came up with the headline "Swine flu: Infections explode! ... even tennis star Thommy Haas falls ill." That could make you afraid if you did not know how absurd the headline is. It cannot be repeated often enough: It has never been proven that even a single person who has been classified as a victim of the so-called swine flu actually died from the so-called swine flu virus.*

The Media Disregards the Patients' Lifestyle Factors and Pre-Existing Illnesses

In the case of swine flu most of the mainstream media acted as a voice for the vaccine manufacturers and readily conveyed their propaganda to millions of readers. Tabloid media outlets such as the German newspaper *Bild-Zeitung* did not consider themselves above spreading inaccurate assessments in a sensationalistic manner and thus added a lot of fuel to the swine flu fire of panic (see two *Bild* headlines). However, it was not only the sensationalism that was once again deplorable—as was previously the case with HIV/AIDS, BSE,

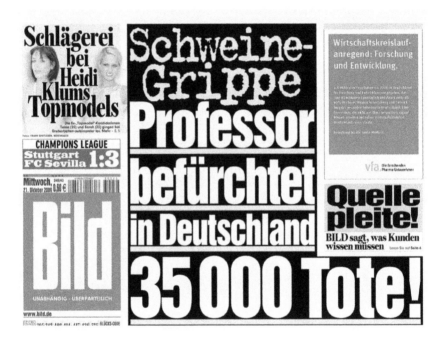

On the 21st of October 2009, Germany's daily newspaper Bild throws a horror headline at its readers. Soon there could be 35,000 swine flu deaths in Germany—an outrageous claim, as that until then there had officially been just two fatalities. Moreover, there is no proof that these poor people really died of the swine flu virus. Not only did those who died have serious pre-existing conditions, but what is called as the swine flu virus has never been proven to be a disease-causing virus.

SARS and bird flu—but also that important factors were simply ignored. The discussion of these factors could have made a decisive contribution to obtaining a much more realistic picture of what really happened to the poor people who were labelled as swine flu victims.

Even if one assumes that there was a pathogenic swine flu virus, around 99.9 percent of people who were diagnosed with the (never-proven) H1N1 infection by means of (highly questionable) tests still did not suffer any complications as a result. But this should not be surprising, no matter how critically or uncritically one looks at virus research. For example, even Luc Montagnier, who is celebrated as the discoverer of HIV, stated in an interview with the Canadian filmmaker Brent Leung that one can easily cope with HIV if the immune system is strengthened by a healthy lifestyle with a nutrient-rich diet.[1169] And as HIV is pretty much considered to be one of the deadliest viruses in human history—one suspects it should be easy for a person with a robust immune system to eliminate the wickedly depicted swine flu virus.

Among the simple measures that you can take to strengthen your immune system are:

- Ensure an adequate supply of vitamin D. If this is not possible (which is the case in sunless regions, especially in the winter months and for those with darker skin), you should also consider using vitamin D supplements to correct potential vitamin D deficiency. Vitamin D is a widely underestimated substance that plays a crucial role in maintaining our health and strengthening our immune system.[1170] [1171]

- Ensure a diet rich in fiber, bases and vital substances with many active enzymes, vitamins, minerals and trace elements—and if possible without toxins (pesticides).

- Eliminate or reduce processed and nutrient-poor "foods" such as refined sugar from your diet. They are robbers of vital substances and burden your immune system.

- Try as much as possible to avoid negative stress and at the same time strive for fulfilling experiences. Exercise or sport is essential for this balance. Sauna sessions, massages and evening basic baths also provide deep relaxation and promote detoxification.

- Measures providing extra support for the immune system include glutathione administration or intravenously administered nutrient and base infusions if indicated.

However, there is practically no mention about any of these measures in the media in connection with swine flu. This is a serious omission. An eloquent example of this

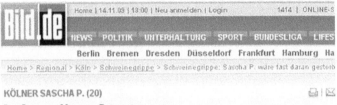

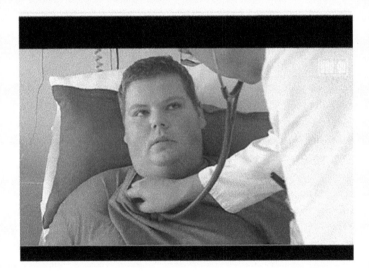

On the 16th of October 2009 Bild.de headlined the (groundless) claim of 20-year-old Sascha P. from Cologne: "I almost died of swine flu."

tunnel vision and blindness by the media is a report in the *Bild* newspaper on the 16th of October 2009 about 20-year-old Sascha P., who, the tabloid was certain, "almost died of swine flu" (see screenshot from the website of Germany' leading tabloid newspaper *Bild*).[1172] "While celebrating at the Ballermann [on Mallorca] Sascha P. caught the H1N1 virus, which almost killed him", *Bild* described the story of suffering with dramatic and moving words. "Lung failure, artificial coma, tracheotomy, 21 days intensive care. Even the doctors had little hope. Now he is healthy again. 'I have been granted a second life', says Sasha." These are exactly the kind of heartbreaking reports that the media likes to give to their millions of readers in order to amplify their circulation and ratings.

Unfortunately, the facts are cast aside all too quickly in these stories. Unproven assertions are sold as facts, because the main point is to stir up the audience emotionally. *Bild* could have easily recognized or should have recognized that even if one considers the "evil" swine flu virus to be real, there are other possible causes for the collapse of Sascha P. Indeed, the tabloid writes about the circumstances leading up to the 20-year-old's collapse in its own article:

"Flashback: On September 14th [2009], Sasha returns from Mallorca with a high fever, aching limbs and a severe cough. Five days later he is admitted to hospital. By then the virus had already attacked his lungs. The doctors put him in an artificial coma. Without artificial respiration he would have died instantly." Alternatively, did a young man have a long party on the Spanish Island of Mallorca and drink himself into a delirium, perhaps for several days? It is well understood that such binge drinking can lead to circulatory collapse and other complications.

Bild should have at least clarified whether Sascha P. was in fact a victim of a substance induced coma and its subsequent course. Just to claim that "the virus had already attacked Sascha's lungs" without being able to present a speck of hard evidence is dubious to say the least.

"Form (*Bild*) your own opinion"– is the slogan with which the tabloid advertises itself. But how can you seriously form a well-founded opinion when the information you are presented with is completely one-sided and unsubstantiated?

Incidentally, *Bild* should also have paid attention to something that was hard to overlook: that Sascha P. suffered from obesity. And "one of the most prominent risk factors for being admitted to the ICU and for dying was obesity", says American physician Russell Blaylock. "Obese people were admitted six times more often to the hospital than those of normal weight. Obesity played a significant role in the risk to children and pregnant women as well, something that has never been discussed by the media, the CDC or the public health officials."[1173] This is all the more incomprehensible when one considers that obesity has been shown to be a risk factor for all sorts of diseases—even for such serious conditions as diabetes[1174] and cancer.[1175] Additionally, a study published

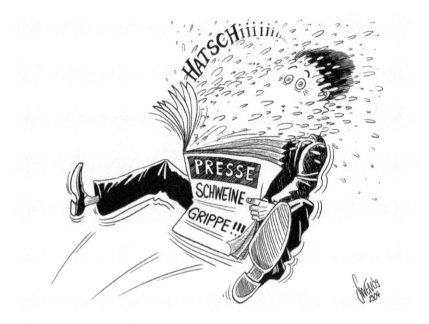

© Silvan Wegmann, www.swen.ch

in the *New England Journal of Medicine* at the end of 2009 showed that obesity increased the risk of contracting secondary diseases among those who were classified as having swine flu.[1176]

It is precisely the fact that those affected usually suffered from obesity and/or other serious underlying diseases that makes it seem so bizaare that the media almost always focused on the nasty swine flu virus. Thus, by the beginning of November, at least five of the six people who were supposed to have officially died of swine flu in Germany actually had chronic pre-existing conditions. Only in one case there had been contradictory statements as to whether a 48-year-old woman from the Rhein-Sieg district suffered from asthma and liver disease or died solely as a result of the H1N1 infection.[1177]

Adjuvants in Vaccinations:
Attack on the Immune System

Despite all the facts described, anyone who still believes that vaccines are a panacea should perhaps remind themselves that it was not the mass vaccinations that succeeded in significantly reducing the incidence of so-called infectious diseases such as tuberculosis, diphtheria, polio, etc. Rather, it was from improved living conditions, such as getting adequate nutrition and enhanced sanitation that were responsible for this. We have outlined this at various points in this book (see also Chapter 11 on measles).

It is also worth remembering the swine flu panic-mongering in the mid-1970s in the USA, which ended in a vaccination disaster—just as it would be with the swine flu panic-mongering in 2009. As described earlier in this book, around 50 million U.S. citizens panicked at the behest of the medical establishment and lined up to be injected with a vaccine that had been hurriedly thrown onto the market. 20 to 40 percent of those vaccinated in good faith developed severe side effects, including paralysis and even death. The resulting claims for damages from this disastrous public health campaign ultimately amounted to $2.7 billion.

An issue that continues to this day is that it is not really known what is contained in the vaccines. Because the manufacturers secretly changed the formulation of the pandemic sample vaccines, ultimately only the manufacturers and regulatory authorities know these classified recipes. This is a scandal in itself and another clear indication of corruption in the health system. After all, we taxpayers have paid for the vaccines, so we should be allowed to know what ingredients they were brewed with.

"Instead of a maximum of 5 micrograms of mercury-containing thiomersal, as stated in the technical information of the sample vaccines, according to the Paul-Ehrlich-Institute, PEI [the German regulatory authority], now suddenly up to 25 micrograms are contained, i.e. five times as much," as Hans Tolzin, editor of the pharma critical journal *impf-report* (*vaccination report*) critically notes. "The PEI press officer, who had the misfortune to take my call, was not allowed to tell me whether any other ingredients had been changed, and I have still not received the desired confirmation by email from him to this day".[1178]

The mercury-containing preservative thiomersal (see also the article "Deadly Immunity" by Robert F. Kennedy Jr. in this book) is not the only additive or booster—called "adjuvant" in technical jargon—that is known to have been included in the swine flu vaccines offered. Mercury is certainly the most alarming ingredient, since the heavy metal is the strongest non-radioactive poison known. Aluminium, a cell and nerve poison, was also an ingredient, as was formaldehyde which can have genetically modifying and subsequent carcinogenic effects. Furthermore, polysorbate 80 was in the mix which has caused infertility and abortions in animal experiments.[1179] [1180]

Another questionable additive is squalene—not least for reasons of animal welfare. Squalene is obtained from sharks, of which some species are endangered. As a natural substance, squalene is also contained in olive oil and when taken orally it is usually well tolerated of course. However, if squalene is injected subcutaneously (under the skin) or intramuscularly (into the muscle), which is more unnatural, it can become an inflammation-promoting and immune-activating antigen/allergen, which provokes the formation of corresponding antibodies and can also result in the development of autoimmune diseases.[1181]

In animal experiments, squalene has caused the clinically apparent picture of arthritis (inflammatory joint disease)."[1182] [1183] Of course there are also positive studies on squalene", says Jürgen Seefeldt, a physician from Paderborn. "But almost without exception it is the vaccine manufacturers who report positive results from their tests." The swine flu vaccine Pandemrix, which was administered to the German population, contained squalene in the form of artificially produced nanoparticles (which in themselves can have cell-damaging effects[1184]) and acts as a so-called adjuvant.

In addition, it's important to understand that a vaccine can only be approved with an adequate so-called vaccination titer level. A vaccination titer is used by the medical establishment as a measure of the body's "immunity" to a certain disease after a previous vaccination. The concentration of antibodies present in the blood following the vaccination is determined. If many antibodies are now found in the blood, it is assumed that the antigen contained in the vaccine (the alleged virus) has triggered this antibody reaction.

However, this is pure speculation and has not been proven at all. According to the "Imp-fkompendium", the most important German standard reference work on vaccinations,[1185] most vaccines don't induce adequate titers without adjuvants (such as mercury and form-

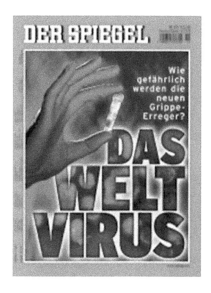

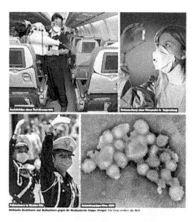

On May 4th , 2009, the German newsmagazine Der Spiegel *declared the so-called swine flu virus a "world virus" in its cover story (see left depiction). However, as with SARS (2002/2003) or the "avian flu" (2004-2006) the super epidemic with countless deaths, which was conjured up by media, never eventuated. The article of the* Spiegel's *cover story had the headline "Attack from the Realm of Shades" (see right depiction), which conveyed the completely unfounded message that the "swine flu virus" was as dangerous for the earth's population as if it was a creature from the underworld. Source: Screenshots from* spiegel.de

aldehyde). The raised titer is probably an immune reaction to the numerous toxins and chemicals present in vaccinations. "So far, neither the PEI nor the RKI, the federal Disease Control Center in Germany, have been able to provide me with scientific evidence that a high titer is a guarantee of no disease", says Hans Tolzin.[1186] In addition, assuming the vaccine could actually "protect" individuals against a pandemic virus, there would still be no meaningful benefit. Even official authorities had to eventually admit that the swine flu in Germany was even milder than a normal flu – which is usually overcome after a few days. The presumed benefit (or probable lack of benefit) of the vaccine was therefore outweighed by the risk of adverse events.

Indeed by August 2009, a few months after the WHO announced the pandemic, reports of suspected vaccine related serious side effects started appearing, including paralysis and death (see also last section in this chapter).[1187]

Of course one must not appear to judge these vaccines too prematurely. In order to realistically assess the amount of "collateral damage" caused by the vaccination, an open-ended comparison of vaccinated and unvaccinated persons (in the form of a

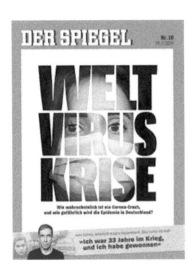
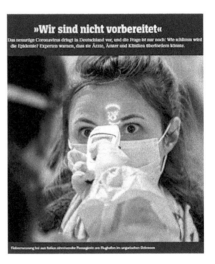

On May 4ᵗʰ, 2009, the German newsmagazine Der Spiegel declared the so-called swine flu virus a "world virus" in its cover story (see left depiction). However, as with SARS (2002/2003) or the "avian flu" (2004-2006) the super epidemic with countless deaths, which was conjured up by media, never eventuated. The article of the Spiegel's cover story had the headline "Attack from the Realm of Shades" (see right depiction), which conveyed the completely unfounded message that the "swine flu virus" was as dangerous for the earth's population as if it was a creature from the underworld. Source: Screenshots from spiegel.de

placebo group) is ultimately required. Such comparative studies, which are basically the only way to estimate health benefits and risks, do not exist—allegedly for ethical reasons.

The appropriate course of action would be to get rid of the antibody titer and measure the actual response of the cellular immune system to the vaccination. But this does not happen, which is tragic because the vaccine titer, the highest criterion for the approval of a vaccination, is so questionable. Not only because there is no immune reaction without "adjuvants" in the vaccines, but also because the antibody reaction has very little to do with the defense against viruses.

"However, this has only been known since the mid-1990s", says the science journalist Michael Leitner. "That is why, in the time before that, people had tried to add something to vaccinations that caused an antibody reaction. And this was only possible by adding metal compounds such as the supposedly 'proven aluminium hydroxide'."[1188]

The immune system is much more complex than most people think, in fact in reality nobody could claim to fully understand it. In any case, pressing it into a simple antigen-antibody model, as the vaccine advocates still like to do, is an over simplification and assumes that the antibodies will react to "evil" viruses.

The situation in the USA also reveals the reservations about the use of novel adjuvants in vaccines. By the end of 2009, not a single vaccine with a novel adjuvant has been approved there by the end of 2009. "The US drug approval agency FDA considers the danger of excessive reactions to be too great," wrote *The Spiegel* in October 2009.[1189]

Judges Confirm: Swine Flu Vaccine Causes Narcolepsy

In the 6th edition of the German version of this book, which was published in 2009, this section was still titled "Especially children and pregnant women should not be vaccinated." However, others like journalist Daniel Schlicht, had quite a different opinion at that time. Mr. Schlicht's article on swine flu, which appeared on the 30th of July 2009 on *www.zeit.de*, was more of an authoritarian pharmaceutical instruction: "Everyone who can, should go vaccinate himself."

313

Shortly afterwards, it was made clear to the general public just how irresponsible this directive was. Only one year later, in 2010, the Swedish Agency for the Regulation of Prescription Drugs started reporting cases of narcolepsy in children and adolescents following swine flu vaccination. Narcolepsy is a long term neurological disorder that leads to a disturbance of the circadian rhythm and often excessive daytime sleepiness. Further analysis confirmed that the Pandemrix vaccine had also caused narcolepsy in vaccinated people in other countries.

The victims' families then began to demand compensation, which was met with fierce resistance from the relevant governments. However, in the summer of 2015, *The Guardian* reported that a 12-year-old boy was awarded £120,000 by a court after the evidence established that the swine flu vaccine had caused narcolepsy in him. The court battle had gone on for over three years because the government persistently claimed that his illness was not serious enough to warrant compensation.

The government representatives initially appeared unsympathetic to his plight, as Peter Todd, the lawyer for the 12-year-old's family, told *The Guardian*. "They were downright offended because their condition was basically dismissed as something pretty trivial." However, the boy's disability was so severe that he was unable to shower unattended or take the bus alone and needed several naps to get through a school day.

Legislators in the USA, for example, have practically shielded the vaccine manufacturers from such claims for damages. This also reinforces the impression that politics is used by the pharmaceutical industry to create profitable conditions for themselves at the expense of the public.

One must not forget: The immune system in early childhood needs time to mature and usually does so under the protection of the maternal antibodies. Any vaccination therefore potentially represents a huge disruption of these natural processes. Especially since vaccinations are not the only stress factors affecting our children today.

As the World Wide Fund for Nature (WWF) showed in its "Generation X" study, for example, our children already have a dangerous chemical cocktail of around 60 industrial chemicals in their blood—"chemicals whose effects we know very little about", says WWF expert Ninja Reineke. These include the flame retardant Tetrabromobisphenol A (TBBP-A), which is used in the circuit boards of electronic devices, so-called non-sticking substances used in pans and synthetic musk compounds used in detergents and cosmetics.

Then there is Bisphenol A, a substance that can affect the hormone system (even in minimal amounts) and used in the manufacture of certain plastics. This chemical has also been detected in high concentrations in children. Many of these detected chemicals are long-lasting and accumulate in the human body over decades and can thus also contribute to the risk of developing cancer.[1190]

This is especially true for the highly toxic heavy metal mercury, which can remain in the body for decades and block important bodily functions. Amalagam fillings are by far the most significant source of mercury exposure.[1191][1192] Gustav Drasch, former professor at the Institute for Forensic Medicine at the University of Munich, has critically demonstrated that mothers transfer the mercury from their amalgam fillings to their fetuses.[1193]

As far as microbes are concerned, they mainly enter the body through mucous membranes, i.e. through our digestive or respiratory organs. An infant's immune system is not fully functional in the beginning: it is supplied with immune components through breast milk. The mother passes on antibodies to the child as well as enzymes that help, for example, in the defense against fungi. Thus, the baby's own lack of defense is replaced by components from the breast milk until it has developed its own immune system, especially during the first year of life.

Injected vaccinations, however, can be a real problem for the child's body. The child's immune system "learns" that injected foreign proteins (which is what the viruses claimed in the vaccines actually are) suddenly appear in deeper tissue. This is the wrong learning environment, since microbes usually penetrate through mucous membranes. Then there are the additives in vaccines, especially the infamous "adjuvants." In order to generate a vaccination reaction, the childhood vaccines use the same quantity of adjuvants as adult vaccines because the childhood immune system is hardly capable of its own antibody formation.

And if one takes into account that until the early 1970s in Germany, children only received one vaccination by the age of one, but today they have up to 30 vaccinations. Children also have to cope with countless environmental toxins and an increasingly unpeaceful world, so one can imagine that this may contribute to increased cases of allergies and autoimmune problems.

What is certain is that none of the swine flu vaccines had been tested on children under the age of three. "That is why the risk is simply too great to use it now unhesitatingly", said Wolfram Hartmann, President of the German Association of Paediatricians. Hartmann accused the federal government of having made "scientifically false statements." And it was also incomprehensible for Hartmann as to why the authorities bought a vaccine that contained significant amounts of adjuvants. "Children have an immune system that tends to overreact, and that is exactly what adjuvants could do."

Hartmann also shook his head over the fact that the mercury-containing preservative thiomersal had also been added to the vaccine. "This stuff has been deliberately left out of current vaccines for infants," Hartmann said.[1194]

Regrettably however, in the period that followed no lessons were learnt from the blatant failure of politicians and mainstream media to convey accurate information.

For this reason, in an interview with the headline "I would like to remove the camera or microphone from such scientists [from the RKI]", statistics professor Gerd Bosbach noted that history was repeating with COVID-19 in 2020 (see also Chapter 12): politicians and the media are speaking to exactly the same people "who have been wrong in the past and who are partly known to be guided by interests. The Robert Koch-Institute already had gained negative attention with the swine flu back then [in 2009]. The swine flu was completely overestimated. [And] one should have reviewed why the swine flu was staged in such a way by the media at that time. One of the lessons to be learned from this was not to listen to a few 'whispering experts.'"[1195]

It also prompted Ulrich Keil, Professor of Epidemiology and Social Medicine at the University of Münster, long-term WHO adviser and previous President of the European Region of the International Epidemiological Association (IEA), along with three others (including the aforementioned Angela Spelsberg) to write an open letter to the North Rhine-Westphalia federal state Government in Germany. The letter written on the 30th of March 2020 stated:

"In 2009 the great fear of the 'swine flu pandemic' was staged in the media. This has been forgotten today, since after the absence of the catastrophe, the mistakes made in the evaluation of the H1N1 flu virus infection were not dealt with in this country. The danger of the 'swine flu' had been completely overestimated; in the end it was milder than many seasonal flues of the previous years. Only 258 deaths were reported, in contrast to the 2017/2018 flu, for example, which killed 25,000 people according to the Robert Koch-Institute. Although demanded by many public health experts at the time, the RKI failed to establish a population-based infection epidemiology. A serious failure, as is currently evident [with COVID-19] and which must not be repeated in this way."[1196]

Chapter 10

Postscript to Chapter 3 About AIDS

> *„We can be exposed to HIV many times without being chronically infected.*
> *Our immune system will get rid of the virus within a few weeks if you have a*
> *good immune system. I would think if you take poor Africans who has been*
> *infected and you build up their immune system it is also possible for them to*
> *get rid of it. It is important knowledge, which is completely neglected. People*
> *always think of drugs and vaccine. There's no profit in nutrition."[1197]*
>
> Luc Montagnier, received the Nobel Prize in Medicine
> in 2008 for his (alleged) Discovery of HIV

Even the Nobel Prize Committee Cannot
Justify the Award for Luc Montagnier

As announced by the Karolinska Institute in Stockholm at the beginning of October 2008, the German cancer researcher Harald zur Hausen received the Nobel Prize for Medicine for the assumption that Human Papilloma Virus (HPV) triggers cervical cancer. He shared the award with the French physicians Luc Montagnier and Françoise Barré-Sinoussi, who are said to have detected the Human Immunodeficiency Virus (HIV).

But just as the hypothesis that HIV causes AIDS has not been scientifically proven, neither has it been established that HPV causes cancer.

Further, in response to repeated requests, the Nobel Prize Committee itself could not even provide direct evidence of HPV and HIV detection. Hence, the awarding of the 2008 Nobel Prize in Medicine reinforced the suspicion that dogmas were being built on un-proven hypotheses — just as we have seen before: for example, with the Nobel Prizes in Medicine for Carleton Gajdusek and Stanley Prusiner.

The Nobel Prize Committee also declared that it wanted to cement the HPV/cervical cancer dogma with the award to zur Hausen and Montagnier. As Nobel Prize jury member, Bjoern Vennstroem, said on Swedish radio: "We hope this will silence those who spread conspiracy theories and who defend ideas that are not founded in research."[1198]

However, no serious critics of the claim that HPV and HIV have been proven to cause cervical cancer and AIDS are spreading conspiracy theories. Behind the term "conspiracy" is the idea that there is a small group of people – conspirators – squatting together with the intention of deceiving a country or sometimes the whole world. But this is not the case with HPV, HIV, hepatitis C, BSE, etc. This has been documented extensively in this book and it should be clear we are not talking about conspiracies here.

Rather, the whole thing is a mixture of many influencing factors, including the profit interests of the pharmaceutical industry, as well as the conditioning of the population to fear microbes and especially viruses. These fears have persisted since the end of the 19th century and are difficult for people today to escape from. As a result, the idea has taken root in people's minds that bacteria, fungi and viruses are the major threat to their health and the primary causes of certain diseases.

However, as discussed in Chapter 1, this ignores the fact that disease-causing bacteria and fungi generally only multiply when conditions are created by factors such as drug and medication consumption, malnutrition or toxins such as pesticides. With alleged viruses such as HPV or HIV, there exists the fundamental problem that even the Nobel Prize committee cannot present a study that proves that what has been designated HPV or HIV is actual formal evidence of HPV or HIV. Despite the fact the Nobel Prize jury is now claiming that critics of virology are "pinning their doubts on scientifically untenable arguments" – unfortunately for them, it is exactly the opposite. Indeed, even after repeated requests the Nobel Prize committee was not able to answer the following questions about evidence-based studies for HIV:

- Don't you think that the article "A critique of the Montagnier evidence for the HIV/AIDS hypothesis" by Papadopulos-Eleopulos et al, published in 2004 in the journal *Medical Hypotheses*,[1199] shows that Montagnier did not prove HIV?

- If not, how do you explain the following facts: Montagnier and his colleagues did not provide direct proof (complete characterization) of HIV, but only claimed on the basis of certain phenomena (surrogate markers) that they had detected HIV in 1983. They based their argumentation mainly on the presence of the enzyme reverse transcriptase in cell culture. However, it is a fact that this enzyme is not specific for retroviruses (HIV is supposed to be a retrovirus), but is present in all cells—something that was not only stated by David Baltimore and Howard Temin, the discoverers of the enzyme reverse transcriptase, as early as 1972, but also by Françoise Barré-Sinoussi and Jean Claude Chermann, Montagnier's most important co-authors, in 1973. In other words: If the enzyme reverse transcriptase is present in all cells, howcan we conclude from its presence in a cell culture, as Luc Montagnier et al. did against their own better knowledge, that a retrovirus or even a special retrovirus is present in the cell culture?

- And even if the enzyme reverse transcriptase were specific for retroviruses, can the discovery of a process even be considered as evidence for the isolation of an object, in this case a virus? If so, can you provide us with the conclusive study?

- Thereupon we were sent the article "Molecuar Cloning of LAV" by Montagnier et al., published in 1984 in *Nature*,[1200] in which, in their opinion, the proof of HIV (previously called LAV by Montagnier) should be found. But in it Montagnier et al. only say "they have sought to characterize LAV by the molecular cloning of its genome." This means that the authors already assume that the genome from which they are making the clones originates from HIV. The argument is circular and therefore worthless to prove the existence of HIV because it is circular. Luc Montagnier just like the well-known AIDS researchers Robert Gallo or even Jay Levy and their colleagues always talk about the purification and isolation of virus particles, but none of them have ever presented any proof of the isolation or purification of retroviral particles or even virus-like particles (which would be the indispensable prerequisite for the detection of a retroviral genome). Or do you see it differently? If so, can you please send us the corresponding study?

- And if such evidence (isolation of retroviral particles or even just virus-like particles) has ever been produced—how do you explain that Montagnier himself (in an interview with the French science journalist Djamel Tahi, conducted at the Institute Pasteur in Paris, recorded on video and published in 1997 in the journal *Continuum*[1201]), admitted that even after „a Roman effort" it was not possible to make particles visible with the help of electron microscope imaging of cell cultures in which HIV was allegedly present, that „have the morphology typical of retroviruses"?

321

In Chapter 3, we have dealt with the subject of HIV/AIDS in detail. At this point it should be added that even the former epidemiological director of the WHO, Professor James Chin, in his 2006 book „The AIDS Pandemic: The Collision of Epidemiology and Political Correctness," published at the end of 2006, clearly admits that the AIDS case figures for developing countries were massively manipulated in order to maintain the flow of billions of dollars. According to Chin, in industrialized countries, on the other hand, according to Chin, the costly prevention campaigns are simply superfluous, because the „epidemic" simply does not want to break out of the risk groups of homosexual men and junkies.

One does not have to be a scientist—and this cannot be emphasized often enough—to realize that AIDS simply cannot be a viral plague. The fact that the disease does not break out from risk groups (poppers and other toxic illicit drugs consuming homosexual men and hard drug taking addicts) in the developed world logically goes against a viral infection. This is especially true for HIV, because, as is often claimed, this is supposed to be one of the most infectious viruses that has ever existed. Therefore we would expect such a virus to affect all people around the world more equally.

Moreover, as explained in detail in Chapter 3, the facts indicate that the well-known diseases classified as AIDS-related are (significantly) caused by factors such as drugs, medications or malnutrition. An excellent critique about the hypothesis that HIV causes AIDS and of Luc Montagnier's Nobel Prize in Medicine can be found on the website of Eleni Papadopulos and Valendar Turner who are Australian researchers and critics of the established AIDS theory (see www.theperthgroup.com/montagniernobel.html).

Nobel Prizes in Medicine for the Solidification of Dogmas

Why was it possible for Luc Montagnier to be awarded this Nobel Prize? One important reason for this is certainly the belief in an evil AIDS causing HIV-Virus that has become so firmly entrenched in people's minds. We need the scientific and media monitoring groups to look into this more closely and ask the really critical questions.

In addition, profit seeking and political power interests are likely to play a decisive role. Let us remember what Roland Scholz (Professor of Biochemistry and Cell Biology in Munich and critic of the prevailing theories of BSE and other pathogens) so aptly expressed: „Depending on the zeitgeist and depending on which authorities dominate, one or the other dogma dominates the scientific scene, often with an exclusiveness that does not allow any other way of thinking and hinders new ideas." The formation of these dogmas can be enhanced by awarding a Nobel Prize in Medicine, since by „ennobling" a theory with a Nobel Prize it receives a further boost in credibility and relevance.

The truth is that the Nobel Prize Committee is far from being a haven of pure wisdom and independence. For example it came to light that Jan Peter Andersson, a member of the Nobel Prize Committee in 2008, had been a scientific advisor to the pharmaceutical giant GlaxoSmithKline since 1999—a company that produces AIDS drugs on a large scale. In addition, Andersson founded the biotech company Avaris in 2001, which develops and produces innovative gene and cell therapy products for use in chronic infections. These significant conflicts of interest make the awarding of the Nobel Prize to Luc Montagnier and Françoise Barre-Sinoussi highly questionable. Such events also illustrate how closely interlinked the pharmaceutical industry is to the Nobel Prize committee.

Additionally, at the end of 2008, Sweden's Sveriges Radio reported that close links existed between the pharmaceutical company Astra Zeneca and the Nobel Prize Committee. Astra Zeneca was the main sponsor of two Nobel Foundation subsidiaries (Nobel Media and Nobel Webb) and at the same time held rights to the HPV vaccines. Astra Zeneca also had several people on its payroll who were involved in the decision making process for the Nobel Prize in Medicine. As a result of this report, not only did the Nobel Prize committee come under increased pressure, but the award of the Nobel Prize in Medicine to Harald zur Hausen also came under the spotlight. It appeared that the award to the German physician may have been a decisive factor in pushing the marketing of HPV vaccines.

The extent to which the Nobel Prize committee can serve as a vehicle for maintaining the power of certain medical interests was demonstrated back in 1949 with the awarding of the Nobel Prize in medicine to Portugese neurologist Egas Moniz for the lobotomy despite increasing criticism. The lobotomy is a crude neurosurgical operation in which the nerve tracts between the thalamus (the largest part of the diencephalon) and the frontal lobe (of the cerebrum) as well as parts of the grey matter (areas containing numerous cell bodies) are severed and thus destroyed.

It should be noted that the Nobel Prize for Medicine was awarded to Moniz without any scientific proof of the safety and effectiveness of lobotomy. Originally, the lobotomy was used as a last resort treatment for schizophrenic patients. However, with the Nobel Prize to Moniz, the lobotomy gained credibility and popularity – especially in the USA. „The lobotomy is an inglorious example of how a Nobel Prize can serve as a promotional tool," says Vera Sharav of the patient protection organization Alliance for Human Research Protection (AHRP).[1202]

In 1946, only 100 lobotomies were performed in the United States – in 1949, the year the Nobel Prize was awarded, the number of lobotomies went up to 5000.[1203] In 1950, just one year later, the then USSR banned lobotomy. Soviet doctors had declared that this radical procedure was „incompatible with the principles of humanity" and „turned mentally disturbed people into idiots," as the *New York Times* wrote in 1953.[1204] [1205] Today, lobotomy is considered as one of the most barbaric „medical treatments" in history.

„The public was fooled from the beginning," says Vera Sharav. „The medical community and the drug regulatory agency, the FDA, have been complicit in this by concealing the tragic consequences of this brain mutilation – for decades. Hospital operators and doctors considered the lobotomy to be a milestone in modern medicine – and so the method was widely accepted, especially after the Nobel Prize cloak was put around it."

The American psychiatrist Walter Freeman (1895-1972) and the neurosurgeon James Winston Watts (1904-1994) had made the method a popular standard technique in psychiatry in the early 1940s. What Walter Freeman was made of is shown by his distorted understanding of his own profession: „Psychosurgery achieves its success by shattering the imagination, dulling emotions, destroying abstract thinking and creating a robot-like, controllable individual."[1206] And the lobotomy – a mutilation of the brain – achieves just that.

Freeman also approached the media with verve. And the media was at his service. The eminent *Washington Star* newspaper described the procedure as „one of the greatest surgical innovations of this generation"; in 1937 the *New York Times* lauded the lobotomy on its front page as a breakthrough „Surgery of the Soul," and claimed that people with symptoms such as tension, anxiety, "crying spells" and insomnia would benefit from it.[1207] [1208]

Nurses and doctors flocked in droves to the lecture halls to learn about lobotomy in theory and practice. The procedure was performed by tens of thousands of practitioners—at the most elite institutions in the country, including John Hopkins University, Harvard Mass General Hospital, Mayo Clinic and Columbia University Hospital in New York, Columbia Presbyterian, where Rosemary Kennedy, the sister of US President John F. Kennedy, was lobotomized.[1209]

In Sweden, according to a report by the Swedish national television station SVT in April 1998, about 4,500 people had been lobotomized by 1963, many of them against their will. At least 500 of them, according to today's diagnostic criteria, were not psychiatrically ill, but actually hyperactive or intellectually impaired children. In Finland, by 1969, about 1,500 people had been lobotomized. In Norway, between 3,000 and 4,000 people were lobotomized between 1941 and 1981.[1210] Worldwide, the number of operations performed is estimated at about one million.[1211] In the 1950s, lobotomies were even used, among other things, to „cure" homosexuality or a communist attitude.[1212]

In 1967, Harvard authors Vernon Mark, Frank Ervin, and William Sweet got carried away with the thesis that the cause of the race riots in Detroit was a „focal brain disorder." In a letter to the editor of the *Journal of the American Medical Association*, the official arm of the American Medical Association, they claimed a neurosurgical solution could prevent further riots.[1213] Unwilling to drop this idea, in 1970, Vernon Mark and Frank Ervin published a book entitled „Violence and the Brain" in which they proposed psychosurgery as the definitive solution to the problem of violence, for example in the case of unteachable prison inmates.

The psychiatrist L.G.West called this approach „biosocial humanism" in a 1969 article. In 1979, the Californian psychiatrist H. Brown recommended psychosurgery for the rehabilitation of juvenile delinquents. Brown's proposals were discussed in the London Times and the *Washington Post*—pointing out that this type of rehabilitation was far more cost-effective, at only $6,000, than lifelong custody, which costs around $100,000.[1214]

Civil rights movements began to take action against lobotomy procedures in the 1960s. Ken Kesey's 1962 novel „One Flew over the Cuckoo's Nest" impressively demonstrated the effects of the surgery on psychiatric patients. The novel was awarded the Pulitzer Prize and made into a film in 1975 by Milos Forman with Jack Nicholson in the leading role (winning five Oscars). In the end, the lobotomy was recognized for what it was: a brutal mutilation that was like a permanent straitjacket for the brain.

However, it is suspected that this procedure was abandoned by the medical establishment, not because it was tantamount to mutilation, but perhaps also because psychotropic drugs that could strongly sedate patients had been appearing since the 1950s.

Just how incorrigible the medical elite can be is shown by the fact that as late as 1998
the Nobel Prize organization defended the Nobel Prize award for Egas Moniz in 1949
with the words: „There is no doubt that Moniz deserves the Nobel Prize for Medicine."[1215]

Meanwhile, the series of mistakes made in connection with the awarding of the Nobel Prize
in Medicine goes all the way back to 1890. Heroically striking for glory, Robert Koch, wanted
to make the world believe that he had discovered a miracle cure for tuberculosis with tuberculin—which later turned out to be a hoax, costing thousands of people their lives.

Experts such as the historian Christoph Gradmann stated that Koch had „skilfully staged" the
market launch of tuberculin. Everything had obviously been planned long in advance. Despite this, Koch was awarded the Nobel Prize in 1905 for his work on tuberculosis. The Nobel
Prize for Koch made a decisive contribution to the fact that microbiology, and subsequently
the hunting of viruses, was able to occupy an extremely dominant position in research with
toxicology being increasingly pushed into the background (see chapter 2).

Other examples of how the Nobel Prize in Medicine has been abused were the awards
to Carleton Gajdusek and Stanley Prusiner, also mentioned in this book, who created the
basis for redefining all sorts of diseases as infectious diseases at will. It was Gajdusek who
helped develop the "breakthrough" concept of „slow viruses", which is a central theory as
to why HIV causes AIDS and HPV cervical cancer. In truth, however, the only thing that can
be said about Gajdusek's slow virus theory and his 1976 Nobel Prize is what Roland Scholz
(Professor of Biochemistry and Cell Biology from Munich, Germany) aptly remarked: „The
scientific world seems to be hornswoggled by a fairy tale" (see also chapter 2).

Gajdusek's erroneous theses about slow viruses was also a decisive prerequisite for the
alleged cattle disease BSE to be declared an infectious disease. In 1982, US physician
and biochemist Stanley Prusiner succeeded in identifying so-called plaques in the brain,
which are characteristic of the nerve damage associated with brain degeneration. These
plaques contain certain proteins, called prions, which are mainly located on nerve cells
and have a pathologically altered structure.

In 1987, Prusiner finally succumbed to the temptation to bring his hitherto little-noticed prions into play as the cause of an epidemic, which earned him an enormous reputation. Ten years later, in 1997, he was „ennobled" with a Nobel Prize, as the German journal *Deutsches Ärzteblatt* put it. The theory of an infectious cause was solidified by declaring the „Prusiner prion" to be the trigger of sponge-like brain diseases. However, the experiments on which this hypothesis and hence the Nobel Prize are based have a number of short-comings which are explained in detail in Chapter 5.

In summary, the claim that prions are infectious is also unfounded. Instead, there is good reason to assume that the so-called cattle disease BSE is the result of a genetic defect due to inbreeding or chemical poisoning from a severely nerve-damaging organophosphate (Phosmet). But if you declare industrial poisons such as pesticides to be the cause of an epidemic, there is no money to be made: on the contrary, this would endanger the sales of powerful industrial corporations. However, with vaccinations as well as gene, antibody and BSE tests based on an „evil" pathogen theory, there is indeed money to be made ...

Strengthening of the Immune System
Instead of Antiviral Drugs

In Chapter 3 we have already gone into the subject of AIDS drugs in detail (among others in the subchapters „AIDS Drugs: The Fable of Life-Prolonging Effects" and „The AIDS Therapy Dilemma"). However, the topic is so important—especially for those affected by it—that we would like to say a few more pertinent things about it:

There are always patients who feel better with or after treatment with so-called antiviral drugs. This is especially the case if the patient is affected by chronic fungal infections. The improvement in health is due to the fact that protease inhibitors were part of the drug cocktail administered and have been shown to have anti-fungal effects.. Just because these patients who have been given the AIDS stamp have done well with these "antiviral" drugs does not confirm the thesis that HIV causes AIDS, or that antiviral drugs should always and exclusively be used.

In particular, many asymptomatic patients are still classified as AIDS patients simply because they tested antibody positive or were diagnosed with a low T-helper cell count or with a high so-called „viral load". These patients should refrain from taking antiviral drugs „prophylactically," as they are associated with potentially severe side effects. Even for those affected with a real ailment (Kaposi's sarcoma, herpes zoster etc.), it is true that the AIDS drugs may be effective in individual cases, but these medications are not a long-term or definitive solution.

The HIV treatments do not address the underlying causes, which are what made the patients fall ill in the first place. As we have described these factors have known immu-nosupressant effects and include drugs like poppers and cocaine, prescription medica-tions with many side effects (AIDS drugs, antibiotics etc.), malnutrition and many other stress factors. As a rule, these factors also tend to act on patients in a cumulative way.

It is extremely important to keep the immune system healthy by means of a diet rich in nutrients, exercise, sunlight, avoiding negative stress and, if necessary, tak-ing restorative supplements such as glutathione and probiotics etc. On this note, in 2009 Luc Montagnierwas interviewed by Brent Leung, in the multiple award-winning documentary „House of Numbers: The HIV/AIDS Story Is Being Rewritten."[1216] In this interview Montagnier made the following statements:

Montagnier: „We can be exposed to HIV many times without being chronically infected. Our immune system will get rid of the virus within a few weeks if you have a good im-mune system."
Leung: „If you have a good immune system then your body can naturally get rid of HIV?"
Montagnier: „Yes."
Leung: „If you take a poor African who has been infected and if you build up his immune system, is it possible for him to also naturally get rid of it?"
Montagnier: „I would think so."
Leung: „That's an important message."
Montagnier. „It's important knowledge that is completely neglected. People always think of drugs and vaccines."
Leung: „There's is no money in nutrition, right?"
Montagnier: „There's no profit, yes."[1217]

In other words, even if one believes in HIV and its disease-causing effects (for which there is demonstrably no reason, see the beginning of Chapter 3), the primary focus should be on doing everything possible to maintain and build up physical health in naturally—and not on throwing toxic drugs „around" with serious side effects into the mix. The degenerative effects of these drugs was also reported by the *New York Magazine* on

November 1, 2009 in the article „Another kind of AIDS crisis: A striking number of HIV patients are living longer but getting older faster." The piece also featured a video [1218] in which those affected talk about how they age much faster when taking HIV drugs, sometimes even go crazy, or suffer from osteoporosis, high blood pressure and dementia or something even go "crazy."

These effects are not surprising, as described in chapter 3, considering how toxic the drugs are on living cells. One of the most important parts of the cell is the mitochondria, also known as cell power stations. They belong to the energy generating system of the body. Their own genetic material can be permanently damaged by a whole range of factors, including heavy metals such as mercury, pesticides and also chemotherapy drugs (AIDS drugs are basically chemotherapeutic drugs, see screenshot of the *Bild* column of drag queen Nina Queer)—and in the end this can lead to serious illness.

It should be noted that, apart from chromosomal damage, the second defining characteristic of cancer cells is that their mitochondria are damaged and their numbers are reduced. Mitochondria not only serve as "energy factories" in cells for living processes, but they are also crucial for cell growth and other central functions. It's tragic that established medicine still largely ignores this fact, because studies have shown that a cancer cell can transform back into a normal cell if its damaged mitochondria are regenerated through natural treatments like detoxification or eating a really healthy diet with plenty of fresh and raw food.

The fact that poor mitochondrial health is related to the extent that AIDS patients become unwell was finally acknowledged by established research at the end of 2008. Unfortunately, however, virus-fixated medicine has not embraced the idea that industrial and drug poisons and other civilizational stress factors negatively affect the mitochondria and thus compromise the immune system and even cause it to crash (which is then referred to as AIDS in the final stage). But without a scapegoat virus, the status quo wouldn't work, because no virus means no reason to administer antiviral drugs and this is a horrible idea from the point of view of the pharmaceutical companies and the AIDS physicians associated with them. Instead they twist the theory around and claim that the damaged mitochondria are involved in the spread of HIV, which in turn causes the immune system to kill itself.[1219]

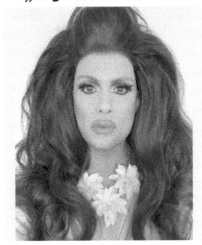

On October 26, 2019 the weekly Bild column featured drag queen Nina Queer with the headline „So dangerous is PrEP!". PrEP stands for „Pre-Exposure-Prophylaxis." The idea behind PrEP is that people who test „negative" for HIV should also take medication as a precaution. But the problem with this according to Nina Queer is that „not only sick people are permanently provided with strong medication, but also the healthy ones. What an ingenious trick to sell drugs to healthy people and to make billions through the desire for unprotected sex. A PrEP pill is nothing more than a kind of 'little chemotherapy' that you expose your body to every day or possibly for years. As with any medication, PrEP has side effects, including diarrhea, fatigue and depression." Less than a week later, the virologist Hendrik Streeck responded to Nina Queer in Bild claiming the effectiveness of PrEP is proven, and „like any drug, PrEP has side effects," but „a depression ... is certainly not one of them"„However, the drug Truvada which was approved as a PrEP in the EU in 2016 is known to cause depression. Additionally, the fact that Hendrik Streeck has received fees and financial contributions from pharmaceutical companies such as Gilead (which earns money with the PrEP-approved drug Descovy) should have been disclosed by the Bild newspaper to its readers. Source: Screenshot of bild.de

But these are groundless speculations. In his book „The Silent Revolution of Cancer and AIDS Medicine," (which has been available in English since 2008,) cancer researcher Heinrich Kremer shows in a well-founded way that AIDS, just like cancer, is a consequence of damage to the energy system — and that no virus is needed for this process. Ultimately, a disrupted energy system leads to a deterioration of every other cell process, which in turn prevents the immune system from working properly. It is therefore vitally important to keep your immune system healthy. If you are already affected by a chronic disease state, it is crucial that the recovery process focuses on bringing your immune system back into shape.

At this point, let us characterize what exactly is meant by an immune system. The immune system comprises a large number of cell types and an even larger number of messenger substances (messenger substances are used for chemical communication in an organism — i.e. to transmit signals or information). It should be noted that about 80 percent of immune cells are located in the intestinal area and combined with the intestinal flora (microorganisms), it is by far the largest and most important immune system in our body.[1220] In total, the intestinal microbes typically weigh a good 1 kg.

Many people are still not really aware of this fact, although even established medicine is increasingly appreciating its importance. The „fitness" of a person's intestinal flora is influenced by a number of factors, especially diet, the amount of negative stress, the amount of physical activity and the amount of drugs consumed, etc. Furthermore, there is much to suggest that the state of the intestinal flora has a significant influence on all sorts of ailments such as obesity and allergies, and also on serious diseases like cancer,[1221] [1222] [1223] [1224] [1225] which is also one of the so-called AIDS-defining diseases (see Chapter 3, subchapter „AIDS: What Exactly Is It?").

In fact, critical experts point out that a shift in the intestinal flora, commonly occurring in industrial societies, is leading to changes in the body that may contribute to the so-called HIV tests turning positive and AIDS patients becoming ill.[1226] [1227] [1228] Also noteworthy in this context are studies showing that it is also beneficial to the health of AIDS patients benefit if they do something to improve their intestinal flora. The best way to do this, of course, is to consume a diet rich in nutrients and fibre, with many enzymes (from raw food). Otherwise beneficial intestinal bacteria can be obtained in the form of preparations such as probiotics.[1229]

Among the multitude of cells that make up our immune system, a distinction is made between so-called lymphocytes, macrophages and granulocytes. All three cell types are white blood cells, which fulfill special tasks in the immune defence system. Lymphocytes are further divided into B-lymphocytes, T-helper cells and T-killer cells; the macrophages are also called scavenger cells. Recent findings have revealed that "the cellular immune system can be divided into two main groups: The TH1 and the TH2-system," according to medical specialist for environmental medicine Joachim Mutter, in his 2009 book „Gesund statt chronisch krank" (Healthy instead of chronically ill).[1230]

The main weapon of the TH1 system is nitric oxide, which can be used to eliminate cancerous cells, among other things. However, when nitric oxide is produced it must be detoxified by the body's own cells through reduced glutathione or sulphur groups (thiols), otherwise it would also destroy the healthy cells. Glutathione is a small „mini-protein" that is present in every cell of the body and is involved in a number of detoxification, transport and biosynthetic functions. The US National Cancer Institute calls reduced glutathione „the primary antioxidant of cells, which plays an important role in neutralizing free radicals and, because it is a co-enzyme containing [sulfur-containing] thiols, in detoxifying foreign substances."[1231]

In a healthy organism, there is usually a balance between reduced glutathione and its oxidized form, whereby only the reduced variant of glutathione develops the nitric-neutralizing effect. If the number of free radicals in the organism increases as a result of toxic influences such as heavy metal poisoning, drug consumption, vaccinations, stress, etc., the amount of reduced glutathione in the cells may decrease. If the organism cannot stop or reverse this decrease (for example, with the help of vitamin E or the amino acid cysteine, which can immediately convert oxidized glutathione back into functional reduced glutathione), a deficiency of reduced glutathione occurs and the aggressive free radicals are thus able to carry out their activities without hindrance.[1232]

This is often observed in cancer patients in particular[1233] as chemo- and radiotherapies usually worsen the phenomenon considerably. These therapies lead to an increased consumption of glutathione, so that the free radicals can do their „mischief" more intensively.

If the levels of reduced glutathione and other antioxidants are insufficient, the immune system switches to the TH2 response, which simultaneously reduces the TH1 immune response. As a result of the suppressed TH1 activity, not only can chronic infections with germs such as Borrelia bacteria or fungi occur—but ultimately also cancer, as cancer cells are destroyed by nitric oxide through the TH1 immune response. In order to compensate for the throttling of the TH1 system, the TH2 immune defense can be easily over-stimulated.

And indeed, the TH2 system is often overactive and the TH1 system is shut down not only in people who suffer from allergies or autoimmune diseases (where the cell's own structures are attacked), but especially in cancer patients.[1234]

„This means that in people suffering from cancer or other chronic diseases, it is advisable to increase the body's own glutathione production by detoxifying the mitochondria and by taking in certain substances", proclaimed the physician Joachim Mutter. „This then leads to the TH2 system being brought down to a balanced level. The significant increase in all kinds of chronic diseases over the past decades suggests that the population in industrialized countries is suffering from a growing glutathione deficit or mitochondrial hypofunction, caused on the one hand by the increasing exposure to more and more toxins and harmful radiation, and on the other hand by the supply of poor-quality food that contains less and less vital nutrients because it is produced using industrial farming methods and on depleted soils."

Cancer researchers Roberto Locigno and Vincent Castronovo from the University of Liège in Belgium also noted in a 2001 review published in the *International Journal of Oncology*: „Reduced glutathione (GSH), a ubiquitous thiol-containing tripeptide, is unanimously recognized to play a central role in cell biology. It is highly implicated in the cellular defense against xenobiotics and naturally occurring deleterious compounds such as free radicals and hydroperoxides. Consequently, reduced glutathione is an essential factor in the prevention and treatment of several human diseases including cancer and cardio-vascular diseases."[1235]

As research shows, glutathione levels in the human body can be greatly increased by consuming raw vegetables and wild herbs. Studies have also shown that foods containing sulphur have antioxidant effects and stimulate glutathione synthesis— and thus can counteract cancer.[1236] [1237] The exotic fruit durian, which is available in Asian food shops in many places, as well as wild garlic and garlic all contain large quantities of these sulphur-containing compounds. Healthy sleep is also said to help regenerate the glutathione reserves of the liver and lead to an increase in melatonin levels as well.

Melatonin is a sleep hormone and, like glutathione, is a free-radical scavenger (some say that melatonin is an even stronger free-radical scavenger than glutathione). However, the formation of melatonin requires that the body is exposed to enough natural light during the day and receives sufficient vitamins and the essential protein component L-tryptophan (which must be taken in with food). Melatonin also protects glutathione from premature degradation, whereas the heavy metal mercury quickly leads to glutathione deficiency and cell damage. Studies have shown melatonin can counteract or prevent cell damage by heavy metals.[1238]

„A central component of a successful therapy must therefore be to strengthen the immune system or to bring the TH1 and TH2-defence systems into a robust condition and thus also to regenerate the damaged mitochondria, i.e. the cell power plants", emphasizes Frankfurt physician Juliane Sacher, who has been treating AIDS and cancer patients for many years. In order to achieve this, it is important to increase the concentration of glutathione in the mitochondria. This can be achieved by supplying the amino acids cysteine, glutamine and glycine. These are transported from the cell plasma to the mitochondria. „As a result, cancer cells can sometimes be transformed back into normal cells", adds Mutter.[1239]

Emergency medicine also makes use of these glutathione pathways. In the case of poisoning with the common painkiller paracetamol, its metabolite N-acetyl-p-benzoquinone imine (NAPQI) is toxic to the liver. Glutathione detoxifies NAPQI, but in cases of overdose the liver's supplies of glutathione are overwhelmed and the NAPQI kills its cells. Hence, this "thief of glutathione" can lead to liver failure and death. Emergency doctors administer high doses of the amino acid cysteine (for example in the form of fluimucil ampoules) in order to stimulate glutathione production to detoxify the cells.

Unfortunately, very few doctors are aware that sometimes only a few variables need to come together to lead to a dicey or even fatal situation. For example, a patient who has already taken a lot of paracetamol for pain, with a background of a poor diet (e.g. compromised by pesticides which is common nowadays) and who perhaps has an unnoticed inflammatory skin disease.

If such a patient undergoes surgery then their glutathione levels can be additionally reduced by the anaesthetics and wound healing process. In this case of glutathione compromise it is not surprising that the patient gets increasingly worse. And if, by chance, they also happen to have the increasingly recognized glutathione S-transferase theta gene defect, they could potentially die in such a situation. Unfortunately, most doctors are at a loss to explain why this has happened and how they could have avoided this drama.

Sacher has found this genetic defect in practice in cancer and AIDS patients. She therefore warns her patients against using paracetamol and instead carries out glutathione infusions a few days before and after operations. In this context, Boyd Haley, Professor and Director Emeritus of the Chemical Institute of the University of Kentucky, has also developed a new remedy that has been shown in animal studies to be practically as non-toxic as water and which he has named Oxidative Stress Relief, or OSR for short. It can effectively increase the glutathione concentration in the brain and spinal cord and can also remove heavy metals.

Initial experiments with humans have shown that people who themselves suffer from serious illnesses such as Parkinson's, Alzheimer's and cardiovascular disease have experienced rapid improvement or at least it has been possible to halt the progression of the diseases. As a dietary supplement, it has been approved by the FDA to raise the body's own glutathione levels.[1240]

It goes without saying that the sooner these substances or procedures are given, the better, unless the person concerned does something else to improve his or her immune system. This includes regular exercise, breathing fresh air, maintaining loving relationships, getting out into the sun sufficiently (to ensure the supply of vitamin D), getting adequate sleep and eating a healthy diet (rich in nutrients and fresh foods, low in toxins), etc.

The importance of the immune system in serious illnesses such as cancer has also been confirmed by studies conducted by Jérôme Galon and his team at the Institute National de la Santé et de la recherche Médicale in Paris. According to these studies, the course of disease in colorectal cancer patients is largely determined by the activity of the body's defenses against the tumor and its immediate surroundings. This applies irrespective of how much the tumor has spread locally or whether metastases have already formed.[1241] Therefore, the assessment of the local immune response to cancer should definitely be included in diagnostic and therapeutic decisions, suggested Galon at the second European Congress of Immunology, which took place in Berlin in September 2009.

Chapter 10

Karri Stokely and Maria Papagiannidou Died from AIDS Medication—and Not from HIV!

Tragically, there are also people who fail in their attempt to get off AIDS medication. Among them is the American Karri Stokely, who died in 2011 at the age of 44. *The Guardian* wrote a rather cynical obituary about her, which stated that Stokely, „a poster girl for a different way to look at health," had died a „death by denial" by stopping her antiviral drugs.[1242] But as always, one has to look at the actual facts in order to avoid jumping to the wrong conclusions.

But jumping to the wrong conclusions is exactly what the *Guardian* article does. The author, Brian Deer who is praised as a great „investigative journalist" should have known

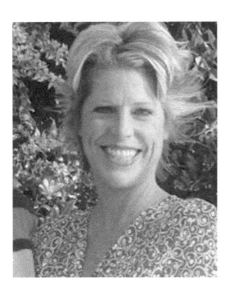

better. Deer quotes the journalist Joan Shenton, who is one of the prominent critics of the HIV=AIDS dogma and who knew Stokely well, as saying: „I think Karri died from the side-effects of the drugs. She'd stopped taking them, but she'd been taking them for about 10 years before."

Immediately following this quote, Deer writes that "there's no answer, of course," to thesis that Shenton's assessment of the Stokely case. So Deer seems to admit that he's uncertain if Stokely died solely as a result of stopping her medication. And to our request to explain this (sent by e-mail on February 12, 2014 and again on March 24, 2020) Deer did not respond. So let us look closely at how

Karri Stokely

Stokely died. Stokely had been on medication for eleven years from 1996 until 2007, when she came across critical reports that eventually led her to stop taking the drugs. After that she experienced a relatively short period of good health, even though it was accompanied by an unpleasant „crisis" including drug-related withdrawal symptoms. But

336

after a while, the problems reappeared again, mainly due to the „invisible" effects of the AIDS drugs. For example, the drugs had contributed to her developing non-Hodgkin's lymphoma, a malignant disease of the lymphatic system.

At the beginning of 2010, she was diagnosed with an anal fissure, which ulcerated in the following months, leading to severe pain. The doctors took a tissue sample in which they claimed to have found cytomegalovirus (abbreviated CMV). The topic of CMV is worth a discussion of its own but will not be dealt with further here. However, it is a fact that there is no peer-reviewed study that proves that the CMV group are infectious viruses.

Unfortunately though, because of viral scaremongering and the unshakable (though unfounded) belief in the effectiveness of the antiviral drugs, the doctors would only agree to operate on Stokely if she took the medications. Finally, she gave in to medical pressure, because the fissure simply had to be removed. Stokely was administered intravenous ganciclovir, a particularly toxic antiviral, whose frequent(!) side effects include liver and kidney dysfunction and retinal detachment. And indeed, shortly afterwards (at the end of 2010) she was affected by massive visual disturbances and loss of vision, among other problems. „The administration of ganciclovir together with a highly toxic antibiotic caused the neurological and visual damage in Karri and ultimately caused her death," concludes David Rasnick, a researcher critical of HIV/AIDS who accompanied Stokely during her final months.

The use of protease inhibitors, for example, which are administered to AIDS patients, can be quite helpful temporarily. However, this is not because they block an „evil" virus, but because they are antifungal, i.e. fungicidal, and probably also have an effect against parasites. And indeed, many AIDS patients also suffer from fungal infections. However, protease inhibitors and HAART (Highly Active Antiretroviral Therapy) only treat symptoms and not the actual causes (i.e. a suppressed immune system allows fungi to grow pathologically). Therefore, when the treatments are discontinued, the fungal infections often reoccur.
Interestingly, there was a 2008 meta-analysis published in HIV Medicine titled „Antiretroviral effects on HIV-1 RNA, CD4 cell count and progression to AIDS or death." The study evaluated 178 papers, and according to the authors is the largest of its kind to investigate how HAART affects the surrogate markers CD4 helper cell count and viral load as well as two clinical endpoints „the outbreak of AIDS" and „death". The scientists concluded that they „were unable to demonstrate a relationship between change in CD4 cell count or viral load and clinical events" [= AIDS outbreak and death]. „Even if one assumes there

are beneficial effects from HAART therapy," says Valendar Turner of the Australian Perth Group, „the fact that no correlation exists between virological and clinical outcomes means the benefits are not the result of an antiretroviral effect."

„I have done intensive research into the damage caused by AIDS drugs," says Rasnick. „And I found that about half of those who take antiretroviral drugs experience vision loss and varying degrees of blindness. That's a tremendous proportion, but how often do you hear about it in the media or from the doctors? Another side effect of these drugs is progressive multifocal leukoencephalopathy or PML for short, a severe disorder of the central nervous system, which has the exact symptoms that Karri Stokely ultimately suffered from and that caused her death.[1243] AIDS physicians know about this as well, but they do their best to avoid educating people about it. Moreover, the autopsy report clearly shows that Karri did not die of 'AIDS' or 'HIV', but of kidney failure followed by multiple organ failure."

It should also be mentioned that shortly before Karri Stokely's death abnormally high levels of highly toxic thallium (the metal between mercury and lead on the periodic table) and other heavy metals were measured in her stool and urine samples. And as incredible as this may sound, it raises a startling possible conclusion: deliberate poisoning ...

Another tragic example of the power of official propaganda is the case of Greek woman Maria Papagiannidou. She tested „positive" for HIV in 1985, at just 20 years of age, and was then treated with AZT from 1987 onwards. 20 years later, when she was just over 40, she stopped taking the medication and published the book „Goodbye AIDS!" In 2011, however, she unfortunately became very ill and in desperation restarted antiviral therapy until she died in spring 2012.

But why had Papagiannidou got into such a health crisis after stopping the medication? The answer is probably two-fold. Firstly, her body had "forgotten" how to keep potentially disease-causing germs in check, since the medication had taken over this role for years. Secondly, the medications she had been taking for two decades had caused massive damage to her mitochondria.[1244] Once she stopped taking the drugs, new resistant germs quickly accumulated, which may not respond to a new antiviral medication successfully. Just like with Stokely, Papagiannidou's death was not—as is often hastily claimed—due to her stopping her medication. Rather, the highly toxic medication itself could be implicated which over time actually destroyed her physically.[1245]

So what could Papagiannidou have done? „An exit from years of AIDS medication is only possible if laboratory analyses are made, on the basis of which specific infusion treatments can be carried out," says Felix de Fries, who has been active in the Gay Rights Movement since the mid-1970s and who has also been a former employee of Alfred Hässig, a pioneer of blood transfusions. „This makes it possible to help the patients be immuno-active again and to rebuild their health, especially with regard to the mitochondria. Anyone who undergoes antiviral therapy simply loses the ability to fend off bacterial, fungal and parasitic infections after a short time. Combination therapy intervenes in a fundamental way in metabolic processes and immune reactions. Protease inhibitors slow down the cell division in organs that, however, depend on increased cell division in order to function."

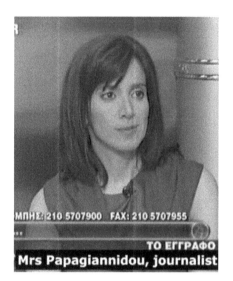

Mrs Papagiannidou, journalist

Maria Papagiannidou on May 19, 2009 on Greek television (Youtube-Screenshot)

De Fries has compiled „Therapy recommendations for HIV positive and AIDS patients."[1246] „For example, it makes sense to give antioxidant plant substances and probiotics to rebuild the intestinal flora and the intestinal mucosa," says de Fries. In addition, the administration of various substances could remedy deficiencies and support the activity of the mitochondria, the formation of their membranes and the repair of mitochondrial DNA damage and thus restore the cell metabolism and the functioning of all organs.

Examples of restorative substances include trace elements, amino acids, vitamins, medicinal mushrooms and plant substances such as co-enzyme Q10, L-glutathione, folic acid, lecithin, lutein, manganese, orotic acid, pangamic acid, selenium, magnesium, humic acid, chromium, zinc, L-arginine, L-cysteine, L-glutamine, L-glycine, L-histidine, L-isoleucine, L-lysine, L-tyrosine, grape seed extract, Ling-Zhi, Agaricus, shitake, yam root and vitamins B1, B2, B3, B5, B6, B12, C, D and E as well as alpha-lipoic acid, reduced glutathione and phosphatidylserines. Many of these have anti-cancer, anti-inflammatory, anti-allergic, antibacterial, detoxifying effects and support defense activity, blood circulation and metabolism in the brain.

In this context, it should also be remembered that the conditions subsumed under the term AIDS are often the result of oxidative substances damaging the body's antioxidant system. And when these oxidative processes, produced by drugs, prescription medications, industrial toxins, stress, etc., act on the body over a long period of time, degenerative phenomena such as Kaposi's sarcoma (one of the most important AIDS-defining diseases in industrialized countries) occur and increased cell decay leads to the increased release of proteins from the cytoskeleton and mitochondria. Against these released proteins and against a large number of different bacterial antigens, the body produces antibodies to a greater extent, which can cause HIV antibody tests to be „positive" above a certain laboratory value, which was set in 1984.

Those who have tested „positive" should have further laboratory tests carried out to show which germs may be causing infections and what kind of antibiotic resistance they exhibit. In addition, assessments should be made of mitochondrial function and general metabolic status. Toxicity from drugs, chemicals and heavy metals—for example from excessive vaccine adjuvants and mercury-containing dental fillings—should be assessed as they can severely impair the immune response.

It's important to remember that it is a long process to get the „cart that is deep in the mud" back onto firm and healthy ground. This can sometimes require a will of iron.

Two Experience Reports: A Life Without AIDS Drugs

Raúl Erichs de Palma

„In the mid-1980s, when I was not even 20 years old, I started injecting heroin intravenously. And after about eight years, I even started mixing it with cocaine. This drug addiction lasted for almost ten years, until 1995, when my health literally collapsed. My kidneys, for example, were only functioning at 20 percent, the damage to my liver left my blood with very few platelets, and even one of my heart valves was broken off and surrounded by several warts, two to three centimeters in diameter. When I was admitted to the hospital, I weighed less than 40 kg—with a height of 1.83 m.

After the admission I tried to breathe, but no oxygen got into my lungs and I had a respiratory arrest. On the way to the heart valve surgery I lost consciousness and woke up three days later. I had to stay in the hospital for another three and a half months for minimal recovery. At this point I decided to change my life completely.

After I left the hospital, I never took drugs again and became a vegetarian. For five years I have even been on a vegan diet, following the philosophy that animals should not be hurt or used. I also studied naturopathy for three years and Gestalt therapy for four years. And still I am constantly trying to acquire knowledge about how to live a healthier life.

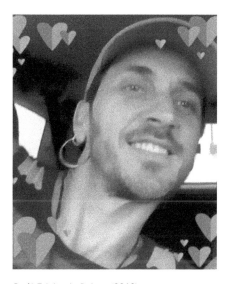
Raúl Erichs de Palma (2018)

I was first tested for HIV in 1995. It was 'negative'. In 1997, I had to go to the doctor to get a prescription for anticoagulants that I had been taking since my heart valve surgery. However, although the only clinical signs that I showed were of recovery, the doctor urged me to have an 'HIV test'. The Explanation: I had been an intravenous drug user, which is why I would have to have such a test every six months. Finally I gave in and took the test. At that time I had no background knowledge about HIV/AIDS. When I got the 'positive' test result, my first thought was: 'This is the beginning of the end'. And I didn't tell anyone about the results for months. But then I thought: The news that I am supposed to suffer from a deadly viral disease does not fit at all with how I was feeling physically and what the doctors told me about my health condition.

And so I started to read various books about how to get healthy. One of the first was '¡Cuídate compa!: Manual para la Autogestión de la Salud' (Take care of yourself, buddy! Manual for the self-management of health) by Eneko Landaburu, which mentions the doubts of solid scientists and doctors about the HIV=AIDS theory.[1247] Then I came across, for example, the book 'Roger's Recovery from AIDS' by Dr. Bob Owen, or 'Poison by Prescription: The AZT Story' by the great gay rights activist and prominent critic of the HIV=AIDS theory John Lauritsen.

Books that have helped me a lot include 'El arte de saber alimentarte' and 'La enferme-dad, qué es y para qué sirve?' by Karmelo Bizkarra Maiztegi, 'Toxemia: The basic cause of disease' by John H. Tilden and also books by Désiré Mérien and Herbert M. Shelton.

I also felt better and better the longer I followed the healthy lifestyle. And also the doc-tors always confirmed that I was very healthy. I never had a so-called 'viral load', by the way—and the value for my CD4 helper cells was always higher than 400. With what I know today, I will always refuse any 'AIDS medication.'"

Raúl Erichs de Palma lives in Spain, his website is http://replanteamientodelasalud.blog-spot.com

The use of protease inhibitors, for exam-ple, which are administered to AIDS patients, can be quite helpful tempora-rily. However, this is not because they block an „evil" virus, but because they are antifungal, i.e. fungicidal, and proba-bly also have an effect against parasi-tes. And indeed, many AIDS patients also suffer from fungal infections. However, protease inhibitors and HAART (Highly Active Antiretroviral Therapy) only tre-at symptoms and not the actual causes (i.e. a suppressed immune system allows fungi to grow pathologically). Therefo-re, when the treatments are discontinu-ed, the fungal infections often reoccur.

Interestingly, there was a 2008 meta-analysis published in *HIV Medicine* titled

„Antiretroviral effects on HIV-1 RNA, CD4 cell count and progression to AIDS or de-ath." The study evaluated 178 papers, and according to the authors is the largest of its kind to investigate how HAART affects the surrogate markers CD4 helper cell count and viral load as well as two clini-cal endpoints „the outbreak of AIDS" and „death". The scientists concluded that they „were unable to demonstrate a relation-ship between change in CD4 cell count or viral load and clinical events" [= AIDS outbreak and death]. „Even if one assumes there are beneficial effects from HAART therapy," says Valendar Turner of the Aus-tralian Perth Group, „the fact that no cor-relation exists between virological and clinical outcomes means the benefits are not the result of an antiretroviral effect."

Nash

„For more than 20 years now (as of 2020), I have been living disease-free without taking the ARV drugs after being told I was HIV 'positive.' I am now 55 years old. I am doing fine, I feel great and look great.

One year ago there was a bad flu virus going on here at work and my colleagues were dropping like flies, I had minor symptoms that lasted one day and I was fine.

I was diagnosed 'positive' in September 1999, then immediately was coerced into taking the drugs. I started the ARV therapy a year later after I initially refused to do so. I took the drugs for just over a year, then against the doctor's advice, I stopped taking them, because I simply couldn't take the horrific side effects anymore. When I first started taking the drugs, I got a burning and stinging sensation in my fingertips and toes, which lasted for about 4 months. The other side effects were the wild crazy dreams every night, and the feeling I got every day like I was drunk or high. I also felt as though my organs were hardening. The later effects lasted until I decided to stop taking the drugs.

The fact that I was suicidal at the time helped me make the decision to stop and just let the 'virus' take its course. But, a wasting disease didn't happen. To my surprise, I immediately started to feel and look better.

Since late 2002, like any other healthy person, I've had cases of the flu and a couple of times serious bouts of pneumonia (which I suffered often as a child). None of those illnesses killed me, I think it made my immune system stronger.

The longest I am down with the flu is two days—no more than three. I can't prove it yet but the drugs may have damaged my arteries (arteriosclerosis) during the time I took it (I now suffer from hypertension which I didn't have before I took the drugs, only during and after).

I am constantly studying the work of HIV/AIDS dissidents on this subject so that I can best defend our point of view.

I'm ready to join in the fight against the HIV-AIDS lie and hopefully, together we can help put an end to the horrific HIV-AIDS machine. Their lie cannot last much longer.

Thanks to the work and time of all those who have fought this battle. May they all have much success and happiness in life."

Nash, born 1965, lives in Houston, Texas, USA. His experience report can also be found at www.livingwithouthivdrugs.com.

The full name of Nash is known to the authors of this book.

US Mortality Rate Make Nonsense of the AIDS Drug Dogma

Raúl Erichs de Palma and Nash, as mentioned earlier, are far from the only ones who have tested "HIV positive" and are doing just fine without medication. According to the CNN report "Left behind: Who's being treated for HIV in the U.S.—and who isn't," released in late 2015, "about 66 percent of the 1.2 million people living with HIV/AIDS in the United States are not in treatment." That is, they are not receiving or taking highly toxic medications, respectively.

At the same time, official U.S. statistics for 2018 show just under 16,000 deaths of peo-ple ever classified as having AIDS—whereby „these deaths may be due to any cause," as the hiv.gov website remarkably states. But even if we put these nearly 16,000 deaths in relation to the estimated 1.2 million people labled as „HIV positive" in the U.S., the mortality rate is just 1.3 percent. And such a low figure is simply inconsistent with the hypothesis that alleged „HIV infection" poses a serious risk to those who do not receive drug treatment—and it makes nonsense of the claim that so-called "HIV infec-tion" will inevitably lead to immune system breakdown if one refuses taking so-called AIDS drugs.

Also noteworthy in this context is the article "AIDS Cocktail", which appeard in the *Times of India* on May 29, 2001. In this piece it says:

"A large number of people from within the general population, that is, those not part of the 'high-risk group' enjoy good health despite testing 'HIV positive' a decade ago. In Mumbai, the 'AIDS capital of India," counseling groups such as Salvation Army and CASA (Counseling and Allied Services), who attend to HIV-positive people from this segment of the population say there is strong evidence to show that the damage caused to the immune system can be reversed. 'This happens when people change their habits of substance abuse, eat nutritious food, involve themselves in community service, practice discipline and hygiene, receive regular counseling, family and social support. Such persons emerge stronger and healthy', says Arun Meitram, a counselor at the Salvation Army clinic.

Incidentally, Salvation Army counselors recall only 15 deaths have occured among the 900 patients they have been following over the past decade. In most cases the cause of death is related to malnutrition or tuberculosis. Says Nagesh Shirgoppikar, a medical consultant to Salvation Army, "Our experience in treating 'HIV positive' persons over the past decade shows that all the components of comprehensive psychological, emotional, physical and conventional medical treatment are very important. If a person is treated wholly, the is fine. Our patients have remained asymptomatic for up to ten years, and enjoy perfect health without anti-retroviral drugs."

Chapter 11

10 Reasons against Measels Vaccination

> *"It is well known that deaths from common infectious diseases declined dramatically before the advent of most vaccines due to improved environmental conditions—even diseases for which there were no vaccines."*[1248]
> Anthony R. Mawson, Professor of epidemiology and biostatistics

> *"[Since the second half of the 19th century,] unquestionably the doctrine of specific etiology has been the most constructive force in the medical research. In reality, however, search for the cause may be a hopeless pursuit because most disease states are the indirect outcome of a constellation of circumstances."*[1249]
> René Dubos, Microbiologist and Pulitzer Prize winner

> *"By the way, I could walk at that time—until I was vaccinated."*
> Boy in wheelchair, series "Big Mouth" (season 1, episode 2)

They are literally bombarding us with recommendations to get vaccinated, whether for cervical cancer, influenza, mumps, measles, etc. If you follow the immunization schedule, a two years old child will be injected with almost 40 vaccines in Germany. In March 2020, Germany made measles vaccination compulsory for children in day-care centres and schools, for teachers and educators, for staff in medical institutions such as hospitals and doctors' surgeries, and for residents and staff in psychiatric centres. But there is no factual substance to support it. Here are the top ten reasons against the measles vaccination:

(1) The Monocausal Mindset—a Virus Causes Measles and Vaccination Is the Only Protective Measure Against It—Is Unrealistic

Waldorf pupils near Stockholm who were not vaccinated against measles, mumps and rubella (MMR) have a lower risk of allergic skin conditions than the vaccinated children from mainstream schools. That was the result of a study published in 1999 in the *Lancet*, one of the world's most respected science journals.[1250] With regard to this study result, vaccination advocates like to retort: Could lifestyle factors such as better nutrition be the actual cause of the reduced risk of allergies in the non-vaccinated Waldorf pupils?

However, the problem with this question is that there are no studies that conversely show that vaccinated children have a reduced risk of allergies compared to their non-vaccinated peers. Also, if there are several possible causes for the development of allergies—including diet and other lifestyle factors as well as the vaccinations themselves—couldn't this also apply to diseases such as measles, which are vaccinated against? But if that's the case, we should also be concentrating on these factors and it would no longer be justified to demand that one should be vaccinated against measles.

The fact that it is unrealistic to assume that only one cause—a virus—could be the primary cause of diseases such as measles has already been discussed in detail in chapter 1 "Society Under the Spell of the One-Dimensional Microbe Theory". Most people who come into contact with someone diagnosed with measles do not develop measles themselves. F

actors other than a "highly infectious" measles virus must therefore determine, or at least play a part in determining, whether or not someone falls ill with the symptoms associated with the term measles.

For example, the health of the intestine, which is teeming with microbes, has been proven to be an important factor when it comes to combatting illness—and its condition is strongly influenced by diet. Additionally, experts point out that the severest cases of measles are usually observed in those affected by previous illnesses, have vitamin A deficiency or are treated with unrestrained fever reduction measures—all factors that are separate from a disease-causing virus.

(2) History Shows: Vaccines Have Nothing to Do with Controlling Measles & Co.

In connection with the fact that aspects such as diet, industrial toxins, lack of exercise, psychological stress, etc. must also be taken into account as causes of measles, Harvard physician Edward H. Kass should be quoted again at this point. He pointed out in a 1971 article in the *Journal of Infectious Diseases*:

„We had accepted some half-truths and had stopped searching for the whole truths. The principal half-truths were that medical research had stamped out the great killers of the past—tuberculosis, diphtheria, pneumonia, puerperal sepsis, etc.—and that medical research and our superior system of medical care were major factors in extending life expectancy. The data on deaths from tuberculosis show that the mortality rate from this disease has been declining steadily since the middle of the 19th century and has continued to decline in almost linear fashion during the past 100 years [till 1970]. There were increases in rates of tuberculosis during wars and under specified adverse local conditions. The poor and the crowded always came off worst of all in war and in peace, but the overall decline in deaths from tuberculosis was not altered measurably by the discovery of the tuberculosis bacillus, the advent of the tuberculin test, the appearance of BCG vaccination, the widespread use of mass screening, the intensive anti-tuberculosis campaigns, or the discovery of streptomycin. It is important that this point be understood in its completeness. The point was made years ago by Wade Hamptom Frost, and more recently by René Dubos, and has been repeatedly stressed through the years by many observers of the public health. Similar trends in mortality have been reported with respect to diphtheria, scarlet fever, rheumatic fever, pertussis, measles, and many others."[1251]

Anthony R. Mawson, professor of epidemiology and biostatistics, echoed this in 2018: "It is well known that deaths from common infectious diseases declined dramatically before the advent of most vaccines due to improved environmental conditions—even diseases for which there were no vaccines."[1252]

For example, the historical course of measles in Germany clearly shows that mass vaccination came at a time when the "measles scare" was essentially over (see diagram 10).

And although the facts are clear, the *Süddeutsche Zeitung* in all seriousness claimed that "vaccination with viruses could almost eradicate measles except for rare outbreaks like the one now [2015] in Berlin."[1253] When asked how the newspaper came to publish such a statement, which clearly contradicts the factual data, the answer was that it was not "the number of deaths but the number of illnesses" that was important for assessing the situation. And these illness figures "were not recorded in West Germany, but they were recorded in the GDR [former East Germany]. There, the number of measles cases fell significantly with the start of vaccinations in 1967."[1254]

But this answer is without substance. First of all, it should be noted that the illness figures are de facto irrelevant when it comes to assessing whether a vaccination against a disease such as measles has worked or is useful. Instead, one must look at the number of deaths, because if no one dies from measles or its complications, or if no serious complications occur there would be no need to vaccinate.

Diagram 10   Measles Deaths in Germany (1961-1995)

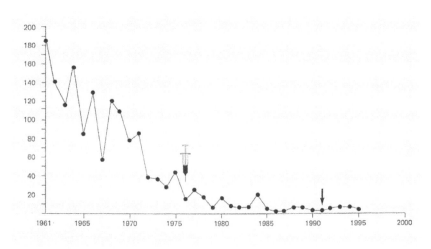

Measles vaccination was introduced in West Germany in the mid-1970s (where the syringe is shown in the graphic), at a time when the "measles scare" was essentially over. The arrow (early 1990s) indicates the combined the data from reunited Germany. Source: Buchwald, Gerhard, Impfen: Das Geschäft mit der Angst (in English: Vaccination: a Business based on Fear), Knaur, 1997, p. 133

Therefore, in his book "Vaccination: a Business based on Fear," the physician Gerhard Buchwald explicitly points out that the vaccination campaigns were started precisely because of serious complications such as encephalitis. And "if the deaths [associated with measles] are decreasing, it means that the complications of this disease, in this case encephalitis, are decreasing, because it is the severe cases that are often fatal." And this decline, as the historical progression curves clearly show, simply cannot be explained by vaccination.

Moreover, the data from the GDR which the *Süddeutsche Zeitung* cites cannot be considered credible. The Enquete Commission of the German Bundestag (of West Germany) concluded that the GDR statisticians as a whole were a "professional gang of counterfeiters" who had deliberately used statistical information as a propaganda tool in the worldwide confrontation between the two opposing social systems (East against West).[1255] Indeed, the GDR Ministry of Health boasted—in propaganda style—that it had been possible to eliminate measles as a widespread disease by using its own vaccine and that this "represented a success that was also highly regarded internationally" (see its "Vademecum für Impfärzte", published in 1972).

We asked the *Süddeutsche Zeitung* to comment on this information twice, but not on both occasions, we did not receive an answer.[1256]

The measles case figures from the GDR, cited by the *Süddeutsche Zeitung*, are also refuted by data from the USA (which can be considered as more reliable than the GDR's data). This shows that in the United States of America both the death rate from measles and the number of measles cases had fallen drastically long before the vaccination was finally introduced.[1257] Moreover, although the German Federal Statistical Office does not have any data on the number of cases of measles, it does have data on the number of cases of diphtheria (see diagram 9 in chapter 8). And this also revealed that vaccinations targeting diphtheria appeared to have nothing to do with the control of the disease.

Vaccination against diphtheria was introduced in Germany in 1925—but subsequently diphtheria diseases actually increased massively and peaked in 1945, the last year of the Second World War, with 250,000 cases per year. Subsequently, the number of cases fell steeply, "although hardly any or very few were vaccinated in the post-war period," as the physician Buchwald writes in his book "Impfen: Das Geschäft mit der Angst" (Vaccination: The Business of Fear). And even the mass vaccination campaigns between 1970 and 1980 had no discernible effect. According to Buchwald, this data also provides clear evidence "that misery, hunger and miserable years are breeding grounds for infectious diseases, as can already be seen from the curves for smallpox, tuberculosis and whooping cough."[1258]

It should be noted that in Germany in the mid-1970s, when measles vaccinations were increasingly rolled out, about 40 measles deaths were reported annually. This number subsequently fell to a few isolated cases per year. However, this does not change the fact that the measles death rate had fallen by around 99.9 percent compared to 1900 and that vaccination cannot, even in the most optimistic light, take credit for this drastic drop. In addition, even after the start of mass vaccination against measles in the 1970s, living conditions in Germany continued to improve gradually, which explains the further drop in the death rate.

(3) Many Vaccinated Persons Get the Disease They Were Vaccinated Against

A study published in the *Journal of Infectious Diseases* in 2013 showed that vaccinations frequently do not offer protection against disease. In 2011, Quebec experienced the largest measles epidemic in North America in a decade. Despite the fact that an estimated 96 percent of the population was vaccinated, the outbreak still occurred and many of the cases were in those who had been vaccinated. The number of measles cases among those who had been vaccinated twice also surprised the investigators. Many of the cases were in the unvaccinated but the study did not address factors apart from vaccination status and as we have already discussed these other factors simply cannot be ignored.[1259]

This example from Quebec shows what is often observed: namely that you can still get the disease that you've had multiple vaccinations against. Indeed, the assertion made by politicians, many doctors and media, almost like a broken record, that high vaccination rates protect against outbreaks of disease is simply not accurate.

This has been proven by several solid reports. For example, in 2008 the journal *Eurosurveillance* reported that in the Czech Republic, despite a programme for vaccination against measles, mumps and rubella (MMR) starting in 1987, thousands of people contracted mumps in 2002 and even more so in 2005. The highest number of cases was in the group of 15 to 19-year-olds, almost 90 percent of whom had been vaccinated twice.[1260]

There are many cases of brain inflammation, specifically subacute sclerosing panencephalitis, or SSPE, in which those affected have been vaccinated once or even several times
before the condition appears.[1261] As Angelika Müller from the organization Eltern für Imp-
faufklärung (EIA) reports in the specialist magazine *impf-report*, even the manufacturer of
a measles vaccine concedes: "There have been reports of SSPE in children who, according
to their medical history, were not infected with the wild measles virus but had received
a measles vaccine. Some of these cases could be the result of an undetected measles
infection during the first year of life or could be due to the measles vaccine.[1262]

(4) There Is No Evidence of the Effectiveness of Vaccination

It is sometimes claimed—such as in the 2018 German film "Eingeimpft" ("Vaccinated")—
that a group lead by the Danish anthropologist and epidemiologist Peter Aaby showed
in several studies in Africa that the live version of the measles vaccine prevented the
disease and reduced infant mortality by about half in a developing country. But Aaby's
data sets were vehemently criticized by orthodox groups—which is not surprising considering that Aaby was based in Guinea-Bissau in West Africa, a region where experience has
shown that obtaining "clean" data is much more difficult than in industrialized countries.

Even the German news magazine *Der Spiegel*, whose reports usually look like a copy
of the press releases of the vaccine manufacturers, wrote the following about Aaby's
live vaccine research: "The vaccination can cause symptoms similar to the disease."[1263]
And Martin Hirte, pediatrician and member of the association Ärzte für individuelle Imp-
fentscheidung (Doctors for Individual Vaccination Decisions), points out that "for dead
vaccines, which are usually administered in infancy, infant mortality actually increases, at
least in African countries."[1264]

Also, Aaby's vaccination studies did not include participants in a placebo group. But that
is what was needed to verify his research results, in order to prove that only the vaccination (and not an improvement in living conditions, for example) was responsible for
the observed decrease in infant mortality. Strictly speaking, he should have carried out a
placebo-controlled double-blind study (see also the chapter on HIV/AIDS). "Placebo-controlled" means that one group of participants (subjects) receives the vaccine and the
control group receives an inactive substance (placebo). And "double-blind" means that

neither those who conduct the study nor the test persons are aware who receives the vaccine and who receives a placebo.

Only a double-blind study, with placebo-control, can determine beyond doubt whether the measles vaccine or any other vaccine is effective and superior to non-vaccination. During a January 2018 deposition, Dr. Stanley Plotkin, one of the world's most influential vaccinologists, acknowledged that researches who try to ascertain vaccine safety without a placebo are in "La La land."[1265] But there are no such studies—not on measles or on many other vaccines. There are a number of studies that claim to be placebo studies, but in most of these studies no inactive placebo substance is used. For example, in the pivotal trial of the cervical cancer vaccine Gardasil, the placebos contained aluminum hydroxide which has its own effects. And in the very few studies where a vaccine was actually compared with a truly inactive placebo, the vaccines came off badly.

One of the most famous examples of this is a large-scale field trial which the WHO implemented in India at the end of the 1960s, on the BCG vaccine (for tuberculosis).[1266] In this trial "a large collective was vaccinated with BCG, while an equally large one remained unvaccinated" (= placebo group). The results: not only did the vaccination show no protective effect against tuberculosis, but significantly more participants fell ill and died in the vaccinated group compared to the unvaccinated group.

Another rare example of a properly controlled trial was in 2012, in which an influenza vaccine was compared with a true placebo in children.[1267] The result was devastating and despite the authors trying to support influenza vaccination they admitted: "There was no statistically significant difference in the risk of confirmed seasonal influenza infection" between the groups. Even worse: the vaccine group "had higher risk of acute respiratory illness," with non influenza infections.[1268]

(5) Studies Show: Unvaccinated People Are Healthier than the Vaccinated

In addition to the few genuine placebo studies mentioned above, there are studies that examine who is in better health: vaccinated or unvaccinated. And the data speaks plainly: unvaccinated people are in noticeably better shape on many measures. For example, an analysis published in May 2020 showed that "vaccination before 1 year of age was associated with increased odds of developmental delays, asthma and ear infection."[1269] The study was unique in that all diagnoses were verified using abstracted medical records from each of the participating pediatric practices. And the lead author Brian S. Hooker from the Department of Sciences and Mathematics at the Simpson University in Redding, California stated:

"The results definitely indicate better health outcomes in children who did not receive vaccines within their first year of life. These findings are consistent with additional research that has identified vaccination as a risk factor for a variety of adverse health outcomes. Such findings merit additional large-scale study of vaccinated and unvaccinated children in order to provide optimal health as well as protection against infectious diseases."

The organization Children's Health Defense, founded by Robert F. Kennedy Jr., reported on this study in an article which stated that "nearly 60 studies have been assembled that find vaccinated cohorts to be far sicker than their unvaccinated peers."[1270]

Moreover, a study published in the journal *Human & Experimental Toxicology* in 2012 revealed that in the USA there was a statistically significant increase in hospital admissions and deaths the more that people were vaccinated.[1271]

A year earlier, the same journal published a paper which revealed that the more vaccinations a country has had, the higher the mortality rate is for babies aged up to one year in that country.[1272] Not less than 34 nations were compared, including several leading industrial nations such as the USA, Germany, Great Britain, France, Denmark, Sweden, Japan, Canada and Australia. Infant mortality was highest in the USA—despite this country having the highest per capita health expenditure and the highest vaccination rates in the world.

Also worth mentioning is the study on the health of children and adolescents in Germany (KiGGS) under the leadership of the Robert Koch-Institute (RKI). The KiGGS data sets include those of unvaccinated persons—and an evaluation showed that vaccinated children and adolescents have many more allergies, suffer more often from developmental disorders and are affected by more infections and chronic diseases than unvaccinated persons. Although—not surprisingly—RKI researchers in the journal *Deutsches Ärzteblatt* 2011 contradicted this evaluation by stating: "Differences in the occurrence of allergic diseases and the frequency of infections between unvaccinated and vaccinated persons are not observed."

There are some objections to this conclusion. First of all, it should be noted that two authors of this paper declared conflicts of interest because they were associated with two large vaccine manufacturers.[1273] In keeping with this, the physicians Martin Hirte and Steffen Rabe began their criticism of the work of the RKI researchers, which is also printed in the *Deutsches Ärzteblatt*, with the following words: "In an article that gives undifferentiated praise to the 'protective vaccinations' in the very first sentence, doubts about objectivity are justified." And they further state that "the unvaccinated children in two of the three age groups investigated tend to have fewer infections and atopic diseases than the vaccinated, and none of the unvaccinated children under ten years of age has bronchial asthma."[1274]

Incidentally, the RKI authors achieved their "desired result" only through unfair trickery. For example, migrants were excluded from the evaluation, which decisively decimated the group of unvaccinated 11 to 17-year-olds in terms of numbers. And this exclusion of migrants was simply justified by claiming that their vaccination documents were often incomplete or missing altogether. But this argument is questionable. Not least because in an earlier publication from the RKI in 2007 they had analyzed the vaccination rates from the KiGGS data—and in this the migrants were included, without the RKI being in any way disturbed by this.

Apart from this, there are further studies that show that unvaccinated people have certain advantages over vaccinated people. These include the Canadian Cohort Study, published in 2008 in the *Journal of Allergy and Clinical Immunology*.[1275] This study investigated whether the timing of vaccination against DTP (diphtheria, tetanus, pertussis) influences the risk of suffering from asthma at the age of seven. Result: The later the vaccination is administered, the lower the risk of asthma.

With all the studies mentioned, you will certainly find fault with something, if you really want to. For example, one could argue that factors that could potentially cause illness or be beneficial to health (smoking, no sport, breastfeeding, nutrition, etc.) were not taken into account in a comprehensive way or that the period of investigation was not long enough.

"Ideally, one would have to carry out a detailed planned study that accompanies a large number of vaccinated and unvaccinated persons over many years and removes all disruptive factors, but such a study has not been carried out so far," says the physician Martin Hirte.[1276]

Therefore, one can only agree with Barbara Loe Fisher, President of the American National Vaccine Information Center (NVIC), who laments that "industry and government agencies have refused to fund sound research to better understand whether there are significant differences in the health status of vaccinated and unvaccinated people."[1277] But why do they refuse to do so? There is enough money and time!

This leads to the suspicion that conclusive studies are not being done for fear that such research might confirm the results suggested by the studies mentioned here. Indeed, such studies that meet acceptable standards and don't support the mainstream pro-vaccine narrative include the 1999 MMR vaccine study with Waldorf pupils in Stockholm, the 1979 WHO trial of BCG vaccines in India and the 2012 placebo-controlled study in children with an influenza vaccine.

(6) Vaccine Manufacturers and Their Studies Lack Credibility

Such suspicion seems all the more justified when one considers that the credibility of the vaccine manufacturers and their studies is already very low. It is further diminished by the fact that there are an increasing number of reports of scientific misconduct, biased reporting, conflicts of interest and downright fraudulent activities by pharmaceutical companies which produce an ever-growing list of vaccines.

The main driver for this development is that there is a lot of potential for profit in the vaccination business. At the beginning of the 21st century, vaccine manufacturers had a turnover of "only" around $5 billion, but by 2014 it was already more than $30 billion— and by 2020 the $60 billion mark will be scratched.[1278] [1279] Klaus Hartmann, who worked for a long time at the Paul Ehrlich Institute responsible for vaccine approval, described in his book "Impfen bis der Arzt kommt: Wenn Pharmakonzernen Profit über Gesundheit geht" (Vaccinate until the doctor comes: When pharmaceutical companies profit over health) how the authorities are being corrupted by the pharmaceutical industry for the purpose of maximizing profits.

This casts even more doubt on the accuracy of the companies' claims about the safety and efficacy of their vaccines—doubts that are confirmed by analyses such as those carried out by the highly regarded Cochrane Collaboration. It has looked at many studies concerning the MMR (measles, mumps, rubella) combined vaccination and it's analysis published in 2012 found that the design of the trials and the presentation of results on the safety of MMR vaccines—both before and after they were launched—were seriously flawed.

In fact, none of the studies included in the review met the methodological criteria of the Cochrane Collaboration. What is particularly noteworthy is what the Cochrane Collaboration stated in relation to the 2001 study by Fombonne and Chakrabarti—a work that was generally considered by medical authorities to be the most convincing refutation to the link between the MMR vaccine and autism. Concerningly, they drew the following conclusion: "The number and possible impact of biases in this study was so high that interpretation of the results is impossible."[1280]

(7) Vaccinations Entail Incalculable Risks

Meanwhile, pivotal studies such as those on measles lack sufficient power because they do not have enough test subjects and were too short-term in duration to be able to record severe side effects with statistical certainty. Therefore, no one can say with certainty how many people are harmed by these vaccinations.

As reported by the *impf-report*, an average of 130 vaccination complications are reported in Germany every year following measles vaccination, including four reports of permanent damage and one death. However, according to an expert estimate quoted by the Paul Ehrlich Institute (PEI) in the *Bundesgesundheitsblatt*, at least 95 percent of adverse reactions are not reported. Therefore, the actual number of annual vaccination complications would be more than 2,600 and potentially 19 deaths—and some estimate the numbers to be even higher. Incidentally, the PEI says it lacks the solid data to refute such estimates.

In this context, Anthony R. Mawson from the Department of Epidemiology and Biostatistics at the Jackson State University wrote in 2018: "Over $3 billion has been paid by the US Vaccine Injury Compensation Program for vaccine-associated injuries and deaths, and only about 1 percent of vaccine-associated injuries are officially reported to the Vaccine Adverse Events Reporting System. The long-term effects of vaccination on children's health remain virtually unknown but are assumed to be limited solely to prevention of the targeted disease. Studies have been recommended by the Institute of Medicine to address this question. However, randomized controlled trials, the 'gold standard' for such research, have been considered unethical because they normally involve depriving some children of the needed vaccines in order to create a control group. Vaccines also have a quasi-religious status as a 'sacred cow' of medicine and public health, which has discouraged scientific inquiry, and critics are often attacked personally and pejoratively labeled as 'anti-vaxxers.'"[1281]

In other words: There is no way to exclude or even calculate vaccination risk across a population. It is often said that there is no evidence of a causal link between the reported complications and the vaccinations. But this claim is irrelevant, if only because the most

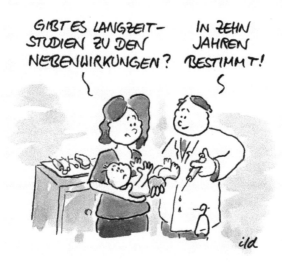

Mother: *"Are there long-term studies on the side effects?"*
Doctor: *"Certainly in ten years!"* © Ingmar Decker, www.achecht.de

359

pertinent question is whether the authorities and manufacturers are able to rule out this link—and they simply cannot.

It should also be borne in mind that a causal link between vaccinations and adverse complications is much less frequently identified or reported than would be appropriate. The reasons for this include the following:

- The vaccine is not compared with an inactive placebo, see "4. There Is No Evidence of the Effectiveness of Vaccination" above.
- Those who carry out the research or studies usually assume that the vaccines are unlikely to or cannot cause adverse effects.
- The studies are not designed to identify vaccination complications.
- Only the administration of one vaccine is investigated, although in reality several vaccines are usually given at once.

And if very poorly tested active ingredients are then given to the most vulnerable population groups—babies, and children for instance—this can hardly be considered ethical. Unfortunately, this is often the approach taken in medical practice when it comes to vaccinations.

(8) Antibody Titer: Surrogat Marker With High Belief Factor

Since the companies refuse to conduct placebo-controlled double-blind studies, the so-called antibody titers (number of antibodies in the blood), i.e. only laboratory values, are used instead in the approval studies. However, as the magazine *impf-report* found, even the federal authorities have been unable to provide evidence that there is a health benefit for people who have a high antibody titer.[1282] And even various orthodox sources confirm that the amount of so-called antibodies in the blood does not reliably predict a person's immunity.[1283] Here are a few voices:

- Ulrich Heininger, member of Germany's Permanent Vaccination Commission (Ständige Impfkommission, STIKO), writes in his book "Handbuch Kinderimpfung" (Child Vaccination Manual): "It is neither necessary nor useful to determine the effectiveness of a vaccination by taking blood samples and determining antibodies after the vaccination has been carried out. On the one hand, even an antibody determination does not provide a reliable statement about the presence or absence of vaccination protection, and on the other hand it is simply too expensive."

- *arznei-telegramm* (April 2001 edition): "Even increases in titer caused by vaccines are unreliable substitute criteria for effectiveness. What benefit or harm the vaccinated person can expect cannot be deduced from such findings. The regulatory authorities are required to review their requirements."

- "Impfkompendium" (Vaccination Compendium), published by Heinz Spiess, 5th edition 1999: "A conclusion from the level of the measured titer on the immune status regarding protection against reoccurrence of the disease is currently not possible."

- *Epidemiological Bulletin* (EpiBull) No. 30 (2012), p. 299: "Antibody levels are not indicative of a possible cellular immunity."

- Answer of the Paul-Ehrlich-Institute to a question (May 13, 2006) from Hans Tolzin, editor of the *impf-report*: "There is no general statement of the Paul-Ehrlich-Institute that a sufficiently high regarded specific antibody titer is a guarantee for non-disease."

(9) The Worthless Measles Infection Experiment from 1911

The world's most important publication by vaccination experts is without a doubt "Vaccines," a compendium of over 1000 pages. If one searches the publication for the historical references that established the currently prevailing doctrine on measles, one is referred to a contagion experiment from 1911. This was carried out by researchers John F. Anderson and Joseph Goldberger in Washington and, according to "Vaccines," represented the pinnacle of measles research until 1954.

After various attempts to transmit measles in small animals had failed, Anderson and Goldberger were the first to carry out experiments with rhesus monkeys. They may have been encouraged by Landsteiner and Popper's famous (but in reality lousy) contagion transmission attempts, which they had made in Vienna in 1908 in the context of polio (see Chapter 2, subchapter "Polio: Pesticides Such as DDT and Heavy Metals under Suspicion").

The aim of the measles contagion experiments was to cause fever in the monkeys as well as a rash typical of measles. Hans Tolzin, editor of the *impf-report*, has analyzed the experiments in detail.[1284] His conclusion: "According to the understanding at the time, the experiment may have been scientifically up to date, but according to today's understanding, it is at best useful as a warning medical-historical example of how not to do it."

A total of nine rhesus monkeys were injected with defibrinated blood (i.e. blood that is free of the glycoprotein fibrinogen) from four human measles patients. Of these nine pitiful animals, four showed measles symptoms (fever and rash). And assuming that nothing was faked in the experiments (which is not in the realm of the impossible, considering that, as described at the beginning of chapter 2, even Koch and Pasteur gained their fame through scientific fraud), this result shows only one thing: that monkeys can produce measles-like symptoms by injecting them with blood from diseased humans.

However, this does not realistically illustrates the infection route as it should occur in real life – namely through sneezing or physical contact.

The natural route of infection (contagion) could easily have been reproduced, for example by spraying the suspected pathogen into the throat and face via an aerosol. But such experiments have not been documented. Since this drastic physical intervention – the injection of patient's blood – was able to produce disease symptoms just in a few of the nine monkeys, it is impossible to postulate any consistent causal relationship and hence build a sound hypothesis on it.

It is also likely that none of the nine monkeys would have developed disease symptoms if they had only been sprayed with an aerosol.

The situation is further complicated by the fact that no control experiments were made. This means that there was no comparison group with monkeys injected with blood from healthy people. This would have made it possible to rule out that the manner of the experiment (i.e. injecting foreign biological material) alone caused the observed symptoms. Moreover, not even the first of Koch's postulates was fulfilled, i.e. no recording of the alleged virus was made. This is not surprising, since in 1911 the existence of viruses was pure conjecture, since the resolution of light microscopes were not sufficient to visualise viruses (see chapter 1, section "Viruses: Lethal Mini-Monsters?").

(10) As a Rule, the Opposite Is True of What the Media Reports About Viruses

In the previous chapters we have already explained in detail how irresponsibly the mass media misses the point when it comes to the subject of viruses. Sadly, the topic of measles is no exception. As an example, let us briefly trace the hysteria that was triggered in early 2015 by sensationalist media coverage. Berlin's then Senator for Health, Mario Czaja, announced in a press release[1285] that boy in Berlin had died of measles while not being vaccinated against it.

The whole thing culminated, among other things, on German television's ARD talk show *hart aber fair* when medical doctor and TV presenter Eckart von Hirschhausen dismissed any debate and called a critical attitude towards measles vaccination "bullshit to the power of 10."

And the physician Werner Bartens, in his function as head of the science department at the German daily newspaper *Süddeutsche Zeitung*, also joined the mandatory measles vaccination chorus led by Justice Minister Heiko Maas.[1286] In his article entitled "Dangerous Ignorance," he wrote to his readers' consciences that such a compulsory vaccination resulted from "responsibility—for oneself, but also for others."[1287]

But again in this case, the media did not show the first signs of having done their job and failed to ask the necessary critical questions. For the whole thing was based on a lie or at least a false report. In the press release by Senator Czaja, which formed the starting point for the triggered panic, it was initially stated that the boy had "no chronic pre-existing conditions" and the mass media carried this message to their audience of millions.

However when pressed, the Berlin authorities had to admit that the boy did indeed have a "previous illness." But the authorities did not want to disclose what kind of pre-existing condition it was.

They were equally reluctant to provide any evidence confirming that, "The measles disease alone was the cause of the child's death" and not the boy's previous illness or any errors in treatment. Likewise, it was not made clear if the poor child would have survived measles if he had not been affected by his previous illness and/or medical treatment.

The question of whether the boy was not vaccinated against measles also needed clarification because it was reported by the deceased boy's kindergarten that he had indeed

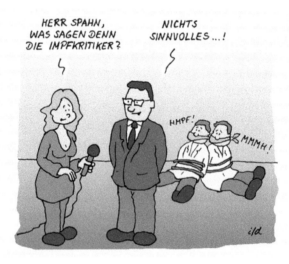

Newswoman: "Mister Spahn, what do the vaccination critics say? Jens Spahn, German Minister of Health: "Nothing meaningful ...!" © *Ingmar Decker, www.achecht.de*

been vaccinated. The fact that the mass media failed to probe into this matter is all the more serious when one considers the comments from physician Steffen Rabe: "Only a complete clarification of this death can restore the credibility of the Berlin health authorities, which was badly damaged by the (dis)information campaigns, and can protect the actually renowned Charité [Clinic] from the suspicion of being misused by political-media-pharmaceutical campaigns."[1288]

The case illustrates just how much media and politics stray from the facts to promote vaccination against measles and other diseases.

Addendum: The Measles Virus Lawsuit

For the sake of completeness, the "measles virus lawsuit" should also be briefly mentioned here, as it caused a lot of attention in Germany and had a remarkable outcome. It started when the microbiologist Stefan Lanka offered a reward of €100,000 in 2011 to anyone who, by means of a scientific publication, could prove the existence of and the size of the measles virus.

In response, the physician David Bardens submitted six publications, but Lanka felt the conditions of his tender had not been fulfilled. Subsequently a disgruntled Bardens sued Lanka. In March 2015, the Ravensburg Land Court ruled that Lanka had to pay the €100,000, including interest. However, Lanka appealed against this ruling and won the case before the Stuttgart Higher Regional Court in February 2016. Although Bardens appealed against this ruling to the BGH (the highest court in Germany), the appeal was dismissed in December 2016.

Lanka then proudly announced: "Five experts have participated in the process and presented the results of scientific studies. All five experts, including Prof. Dr. Dr. Andreas Podbielski, who was appointed by the court of first instance, agreed that none of the six publications submitted to the trial contained scientific evidence of the existence of the alleged measles virus." This is all the more remarkable when one considers that "the six publications presented in the trial are the authoritative publications on the 'measles virus'" and that "apart from these six publications, there are demonstrably no other publications in which scientific methods have been used to attempt to prove the existence of the measles virus."[1289]

Strictly speaking, the judgement does not mean that there is no scientific evidence for the existence of the measles virus. The court "only" ruled that the six scientific publications submitted by Bardens did not meet the conditions of Lanka's offer of a reward—because they required the submission of "one" single scientific publication with complete proof. The judgement thus allows the conclusion that "the one" publication with complete proof of the existence of a specific disease-causing measles virus does not exist.

But one should actually expect there to be a single(!) conclusive study on a virus, because otherwise—whether with HIV or with SARS-CoV-2—individual studies are usually cited from which the existence of the virus is supposed to have been established. No more than one study is needed in order to show the processes that are or would be necessary to detect a virus.

So the question arises: Why not simply carry out an individual study proving the existence of the measles virus to dispel any lasting doubts? There would undoubtedly be more than enough funds and time for this ...

Chapter 12

Total Corona Mania: Worthless PCR Tests, Lethal Drugs – and Mortality Data that Makes a Viral Cause Impossible

"The PCR test doesn't tell you that you are sick.[1290] *These tests cannot detect free, infectious viruses at all."*[1291]
Kary Mullis, who Ggot the 1993 Nobel Prize
in Chemistry for the invention of PCR

"There is very little conclusive evidence as to whether measures such as school or restaurant closures are actually effective. Not every question or doubt is trivialization or conspiracy mania. It would be worthwhile to deal with the arguments."[1292]
Jürgen Windeler, Head of the IQWiG, Germany's most important
independent institution for evaluating health care measures

"We are in the field of speculation. Basic rights are restricted without having exactly usable numbers, and I consider this to be an absurdity. The daily infection figures [of the Robert Koch-Institute] are worth nothing."[1293] [1294]
Matthias Schrappe, Professor of medicine and former
CO-head of the German Advisory Council on Health

Virology, Politics and the Media vs. Common Sense

In 1882, the German philosopher Friedrich Nietzsche wrote in aphorism 224 of his book "Die fröhliche Wissenschaft" ("The Joyous Science"): "I fear that animals regard humans as beings of their own kind, who have lost their common "animal" sense in a highly dangerous way."

Almost 140 years later when total corona madness broke out worldwide in 2020, how prescient he seemed with his uneasiness about human nature. In fact, the whole world was de facto more or less put into quarantine, although there was (and still is) no scientific proof whatsoever for the theory that in December 2019 a new and highly dangerous subtype of a corona virus (SARS-CoV-2) started to cause lung diseases (COVID-19) in hu-mans in the Chinese city of Wuhan, a city of 11 million people, and then spread practically all over the world.

A pivotal point in this context is that the so-called polymerase chain reaction (PCR) tests, which were claimed to be rock-solid in their ability to detect SARS-CoV-2 infections, were (and still are) without validity and thus worthless in reality. That the so-called SARS-CoV-2 PCR tests cannot detect such an infection was even confirmed by a *Lancet* study in mid-November 2020[1296] – and a few days later by a German court.[1297]

The phony nature of the official narrative is exposed by the fact that central figures in the "play", including the Robert Koch Institute (RKI) and the Charité virologist and advisor to the German government Christian Drosten, were unable to answer the most fundamental questions which we had asked in March 2020, even after repeated requests (four of the questions asked and the complete list of those contacted are listed in the box on pages 436/437).

This is incomprehensible. After all, the official theory on SARS-CoV-2 can only be correct if the aspects we are addressing with our questions have been properly clarified. And if the aspects had actually been clarified, answering the questions should have been easy for all the authorities we contacted. The science historian Horace F. Judson writes about this "model of how not to respond" in his book "The Great Betrayal. Fraud in Science":

„Central to the problem of misconduct is the response of institutions when charges erupt. Again and again the actions of senior scientists and administrators have been the very model of how not to respond. They have tried to smother the fire. Such flawed responses are altogether typical of misconduct cases."[1298]

We have already quoted Judson in Chapter 3 on HIV/AIDS and with HIV/AIDS, we have indeed come full circle. The irrational mega-panic of SARS-CoV-2/COVID-19 was only possible because HIV/AIDS had already set the stage. The importance of this point cannot be stressed enough.

It is important to bear in mind what we discussed at the end of Chapter 2 in the section "The Virus Disaster of the 1970s – and HIV as Salvation in the 1980s". At the end of the

„When an experiment is challenged no matter who it is challenged by, it's your responsibility to check. That is an ironclad rule of science ... One of the great strengths of American science ... is that even the most senior professor, if challenged by the lowliest technician or graduate student, is required to treat them seriously and to consider their criticisms."

Howard Temin, Biologist and Nobel laureate in medicine

— —

Neither the Robert Koch-Institute, nor the virologist Christian Drosten (Charité Berlin/Advisor to Germany's Government), nor the physician Alexander S. Kekulé (University of Halle), nor Hartmut Hengel and Ralf Bartenschlager (Society for Virology), nor Thomas Löscher (member of the Federal Association of German Internists), nor Ulrich Dirnagl (neurologist/Charité Berlin), nor the virologist Georg Bornkamm were able to answer the following questions—even after repeated requests:

1. The *Süddeutsche Zeitung* article "Too good to be true" (March 24, 2020) states: "Ulrich Dirnagl says that the thesis that without the tests no one would possibly be interested in this virus has been disproved with regard to [the horrible TV pictures from] Italy."

But even if we assume that the mortality in Italy has risen significantly, how can we rule out the possibility that people have died prematurely as a result of non-microbial factors such as the administration of drugs?

A *Lancet* study, for example, shows that out of 41 patients who tested "positive" when they came to hospital in Wuhan, China, at the beginning of the crisis, all received antibiotics and 38 (i.e. almost all) of them

received the highly toxic antiviral drug oseltamivir. Six of the patients (15 percent) subsequently died.

2. If there are "no unmistakable specific symptoms" for the COVID-19 disease and a "differentiation of the various pathogens is clinically not possible," as the physician Thomas Löscher concedes—and if, in addition, non-microbial factors (industrial toxins, drugs, etc.) come into question as the cause of the most severe respiratory disease such as pneumonia, how can we be sure that only what is called SARS-CoV-2 can be considered as the cause of the symptoms of COVID-19?

3. Also leading virologists such as Luc Montagnier as well that complete cleaning of particles (‚‚purification") is an indispensable pre-requisite for the detection of a virus (see quotes in the section "Lousy, More Lousy, Corona PCR Test" later in this chapter).

However, the authors of two significant papers, which are mentioned in connection with the detection of SARS-CoV-2, concede on request that the electron microscope images shown in their work do not depict completely purified particles. But how can one then conclude with certainty that the RNA gene sequences „pulled" from the tissue samples prepared in these studies and to which the PCR tests are then „calibrated" belong to a very specific virus—in this case SARS-CoV-2? Especially since studies also show that the very substances (including antibiotics) used in the test tube experiments (in vitro) can „stress" the cell culture in such a way that new gene sequences can be formed that were previously undetectable?

4. If the PCR test is not sufficient to detect an HIV infection, why should it be good enough to detect a SARS-CoV-2 infection?

1970s – not least as a result of the swine flu disaster at that time – the US Centers for Disease Control and Prevention (CDC) and the National Institutes of Health (NIH) came under massive political pressure. In order to rehabilitate themselves, a new "war" would need to be waged. Ideally this would be against a microbe, because "infectious diseases" remained – despite the recent setbacks – the most effective way to catch public attention, gain blind loyalty and open government pockets.

In fact, Red Cross officer Paul Cumming told the *San Francisco Chronicle* in 1994 that "the CDC increasingly needed a major epidemic" at the beginning of the 1980s "to justify its existence."[1299] And the HIV/AIDS theory was a salvation for American epidemic authorities.

Since the establishment of the HIV=AIDS dogma, the virus hunters have enjoyed an almost Godlike status. And gods are not to be questioned. The "big bang" for this HIV=AIDS narrative was when Hollywood actor Rock Hudson was presented to the world as the first megastar with AIDS in the mid-1980s. In order to do justice to the immeasurable significance of this event – ultimately also for SARS-CoV-2 – we sketch the deceptive AIDS legacy surrounding Rock Hudson in the epilogue of this book.[1300]

With the already unbelievable idea of the HIV=AIDS dogma that sex could mean certain death, in 2020 the even more perverse message spread with the corona panic, namely that even a contact-free encounter can lead to infection and death.

And once again a completely unfounded scientific theory (that a new coronavirus threatened all of mankind) was the basis for influential articles being published in medical journals. This fuelled a panic of undreamt proportions. Numerous papers were printed in which the published data was interpreted in terms of the completely unproven virus hypothesis, even though most of the time the data actually contradicted this theory.

Despite the absolute lack of evidence for the SARS-CoV-2=COVID-19 dogma, the political policymakers did not shy away from draconian restrictions launching attacks on liberty and basic human rights. Entire cities were quarantined Wuhan-style and even nationwide curfews were imposed. French President Emmanuel Macron, for example, ordered a lockdown for his country on 17 March 2020.

Following this, citizens were generally not allowed to leave their houses—unless they had compelling reasons, for example because they had to go to work, the doctor or to buy food. Brief periods of exercise were "permitted" close to home, but only if one was alone, or was walking the dog. Additionally, hundreds of thousands of policemen and gendarmes were supposed to control the curfew (see the report in the box "*Mopo* reporter in the restricted zone: How the holidays in Italy turned into a nightmare").

According to official figures, only 150 people had died of corona in France by then i.e the common sense of a normal citizen is quite sufficient to realize that the actions of the policymakers were completely unfounded. This is true even if it is assumed that the people concerned were killed by a new virus called SARS-CoV-2, as the virologists, politicians and mass media were never tired of pointing out.

There is no question that it is always a sad event when a person dies. But this happens countless times every day, because human life is finite with high-tech medicine or not. So it is crucial that we put the number 150 into realistic context. For example, the 150 or so deaths ascribed to SARS-CoV-2 happened over a period of about 30 days-that would be five corona deaths a day. In France, however, a total of almost 620,000 people die every year—around 1,700 every single day. With this in mind, five SARS-CoV-2 deaths per day seems trivial.

And even if you take the 860 deaths that were ascribed to the alleged "horror virus" in the statistics up to the 23rd of March 2020, this results in a daily average of 23 corona deaths. And even this number is still "puny", both in absolute terms and in comparison to the 1,700 total deaths per day in France.

It is also revealing to see parallels in other areas. According to analyses, particulate matter is responsible for the premature death of around 50,000 people in the Grande Nation every year—around 130 people a day. A 2019 study by the Max Planck Institute for Chemistry revealed that the number of people who die prematurely in Germany due to particulate matter is as high as 120,000 (the equivalent of about 330 people a day). In 2015, the French Senate classified the particulate matter problem as extremely precarious, partly because it generates just over €100 billion in increased health costs, reduces economic productivity and lowers agricultural yields. It would also leave Paris in a very bad position vis-à-vis the EU.

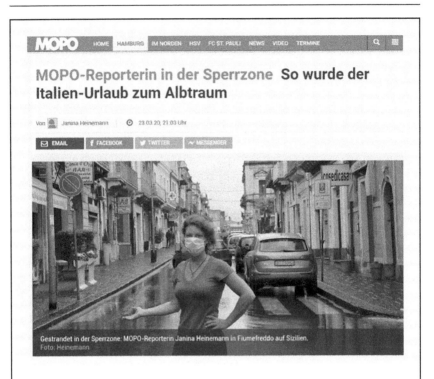

MOPO | HOME HAMBURG IM NORDEN HSV FC ST. PAULI NEWS VIDEO TERMINE | 🔍 ☰

MOPO-Reporterin in der Sperrzone So wurde der Italien-Urlaub zum Albtraum

Von 🖼 Janina Heinemann | ⏱ 23.03.20, 21:03 Uhr

✉ EMAIL | f FACEBOOK | 🐦 TWITTER | ~ MESSENGER

Gestrandet in der Sperrzone: MOPO-Reporterin Janina Heinemann in Fiumefreddo auf Sizilien.
Foto: Heinemann

On 23 March 2020, Janina Heinemann from the Hamburg newspaper Morgenpost (Mopo) reported on how she was caught off-guard during her working holiday in Sicily on the 10th of March when the „zona rossa," the restricted „red zone," was extended to the whole of Italy. „What was initially just annoying turned out to be a nightmare," writes Heinemann. She tried to leave— but the next available flight was a week after the new decree. „A long week ... during which there were always new, stricter rules implemented", Heinemann groans. „For example, you need an ‚Autocertificazione,' a self-declaration, to leave the house. Name, address, identity card and telephone number must be on it. And the most important thing: the reason why you are on the road. Shopping and doctor's visits are okay, going for a walk is not."

"Psychological ordeal"

When she managed to reach the airport with difficulty, it was particularly „spooky." „Empty aisles, dark restaurants and worst of all, just a handful of people. All cleaning staff. None of the check-in counters were manned. I felt panic rising up, but then calmed down because my flight was still displayed normally on the destination board. But then it was canceled ... [Finally] I stood alone at the airport and cried." Further, the two days in the hotel „were a psychological ordeal," especially because of the „imprisonment." A hotel room, a balcony, no other people."

Like "a disaster film"

Getting a flight seemed almost impossible, even after Heinemann asked the German embassy in Italy for help. „The flights were ... all fully booked. In the meantime I've become resigned ... even if I'm in a kind of paradise here: A Paradise that you cannot leave is a prison. No matter how beautiful it is."

On the 3rd of May, Heinemann then reported in the Mopo how, after a real odyssey, she got „through all of Italy and Switzerland to northern Germany", where she lives—and that "this longest journey" of her life "was like a disaster film."

One of the main causes of life-shortening air pollution is the transport sector in France, which is responsible for 59 percent of nitrogen oxide emissions and almost 20 percent of the particulate matter emissions. In 2015, there were calls for increased efforts to combat air pollution, but not much has happened since than. Certainly the attempt to bring all the polluters to a halt paled in comparison to the measures that were taken against whole societies regarding corona.

Of course, the means of transport—cars, trains and planes—as well as other sources of fine dust such as power stations, waste incineration plants and heating systems in residential buildings are a result of coexistence in highly industrialized societies. Correspondingly it is difficult to take measures that actually reduce fine dust significantly and at the same time not destroy the economy and social fabric of society.

Instead of politicians slamming on the brakes of society and the economy, they should have looked at the bigger picture with regards to corona. The resulting collateral damage led to the destruction of livelihoods and even suicides, such as that of 19-year-old Emily Owen on the 18th of March and Finance Minister of Hesse Thomas Schäfer on the 28th of March. Politicians would never have accepted these casualties if they were the result of the air pollution/particulate matter problem.

The fact that such a course of action is not based on any rational logic is also evident when one looks at other areas. For example, in 2016 world hunger increased again.[1304] Nine million people per annum die of hunger and its consequences—and thus officially, more than AIDS, malaria and tuberculosis combined. Hunger kills a child every ten seconds on this planet—and according to Jean Ziegler, the world-famous critic of capitalism and former UN Special Rapporteur on the Right to Food, it's worse: a child dies every five seconds.[1305]

Poor nutrition is responsible for almost half of all deaths among children under five years of age.[1306] In total, the world records nine million starvation deaths per year - that means about 25,000 tragic deaths per day.[1307] In comparison, according to official data on the 23rd of March 2020, 240 people worldwide died from SARS-CoV-2 in a day (a number without scientific basis as we shall see). That is one hundredth of what can be ascribed to hunger.

Here it is also incomprehensible that the efforts being made to combat hunger, which is associated with unimaginable suffering and above all affects those most in need of protection, namely babies and children, are insignificant compared to the corona responses. Jean Ziegler puts it in an even more scandalous way by saying: "Every child who dies of hunger is murdered." And the perpetrators would be "all of us, if we remain silent, and definitely the bandits in the banks and hedge funds who speculate in agricultural commodities on the commodity exchanges and drive up prices." As a result, the well over 1 billion people in the slums, who would have to live on less than $2 a day, could no longer buy enough food. These speculators are "mass murderers."[1309]

This also means—and this makes the situation even more scandalous—that it would be easy to eliminate hunger, for example, by fairly distributing the available food in the world in sufficient quantities. At the same time, food price speculation, which benefits almost no one but the speculators themselves, needs to be curtailed. Or we could simply "skim" funds from the exorbitant pot of global military expenditure, which in 2019 was brimming at record levels with a little more than US$ 1.8 trillion.[1310]

And we wouldn't even hav e to skim off that much. "With a fraction of the global military expenditure, hunger in the world could be eliminated and poverty fought," stated Sevim Dagdelen, deputy chairman and disarmament policy spokeswoman of the parliamentary

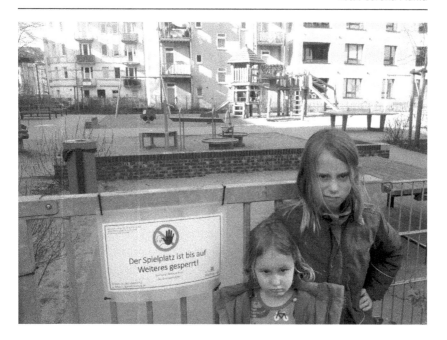

Children, with their strong drive for play and freedom, were particularly severely hit by the draconian political measures. Many parents, out of panic of infection, forbade their children to meet with their friends. Schools and kindergartens were closed down and even playgrounds were forbidden to be entered (the photo above is from March 25, 2020 and shows a playground in the Winderhude district of Hamburg). All this in a time when it's already harder than ever to experience open spaces and wild zones, where a child may just be a child and can go on voyages of discovery. Even a Lancet study came to the conclusion that there is "no data on the relative contribution of school closures to transmission control", whereby „Data from the SARS outbreak on the mainland of China, Hong Kong, and Singapore [in 2002] suggest that school closures did not contribute to the control of the epidemic."[1308]

group of the German Left Party in April 2019.[1311] Only 0.5 percent of the 1.8 trillion US dollars, i.e. a "paltry" 9 billion US dollars,[1312] would be enough. Meanwhile, aid organisations warned in early April 2020 that "far more people" would die from the consequences of lockdowns than from Covid-19 itself. The resulting global recession from lockdowns could plunge 35 to 65 million people into absolute poverty and many of them will be threatened with starvation.

This is not a new idea after all. Former German Chancellor and Nobel Peace Prize Laureate Willy Brandt wrote in his book "Organized Madness: arms race and world hunger," first published in 1985:

"We don't have to put up with the cold-blooded political and economic bureaucrats arguing away simple truths or suffocating them in a tangle of trivialities ... [The question arises] why is it not possible and why should the states of the world not be able to redirect a few percent of the military expenditure. And in such a way that the branched off, diverted funds are used for meaningful, peacekeeping purposes and for mass hunger and blatant misery to disappear."[1313]

How has it come to pass that such a serious problem, which brings so much misery and suffering, has not been actively tackled by policymakers for decades? Why isn't the media "sounding the alarm" to draw attention to it? It brings to mind what Amartya Sen, Harvard economist and Nobel Prize winner, said:

"Famines do not happen in countries with a free press. For famine results from a problem of food distribution, not from an absolute lack of food. A free press would create such a furore that the government would act accordingly."[1314]

If these words are taken seriously, it follows that not only politics but also the media have failed humanity blatantly. Of course, this is not only true with regards to world hunger, but especially with regards to the reporting on corona/COVID-19. In a sick twist, the action of politicians regarding corona even threatened to "expand the world food crisis," as the group of experts of the UN World Food Council Committee on World Food Security (CFS) reported on the 1st of April, 2020. Once more, the media did not act as an impartial critic of the powerful, but only as a propaganda magnifier for politicians and favored virologists.

One example of this is how the media passed on completely unsubstantiated prophecies of doom by so-called experts, such as British epidemiologist Neil Ferguson of Imperial College in London, to their audience of millions.

On 16 March 2020, Ferguson published a study in which he claimed that without a lockdown, corona deaths in the UK would be close to 510,000 and 2.2 million in the USA. This prompted the British government to order a lockdown just one day later. The USA and France also relied on Ferguson's data—and Christian Drosten, corona consultant to the German government, and the health policy expert Karl Lauterbach of the German Social Democratic Party also referred to "Professor Lockdown's" models. This is astounding, if one considers that Ferguson's predictions in the past had been complete flops—and yet they have repeatedly served as a basis for political decisions.

In 2001, a team led by the 1968-born researcher created models of foot-and-mouth disease that prompted the British government to order the culling of around 7 million cattle, sheep and pigs. This not only caused incredible suffering for the animals affected, but also cost the British economy an estimated 12 to 18 billion pounds. Later on an analysis by Michael Thrusfield, Professor of Veterinary Epidemiology at the University of Edinburgh, made scathing criticism of Ferguson's forecasting models.

Nevertheless, Ferguson was appointed a member of the Order of the British Empire in 2002. And he was allowed to continue with his prophecies. In the same year, the epidemiologist predicted that up to 50,000 people in Great Britain would probably die of Creutzfeldt-Jakob disease, allegedly caused by the consumption of BSE-contaminated beef (see Chapter 5 on BSE)—and that this number could possibly rise to 150,000. In the end, 177 deaths occurred on the island according to official figures.

Three years later, in 2005, Ferguson predicted that up to 200 million people worldwide could die from "bird flu." In the end, the WHO counted 440 deaths (for the period 2003 to 2015). And in 2009, when the "swine flu" panic was being frenetically stirred up by politicians and the media worldwide, Ferguson was also involved. Based on his analyses, the British government estimated that a "reasonable worst-case scenario" for "swine flu" would result in up to 65,000 deaths in Great Britain. But in the end, only 457 people officially died of it.

So it is hardly surprising that Ferguson's calculations lacked any medical-scientific basis when it came to corona and the whole thing had the taste of bought science. Not only did Ferguson receive research funds from the government immediately after his prophecies of doom. His activities at the Imperial College in London were also funded by the Gates Foundation, which is closely linked to Big Pharma. In fact, the Imperial College itself received almost $80 million from the Gates Foundation in 2020 alone.

But that is not all. The epidemiologist also acted duplicitously when he allowed his lover to visit him at home during the time he was lecturing the public on the need for strict social distancing (see screenshot from page 1 of *The Sun* newspaper from 5 May 2020).[1315]

The media would only have to rummage through their memory a little to realize that one must assess the statements of the world's "top" virologists very critically. "On the

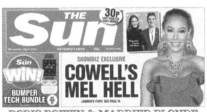
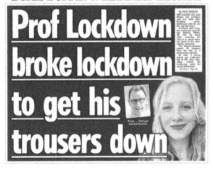

In mid-March 2020, British epidemiologist Neil Ferguson predicted there would be around 510,000 corona deaths for Great Britain and around 2.2 million for the United States if the countries did not implement the strictest control measures. This prompted lockdowns in both countries as well as many others. But Ferguson's calculations not only lacked any medical-scientific basis, but also had the taste of bought politics. "Professor Lockdown" was consulted by the British government for emergency coronavirus research after his prophecies of doom and received huge amounts of tax payer funds. In addition, the work of 1968 born Ferguson at the Imperial College in London was financed by the Gates Foundation; the Imperial College received almost $80 million from the multi-billionaire's foundation in 2020, which is closely linked to Big Pharma. Incidentally, Ferguson did not care about his own instructions as he allowed his beloved to visit him at home while he was teaching the public about the need for strict social distancing, as The Sun *(and other media) reported on the 5th of May 2020.* Source: Screenshot of The Sun

whole, however, the media's memory simply does not seem to be good enough," commiserates the German internist Wolfgang Wodarg, who publicly argued that the solution to the corona problem was to isolate the alarmists[1316] and thus came under fire from mainstream media.

"For example, it had been forgotten again that the 'swine flu pandemic', which the WHO predicted in 2009 in conjunction with the mass media, was in fact one of the mildest flu waves in history," according to Wodarg. "And in the end, it mainly had been the side effects of the vaccines that caused great suffering in the form of narcolepsy and even led to lawsuits for damages" (see end of chapter 9).

The fact that media outlets such as Der Spiegel and The Guardian have received millions from the Gates Foundation has not exactly strengthened their desire to take a critical look at the extremely poor forecasting performance of the supposed experts.[1317]

And the chief promoter of these shocking scenarios in Germany was Christian Drosten, the director of the Institute for Virology at the Charité and advisor to the German government. On 6th March, he told the *Osnabrücker Zeitung* that in Germany "278,000 corona deaths can be expected."[1318]

But the data available at that time was so lousy that such prophecies of doom were not justified in the slightest. After all, "We don't even know if the risk of dying if you get infected with coronavirus is higher than with influenza or many of other virus infections, and most of those who die are old and suffer from comorbidity, just like with influenza," wrote Peter C. Gøtzsche, professor of medicine and co-founder of the Cochrane Collaboration, on the 21st of March 2020 in his personal blog *Deadly Medicine & Organized Crime*. "The panic looks like an unfortunate overreaction."[1319]

John P. A. Ioannidis, Professor of Medicine and Epidemiology at Stanford University, also advised caution: "The data collected on SARS-CoV-2 so far are utterly unreliable," he stated. "The current coronavirus disease, Covid-19, has been called a once-in-a-century pandemic. But it may also be a once-in-a-century evidence fiasco."[1320] [1321]

Incidentally, caution would have been advisable, if only because practically all super-virologists had repeatedly been wrong with their forecasts in the past. For example, at the end of 2004, Klaus Stöhr, then coordinator of the influenza programme at the World Health Organisation (WHO), said in connection with the avian flu that even in the most optimistic scenario, between two and seven million people would die and billions would fall ill worldwide. But in the end, this was a ridiculous overestimate (see chapter 7 about "Avian Flu").

Previously, the magazine *Der Spiegel*, had recklessly promoted Stöhr's avian flu statements with the headline "Millions of deaths: WHO considers global epidemic unavoidable."[1322] Such a line would be disqualified as "fake news" today. Interestingly, Stöhr moved to the pharmaceutical company Novartis shortly afterwards to head their vaccine department—a move that raised a few eyebrows, but which was not worth a a mention from the *Spiegel* or any other major media outlet.

Gerd Gigerenzer, psychologist and Director Emeritus at the Max Planck Institute for Educational Research, in an interview published in the Austrian magazine *Profil* on the 8th of March 2020: "Fear is a market. To instill fear in people, also has advantages. Not only in terms of drug use. Anxiety-driven people are easier to rule. Abstinence from media cannot do any harm with the current corona excitement."[1323] Statistics professor Gerd Bosbach was even clearer: "The Robert Koch Institute had already attracted negative attention at the time [2009] with the swine flu ... The swine flu was completely overestimated ... We should have reviewed why the swine flu was staged in such a way in the media at the time ... One of the lessons to be learned from this would have been not to listen to a few 'whispering experts' ... I would gladly take the camera or microphone away from such scientists."[1324]

And Peter C. Gøtzsche resignedly noted: "The world has gone completely crazy and the media profits from this hysteria. It's like the Middle Ages." But he added a relevant joke concerning politics and media: "'Why do you blow the horn?' 'To keep the tigers away.' 'But there are no tigers here.' 'There you see!'"[1325]

Indeed, even the data on the so-called basis reproduction number, in short R_0 (pronounced "R zero"), show that the lockdown was all for nothing. This reproduction number, which was regularly determined in Germany by the Robert Koch-Institute, is supposed to indicate the expected number of cases directly generated by one case in a population where all individuals are susceptible to infection. If the value is above 1, this is supposed to indicate that the number of new infections is increasing—if it is less than 1, there are supposed to be fewer and fewer new infections.

But the R-value was already falling in Germany from March 10/11, 2020, and thus a good two weeks before the start of the lockdown, which did not occur until March 23, and slipped "as if by magic" from around 3 to about 1 in those 14 days. This is all the more remarkable when you consider that during this period, for example, close to 30 million people in Germany also used public transport every day(!), and they did so without covering their mouths. This is because the mask requirement was only introduced on April 29. These figures alone make the virus hypothesis absurd!

Unexplained Paths of Virus Transmission

The basic assumption in the corona/COVID-19 panic was that contact or even just proximity between people transmitted the virus and those who were infected had a "positive" PCR test result—potentially meaning a death sentence. In order to get this assumption deep into people's minds, it was repeated mantra-like to the population via the mass media—with the goal of presenting the draconian "lockdown" measures as the only reasonable way to go.

To the regret of the political policymakers, however, on the 24th of March 2020, as reported by *focus.de*, there was still disagreement among the population as to whether these measures were actually effective.[1326] But then, as chance would have it, a paper from Hong Kong appeared to help convince more people that the official virus theory was correct. The theme of the study was that "many infected people infect others before they feel sick themselves," as was stated in the aforementioned *focus.de* article.

Even without being really ill, you were still contagious—which sounded particularly frightening. And *focus.de* acted like a PR agency for the politicians and ruling virologists broadcasting: "Germany is resisting the spread of the corona virus and is reducing social life to a minimum. The results of a study from Hong Kong show that these measures are exactly right to counteract the pandemic."

Subsequently, no matter what happened, the media turned everything in exactly one direction: that the virus hypothesis was irrefutable and there was no alternative to the draconian restrictions on freedom. However, between 1985 and 2008, long before the corona virus "appeared," 3 to 17 million people died in China every year as a result of pneumonia.[1327] And it was precisely this disease that affected the first 41 patients who were said to have been infected with SARS-CoV-2 at the Huanan Seafood Market in the Chinese metropolis of Wuhan.

But in fact there does not need to be a SARS-CoV-2 virus at all to plausibly explain what is called COVID-19. Indeed, a study in the *New England Journal of Medicine* that examined the first 425 corona cases revealed that 72 percent of those who tested "positive" for corona on the 1st of January 2020 or later had "no exposure to neither the [Huanan Seafood] market [in Wuhan] nor a person with respiratory symptoms."[1328]

Studies in the prestigious *Lancet* journal, which examined the first Chinese cases, pointed in the same direction. One of these studies showed that only 27 of the first 41 patients had contact with the Huanan Seafood Market. This means: 14 (34 percent) had no such contact. This paper also showed that the first patient to whom the COVID-19 label was attributed developed symptoms on the 1st of December 2019. However, none of his family members developed fever or any respiratory problems. And in any case, no epidemiological link could be found between the first patient and later cases.[1329] Another study revealed that only 49 of 99 pneumonia patients who tested "positive" had been to the said market in Wuhan; in other words, about 50 percent never went there.[1330]

In another analysis, a family (two grandparents, their daughter and son-in-law as well as their 10-year-old grandson and 7-year-old granddaughter) travelled from Shenzhen near Hong Kong to Wuhan on the 29th of December 2019 and returned on the 4th of January—all of whom were found "positive" on the 9th /10th of January. Despite the authors of this study attempting to confirm the official virus narrative about COVID-19 using their data, there are multiple inconsistencies undermining the theory.

For example, none of the family members had any contact with the Wuhan markets or with animals (which are purported to be the original source of the alleged SARS-CoV-2 virus). In addition, no one had eaten game meat in restaurants. Meanwhile, the grandparents were already in poor health. The grandmother had previously been treated for a brain tumour, and both of them suffered from high blood pressure. In Wuhan, both developed fever, dry cough and weakness—and later laboratory tests revealed various abnormal values. So indeed they were frail and unwell.

It was reported that the grandson was a "naughty" boy, as he had refused to wear a face mask in Wuhan. That is why his parents insisted that he should be taken for a CT scan. And although the boy was completely symptom-free, i.e. not ill, he was diagnosed with pneumonia simply because the CT scan showed slight clouding of the lungs. In the case of the daughter, although she was subjected to 18 PCR tests, none of them showed a "positive" result. Nevertheless she has been classified as an "infected case," on the absurd grounds that she had a strong epidemiological link to the Wuhan hospital and her Chest X-rays had shown abnormalities.

The fact that the authors of this study also failed to take into account any other possible cause of disease such as chemicals, environmental pollution, contaminated food, etc. proves how narrow their perspective was. The intention of this study seemed suspiciously designed to show that the suspected corona virus was infectious, and omitted other possible explanations, hence failing in their duty as genuine scientists.

It is therefore clear from these and other reports that the official theory of transmission of SARS-CoV-2 was never established. If you want to learn more about this, we recommend reading the paper "Is the 2019 Coronavirus Really a Pandemic?" by Canadian David Crowe[1331] who died quite suddenly (from cancer) on July 12, 2020.

Lousy, More Lousy, Corona PCR Tests

In 2007, science journalist Gina Kolata described in the *New York Times* how problematic it is to declare virus pandemics on the basis of PCR tests, which also played a crucial role in the rapidly spreading corona panic in 2020. The title of her article was "Faith in Quick Test Leads to Epidemic That Wasn't."[1332] The bottom line of the article was that epidemiologists and infectious disease specialists had declared an epidemic without any foundation by placing far too much trust in molecular biological diagnostic methods such as the PCR test. But these cautionary tales were completely ignored in the context of corona.

A typical example was that of virologist Hendrik Streeck— an "expert" who has received funds from pharmaceutical companies, including Gilead Sciences, whose drug remdesivir was the first drug worldwide to receive emergency approval for the treatment of so-called COVID-19 patients on May 2, 2020 in a highly dubious manner (see end of this chapter). He was able to claim in all seriousness in an interview with the German newspaper *Frankfurter Allgemeine Zeitung* (*FAZ*): "Almost all infected persons whom we interviewed, and this applies to a good two thirds, described a loss of smell and taste lasting several days."[1333] But even with the best will in the world, you cannot equate "two thirds" of a patient group with "almost all," even if this 'rounding error' suits your purpose. In any case: "loss of smell and taste" cannot really be called "new" symptoms.

Nevertheless, the *FAZ* was happy to make their headline "We have discovered new symptoms [for COVID-19]". So this was more fake news based on statements of a virologist who was either craving recognition or lacking basic medical knowledge, or both. But the motivation behind this article was obvious: They wanted to break a big news story, and be the first to tell the world that COVID-19 was indeed a new disease.

But this was and is medically untenable, as confirmed by Thomas Löscher,[1334] an infectious diseases physician who responded to *focus.de* in the "Corona crisis".[1335] This is because "for most respiratory diseases there are no unmistakable specific symptoms," says Löscher. "Therefore a differentiation of the different pathogens is purely clinically impossible." According to Löscher, the pathogen SARS-CoV-2 alone was novel.[1336]

But the narrative was being established that COVID-19 *and* the SARS-CoV-2 virus were both something completely new. But even if one assumes that SARS-CoV-2 is a potentially disease-causing virus, solid data from Scotland collected from 2005 to 2013 showed that even a slight "flu-like" infection has a 7 to 15 percent chance of corona viruses being detected.[1337] It is therefore apparent that corona viruses were widely prevalent in the population before becoming "famous" in 2020. According to the physician Wolfgang Wodarg, corona is ultimately only a test epidemic.

"The horror reports from Wuhan were something that virologists all over the world are waiting for," said Wodarg. "This would have meant looking only at test results and not at clinical findings."[1338] Indeed, it quickly became apparent that as more tests were performed, more cases were found.[1339] So of course the tests came onto the market en masse, and we had a "PCR pandemic," rather than a real pandemic.

Germany's chief virologist Christian Drosten, who together with his team, had developed the world's first COVID-19 PCR test protocol approved by the WHO,[1340] [1341] told Deutschlandfunk radio on 23 January that they had "immediately set about doing what we are particularly good at: Developing diagnostic test procedures in a very short time. And then above all, making them available worldwide." And as Deutschlandfunk further reported, "there would have been great interest among the Southeast Asian nations in Christian Drosten's test. And there are also many enquiries from Europe. Padded envelopes containing the reagents are piled up in the corridor—financed by EU subsidies. Wherever a traveller from Wuhan arrives with breathing difficulties and high fever, the new test can be used."[1342]

About two months later, the Swiss pharmaceutical company Roche received emergency approval in the USA for a highly automated test for SARSCoV-2, which could test up to 4,000 samples within 24 hours.[1343]

On 28th March 2020, *Multipolar magazine* reported in the article "Coronavirus: Misleading case numbers now proven," that official data showed there was a massive increase in testing, while the proportion of infected people themselves—or rather the number of "positive" test results—did not actually grow at all, let alone exponentially.

In order to understand this, the following must be made clear: According to the RKI situation report, the number of people testing "positive" (who are officially referred to as "infected," though of course this is not factually correct) was 7,582 in the second week of March 2020, and 23,820 in the third week of March. This quickly gives the uninitiated observer the scary impression that there has been an increase in the number of "infected" people in Germany of around 300 percent within one week. But this is completely wrong, because in the third week of March, around three times as many tests were carried out compared to the second week of March. The bottom line is that the increase in the proportion of "positive" results was ultimately negligible.

"If we had not started testing wildly in Wuhan, China, but in Beijing, we would have found the corresponding corona case numbers there," said Wolfgang Wodarg in early March 2020. In this context, one would simply have to realize that people in China have relatively homogeneous lifestyles. So why would a new virus spread from animals to humans in Wuhan in particular? "And what a coincidence," said Wodarg, "that the 'epidemic' just started in Wuhan—a metropolis of millions that is a kind of center of virology in China. This is where the country's largest laboratory for research into pathogens is located with the highest level of security, and it is also where the people who work most with viruses are based."[1344]

The virologist Georg Bornkamm also agreed with Wodarg on one point, as was reported in the newspaper *Süddeutsche Zeitung*: "Coronaviruses have always been around, and in part they are responsible for the respiratory tract infections including pneumonia during every flu season. That much is true about Wodarg's thesis. But the new coronavirus is by no means similar to the previous viruses." And even if all corona viruses belonged to one virus family, the former professor from Helmholtz Zentrum München said, they could differ from each other like a "shark from a stickleback," both of which are fish. According to

Bornkamm, the new SARS-CoV-2 is genetically only a distant relative of the other corona viruses, which is why it cannot be confused with the older viruses when tested. "The thesis that the pandemic exists only because testing is carried out is absolutely untenable," said Bornkamm.[1345] But his conclusion is without any scientific substance. SARS-CoV-2 can still be confused with other viruses – assuming they have been proven – when tested.

Comments of world-famous experts on the topic "Complete particle purification as an essential prerequisite for the detection of a virus":

Luc Montagnier: „Analysis of the proteins of the virus demands mass production and purification. It is necessary to do that ... to prove that you have a real virus."

Robert Gallo: „You have to purify ... Conclusive serological testing, in our view, required finer, more specific assays based on using purified virus particles or proteins obtained from the virus instead of whole cells infected with virus."

Françoise Barré-Sinoussi: „You have to purify the virus from all this mess ... Because we wanted these diagnostic kits [the antibody tests] to be as specific as possible. If you use a preparation of virus which is not purified of course you will detect antibody to everything not only against the virus but also to all the proteins that are produced in the supernatant."

Jean-Claude Chermann: „[To identify the HIV proteins and RNA they had to extract them] from the virus which we had concentrated and purified."

David Gordon: „It's a natural step from obtaining the virus in cell culture to then obtain purified virus ... because purification of virus is then very useful for further studies for the nature of the virus and the nature of the immune response against the virus."

Dominic Dwyer: „The purification, as far as one can go, is important in analysis of any virus or bacteria, for that matter well."

Source: The Emperor's New Virus?, www. theperthgroup.com, July 12, 2017, pp. 37-38

This fact is even stated in the information accompanying the COVID-19 PCR test from CD Creative Diagnostics, which clearly states that the test may not only react to SARS-CoV-2, but also to other viruses and even bacteria.[1346]

Virologists can of course speculate long and hard in metaphors about whether certain coronaviruses are as dangerous as "sharks" or as harmless as "sticklebacks" – but this does not change the fact as can be read in the *Süddeutsche Zeitung* article itself: that "nobody knows at the moment how dangerous SARS-CoV-2 is." Or in the words of Bornkamm himself: "The [SARS-CoV-2] virus may not be as dangerous, that may be true."[1347] And on March 19, a study entitled "SARS-CoV-2: Fear versus Data" was published (previously online) in the *International Journal of Antimicrobial Agents*. Result: SARS-CoV-2 does not differ from other coronaviruses in terms of its dangerousness.

That is to say, if it is clear …

(a) that here are no indicative specific symptoms for COVID-19 disease
(b) that it is not clinically possible to differentiate between pathogens,
(c) that no one has evidence that SARS-CoV-2 is exceptionally deadly
(d) and that non-viral factors such as industrial poisons[1348] and various drugs such as an-tipsychotics, opioid analgesics, anticholinergics or antidepressants[1349] may be a cause of severe respiratory diseases such as pneumonia and thus also of so-called COVID-19

… then it is impossible to conclude that so-called SARS-CoV-2 can be the only cause of symptoms in patients who have the "COVID-19" label attached.

Lack of Detection of So-Called SARS-CoV-2

Incidentally, the virus hunters have conveniently ignored a pivotal scientific principle in their argument. Complete purification is an indispensable pre-requisite for virus identi-fication as stated by textbooks[1350] [1351], virus researchers such as Luc Montagnier (see box with quotes from well-known experts) and the second of Koch's postulates (see chapter 3, subchapter "Where Is the Proof of HIV?").

"Purification", mind you, means the separation of an object from everything that does not belong to it—as, for example, Nobel Prize winner Marie Curies isolated radium from tons of pitchblende in 1898. Only on the basis of such a complete purification can it be proven that the nucleic acid sequences found in the particles in question originate from a new virus.

For this, one must remember that the PCR is extremely sensitive. This means that it can "pick up" even the smallest genetic fragments—i.e. DNA or RNA fragments. But it is not possible with the PCR to determine where these nucleic acid sequences come from. This must be determined beforehand in a separate process. And since PCR tests are "calibrated" to nucleic acid sequences, in this case RNA sequences (since it is assumed that SARS-CoV-2 is an RNA virus), it must of course be clearly proven that these genetic fragments are actually part of the claimed virus. And in order to prove this beyond any doubt, the correct isolation and complete purification of the suspected virus is an indispensable pre-requisite.

To make this quite clear once again, it is worthwhile to employ a paternity suit analogy. Here, in order to compare the DNA of the suspected father and the child, one must ensure that the DNA is extracted from the bodies of the alleged father and the child. The same standard undoubtedly applies to determining whether RNA belongs to a virus or not. In a paternity suit, the genome can, mind you, be extracted from a single "particle" (father/child). This is different for particles suspected of being viruses. The viral genome cannot be obtained from a single particle due to its extremely small size. This means that it must be obtained from a large mass of identical, i.e. completely purified particles, or at least from material that does not contain any foreign RNA.

Thus, when cells, cell debris and particles are mixed in a laboratory culture, the only way to determine which RNA (or even proteins) are viral is to separate the particles from all non-viral material. However, some researchers use the term "isolation" in their work to give the impression to the uninitiated reader that a virus has been isolated in pure form. In fact, however, this has not happened, because the procedures described in these works do not represent a proper process of isolation including complete purification. Consequently, they misuse the term "isolation" in their publications.

And so we decided to be the first in the world to ask the research teams of the relevant papers cited in connection with the alleged detection of SARS-CoV-2 whether the electron microscope images shown in their in vitro studies depict completely purified viruses. However, not a single team of authors—including those of two pivotal studies (Zhu et al., Wan Beom Park et al.)—could answer this question with a yes. And it should be noted that no one wrote back suggesting that complete purification is *not* a necessary step for solid virus detection.

We only received answers such as "our electron microscope image does not show a completely purified virus" (see table, which has been published in the article that appeared in the *OffGuardian* on June 27, 2020 and was the first in the world to fundamentally demonstrate that SARS-CoV-2 PCR is without substance: "COVID-19 PCR-Tests Are Scientifically Meaningless" by Torsten Engelbrecht and Konstantin Demeter).[1352] Altogether, the authors of five relevant papers (Zhu et al.,[1353] Wan Beom Park et al.[1354]), which are mentioned in connection with the detection of SARS-CoV-2, conceded on request that they did not complete purification.

We also contacted Charles Calisher, who is a seasoned virologist. In 2001, *Science* published an "impassioned plea ... to the younger generation" from several veteran virologists, among

Responses from Study Authors to the Question: Do your electron micrographs show the purified virus?

Study	Replying Author	Answer	Date of Answer
Sharon R. Lewin et al. Isolation and rapid sharing of the 2019 novel coronavirus (SARS - CoV - 2) from the first patient diagnosed with COVID - 19 in Australia, *The Medical Journal of Australia*, June 2020, pp. 459-462	Jason A. Roberts and Julian Druce	"The nucleic acid extraction was performed on isolate material recovered from infected cells. This material was not centrifuged, so was not purified through sucrose gradient to have a density band as such. The EM images were obtained directly from cell culture material."	October 5, 2020
Leo L. M. Poon; Malik Peiris. Emergence of a novel human coronavirus threatening human health, *Nature Medicine*, March 2020	Malik Peiris	"The image is the virus budding from an infected cell. It is not purified virus."	May 12, 2020
Myung-Guk Han et al. Identification of Coronavirus Isolated from a Patient in Korea with COVID-19, *Osong Public Health and Research Perspectives*, February 2020	Myung-Guk Han	"We could not estimate the degree of purification because we do not purify and concentrate the virus cultured in cells."	May 6, 2020
Wan Beom Park et al. Virus Isolation from the First Patient with SARS-CoV-2 in Korea, *Journal of Korean Medical Science*, February 24, 2020	Wan Beom Park	"We did not obtain an electron micrograph showing the degree of purification."	March 19, 2020
Na Zhu et al. A Novel Coronavirus from Patients with Pneumonia in China, 2019, *New England Journal of Medicine*, February 20, 2020	Wenjie Tan	"[We show] an image of sedimented virus particles, not purified ones."	March 18, 2020

Source: Engelbrecht, Torsten; Demeter, Konstantin, COVID-19 PCR Tests Are Scientifically Meaningless, OffGuardian, 27. June 2020; research by Torsten Engelbrecht

them Calisher, saying that "[modern virus detection methods like] sleek polymerase chain reaction ... tell little or nothing about how a virus multiplies, which animals carry it, [or] how it makes people sick. [It is] like trying to say whether somebody has bad breath by looking at his fingerprint."[1355] And that's why we asked Calisher whether he knows of a single paper in which SARS-CoV-2 had been isolated and then truly purified. His answer: "I know of no such a publication. I have kept an eye out for one."[1356]

Some time later, Canadian biostatistician Christine Massey and Michael Speth from New Zealand submitted Freedom of Information (FOI) applications to institutions around the world to obtain documents describing the complete purification of a so-called SARS CoV-2 virus from an unaltered sample of a sick patient. However, as of January 22, 2020, all 46 responding institutions/offices utterly failed to provide or cite any describing "SARS-CoV-2" isolation; and Germany's Ministry of Health ignored their FOI request altogether.

Even Michael Laue from the RKI wrote in an email that we received on September 4, 2020: "I am not aware of a paper which purified isolated SARS-CoV-2," and the U.S. CDC also wrote in a document updated on July 13, 2020: "Since no quantified virus isolates of the 2019-nCoV are currently available."[1357]

If no such particle "purification" has been done anywhere, how can one claim that the RNA obtained is part of a viral genome? And how can such RNA then be widely used to diagnose infection with a new virus? We have asked these two questions to numerous representatives of the official corona narrative worldwide, but nobody could answer them.

The fact that the RNA sequences that the scientists extracted from the tissue samples and which the SARS-CoV-2 RT-PCR tests were finally "calibrated" belong to a new pathogenic virus called SARS-CoV-2 is therefore based on faith alone, not on sound research. Consequently, it cannot be concluded that the "pulled" RNA genetic sequences in these studies, belong to a very specific virus, in this case SARS-CoV-2, which can then be "detected" by the developed RT-PCR test.

We have also looked at all the studies claiming to have isolated and even tested the virus. But in all of them, they actually did something very different: the researchers took samples from the throat or lungs of patients, ultracentrifuged them (spun them at high speed) to separate the larger/heavy from the smaller/lighter molecules, and then took the supernatant, the upper part of the centrifuged material. And this is what they called their "isolate," to which they then applied the PCR.

But this supernatant contains all kinds of molecules, billions of different micro- and nanoparticles, including extracellular vesicles (EVs) and exosomes, which are produced by our own body and are often indistinguishable from viruses: "Nowadays, it is an almost impossible mission to separate EVs and viruses by means of canonical vesicle isolation methods, such as differential ultracentrifugation, because they are frequently co-pelleted due to their similar dimension," as it said in the study "The Role of Extracellular Vesicles as Allies of HIV, HCV and SARS Viruses," published in May 2020 in the journal *Viruses*.

So how do you extract a specific virus from this huge mixture of billions of indistinguishable particles, including naturally occurring exosomes? Well, you simply cannot, it is impossible, unless you have purified the particles of whom you think they belong to a new virus beforehand (and then you have to define its genetic structure and disease-causing properties).

In fact, the scientists "create" the virus by PCR: They take artificial and entirely hypothetical primers (previously existing genetic sequences available in genetic banks) and put them in touch with the supernatant of the pharyngeal or broncho-alveolar fluid of the patient, that is with tens of billions of RNA and DNA molecules; and if, as it is likely, the primers attach to something in that broth, they conclude that whatever attached to the primers, then forming a DNA molecule with the help of the enzyme reverse transcriptase, it is the new and unknown SARS-CoV-2.

As if that weren't enough, the primers used are just an infinitesimal fragment of the alleged genome of the virus; they are in factmade up of only 18 to 24 bases (nucleotides) each; while the SARS-CoV-2 virus is assumed to consist of 30,000 bases, that is to say the primers represent only 0.07 percent of the virus genome. How is it possible to select the specific virus you are looking for with such a minute sequence, and moreover in a sea of billions of virus-like particles? Again, it is just impossible! As the virus you are looking for is new, there are clearly no ready "off-the-shelf" genetic primers to match the specific fraction of the new virus. Instead, you take primers that you believe may be close to the hypothesized virus structure, but it's only a rough guess. When you apply the primers to the supernatant broth, they can attach to any one of the billions of molecules present in it, and you have no idea if what you generated is from the virus you are looking for.[1358]

Let's imagine that all English literature, including many poems and short stories unknown to the public, are collected in a huge database, and that you want to look for an unknown poem which, however, you believe was important at a certain historical period. You don't know anything about this poem, except that it is a love poem. You will therefore have to enter keywords in the computer that make you find the poem, but you can't use more than 18 to 24 letters. So you type "my love I miss you", a phrase of 18 characters, and with this phrase you should find your poem among the about 28 billion poems contained in the database, half of which love poems. What are the chances of bringing out the specific poem you are looking for and not one different from what interests you? We would say next to zero … and this is what happens with RT-PCR in relation to a presumed virus that is said to be new and is therefore unknown.

Incidentally, SARS-CoV-2 was "pieced together" on the computer. The physician Thomas Cowan called this "scientific fraud." He wrote on October 15, 2020: "This week, my colleague and friend Sally Fallon Morell brought to my attention an amazing article put out by the CDC, published in June 2020. The article's purpose was for a group of about 20 virologists to describe the state of the science of the isolation, purification and biological characteristics of the new SARS-CoV-2 virus, and to share this information with other scientists for their own research. A thorough and careful reading of this important paper reveals some shocking findings." In fact, the article section "Whole Genome Sequencing" shows that rather than having isolated the virus and sequencing the genome from end to end, that the CDC "designed 37 pairs of nested PCRs spanning the genome on the basis of the coronavirus reference sequence (GenBank accession no. NC045512)."

Cowan draws the following analogy: "A group of researchers claim to have found a unicorn because they found a piece of a hoof, a hair from a tail, and a snippet of a horn. They then add that information into a computer and program it to re-create the unicorn, and they then claim this computer re-creation is the real unicorn. Of course, they had never actually seen a unicorn so could not possibly have examined its genetic makeup to compare their samples with the actual unicorn's hair, hooves and horn."[1359]

Consequently, it cannot be concluded that the RNA gene sequences "pulled" from the tissue samples prepared in these studies and "calibrated" to the PCR tests belong to a very specific virus, in this case SARS-CoV-2. Especially since the electron microscope images, which are supposed to represent SARS-CoV-2, actually show particles that vary greatly in size. In one paper, the particles range from 60 nm to 140 nm. A specific virus that has such extreme size variation cannot exist by definition.

Total Failure of the PCR Test: No Gold Standard, No "Viral Load" Measurement, Not for Diagnostic Purposes

The PCR tests used to identify so-called COVID-19 patients presumably infected by what is called SARS-CoV-2 do not even have a valid gold standard to compare them with.

This is a fundamental point. Tests need to be evaluated to determine their preciseness—strictly speaking their "sensitivity" and "specificity—by comparison with a "gold standard," meaning the most accurate method available.

Sensitivity can be defined as the proportion of patients with disease in whom the test is "positive," while specificity is the proportion of patients without disease in whom the test is "negative."

As an example, for a pregnancy test the gold standard would be the pregnancy itself. But as Australian infectious diseases specialist Sanjaya Senanayake stated in an ABC TV interview in an answer to the question "How accurate is the [COVID-19] testing?": "If we had a new test for picking up [the bacterium] golden staph in blood, we've already got blood cultures, that's our gold standard we've been using for decades, and we could match this new test against that. But for COVID-19 we don't have a gold standard test."

Jessica C. Watson from Bristol University confirms this. In her paper "Interpreting a COVID-19 test result", published in May 2020 *The BMJ*, she writes that there is a "lack of such a clear-cut 'gold-standard' for COVID-19 testing." But instead of classifying the tests as unsuitable for SARS-CoV-2 detection and COVID-19 diagnosis and pointing out that only an isolated and purified virus can be a solid gold standard, the article claims in all seriousness that "If your swab test comes back positive for covid-19 then we can be very confident that you do have covid-19". Watson also states that "clinical adjudication may be the best available 'gold standard'," including "repeat swabs". But this is not scientifically sound.

Apart from the fact that it is downright absurd to take the PCR test itself as part of the gold standard to evaluate the PCR test, there are no established specific symptoms for COVID-19, as mentioned. And if there are no established specific symptoms for COVID-19—contrary to Watson's statement—COVID-19 clinical diagnosis cannot be suitable for serving as a valid gold standard either.
In addition, "experts" such as Watson overlook the fact that only virus isolation, i.e. unequivocal virus proof, can be the basis of establishing a gold standard. (Keep in mind, even proof of a SARS-CoV-2 virus would not necessarily determine disease causality—but that's another matter!)

That is why I asked Watson how COVID-19 diagnosis "may be the best available gold standard," if there are no distinctive specific symptoms for COVID-19, and also whether the virus itself, that is virus isolation, wouldn't be the best available/possible gold standard. But she didn't answer these questions—despite multiple requests. And she has not yet responded to our rapid response post on her article in which we address exactly the same points, either, though she wrote us on June 2, 2020: "I will try to post a reply later this week when I have a chance."

Even if one were to theoretically assume that these PCR tests could really detect a virus infection—which, as outlined, is demonstrably not the case—the tests would be practically worthless and would thus only cause unfounded panic among "positively" tested people. This also becomes clear when one takes into account a test's "Positive Predictive Value," or PPV for short. The PPV indicates the probability that a person with a "positive" test result is really "positive," i.e. in this case actually infected with the alleged virus.

The PPV depends on two factors: The prevalence of the alleged disease in the general population and the specificity of the test. Specificity, again, is defined as the percentage of people who are not actually ill and who are correctly tested "negative." For example, if a test has a specificity of 95 percent, this means that 5 percent of healthy people are falsely tested "positive."

Based on a fixed specificity, the higher the disease prevalence, the higher the PPV. In this context, the journal *Deutsches Ärzteblatt* published an article on June 12, 2020, in which the PPV was calculated using three different prevalence scenarios. The results must be viewed very critically. Firstly, because it is not possible to calculate specificity without a gold standard, as we have shown is the case with SARS-CoV-2 PCR tests. And secondly, because the calculations in the *Ärzteblatt* article are based on the specificity determined in the above mentioned study by Jessica Watson. But as we have explained, this is a worthless "study".

But even if you dismiss these two points and assume that the underlying specificity of 95 percent is correct and that we know the disease prevalence, the mainstream medical journal *Ärzteblatt* still concluded that the alleged SARS-CoV-2 RT-PCR tests can have "a frighteningly low" PPV. In one of the three scenarios played out in the

Ärzteblatt article, in which a prevalence of 3 percent was assumed, the PPV is just 30 percent. According to this scenario, no less than 70 percent of those tested "positive" would then be falsely "positive."

Nevertheless, all of the people who tested positive would be "quarantined," as even the *Deutsche Ärzteblatt* critically noted. In a second scenario, a disease prevalence of 20 percent was assumed. In this case, the PPV would be 78 percent, meaning that 22 percent of the "positive" tests would be false positives. Transferred to reality this would mean: Out of 10 million people who have tested "positive," a striking 2.2 million would be falsely positive. All this fits in with the fact that even the American CDC and the Food and Drug Administration (FDA) admit that the "SARS-CoV-2 RT-PCR tests" are not suitable for the diagnosis of SARS-CoV-2 infection. And indeed, even the instructions for use of the PCR tests explicitly state that they are not intended for what they are overwhelmingly used for: diagnosis.[1360]

In the Netherlands, this was even brought up in court, as entrepreneur Jeroen Pols testified on November 6, 2020 in an interview with the German Corona Committee (Corona-Ausschuss) headed by lawyer Reiner Füllmich. According to Pols, the focus of the evidence was on 27 user manuals from different PCR test manufacturers, all of which contained the same description: "Research Use Only (RUO), not for diagnostic purposes."[1361]

Moreover, the product descriptions of the RT-qPCR tests for SARS-COV-2 state they are "qualitative" tests, contrary to the fact that the "q" in "qPCR" stands for "quantitative." And if these tests are not "quantitative" tests, they won't show how many viral particles are in the body, or the "viral load".

That is crucial because, in order to even begin talking about actual illness in the real world not just in a laboratory, surely a patient would need to have millions and millions of viral particles actively replicating in their body. That is to say, the CDC, the WHO, the FDA and the RKI may assert that the tests can measure the so-called "viral load," i.e. how many viral particles are in the body. "But this has never been proven. That is an enormous scandal," as the journalist Jon Rappoport points out. However, even the term "viral load" is deceptive. If you asked the question "what is viral load?" at a dinner party, people take it to mean viruses circulating in the bloodstream. They're surprised to learn it's actually RNA molecules.

In truth to prove beyond any doubt that the PCR can measure how much a person is "burdened" with a disease-causing virus, the following experiment would have to be done (which has not happened to date):

One would need to take tissue samples from a few hundred or even a thousand people, making sure the people who take the samples do not perform the PCR test. Then the testers, who are not allowed to know anything about the test subjects, carry out their PCR test on the tissue samples. Then, let's say, they find quite high loads of the target genetic material in patients 29, 86, 199, 272 and 293. Now we un-blind those patients. They should all be sick, because they have so much virus replicating in their bodies. But are they really sick—or are they fit as a fiddle?

With the help of Berlin lawyer Viviane Fischer, we were able to get the Charité in Berlin to answer whether the PCR test protocol developed by Corman et al., essentially by their "in-house" team including Christian Drosten, is a quantitative one. But the Charité were not willing to answer this question with a "yes." Instead, the Charité wrote: "If real-time RT-PCR is involved, to the knowledge of the Charité in most cases these are [...] limited to qualitative detection."

Furthermore, the "Drosten PCR test protocol" outlined in the Corman et al. study, used the unspecific E-gene (i.e. present in other coronaviruses) assay as the preliminary assay. The excuse to use the unspecific E-gene?—they claimed that "early reported cases implicates the possibility of independent zoonotic infections with increased sequence variability." Meanwhile, the Institut Pasteur used the same assay as a confirmatory assay. According to Corman et al., the E-gene assay is likely to detect all Asian corona viruses, while the other two assays are supposed to be more specific for sequences labelled "SARS-CoV-2."

Besides the questionable purpose of having either a preliminary or a confirmatory test that is likely to detect all Asian corona viruses, the WHO changed the algorithm at the beginning of April 2020, recommending that from then on a test can be regarded as "positive" even if just the E-gene assay (which is likely to detect all Asian viruses!) gives a "positive" result.
This means that a PCR test known to be unspecific was officially sold as specific. That change of algorithm dramatically increased the "case" numbers. Examples of tests using the E-gene assay are produced by Roche, TIB Molbiol and R-Biopharm.

High Cq Values Make Nonsense of the Test Results

Another major problem is that many PCR tests have a Cq of over 35 — and some, for example the PCR protocol developed by Corman et al., even have a Cq of 45. "Cq" stands for "Cycle quantification" value (sometimes also called "Ct"), and it indicates how many cycles of propagation (replication) of DNA (genetic material) are required to obtain a real signal from a biological sample by PCR. And "Cq values higher than 40 are suspect because of the implied low efficiency and generally should not be reported," as it says in the MIQE guidelines.

In fact even the *New York Times* featured a story on August 29th, 2020 suggesting that the "COVID-19" PCR Ct values were far too high. Harvard epidemiologist Michael Mina was quoted as saying he would, "set the figure at 30 or even less".[1362] MIQE stands for "Minimum Information for Publication of Quantitative Real-Time PCR Experiments", and is a set of guidelines that describe the minimum information necessary for evaluating publications on Real-Time PCR, also called quantitative PCR, or qPCR.

The MIQE guidelines have been developed under the aegis of Stephen A. Bustin, Professor of Molecular Medicine, a world-renowned expert on quantitative PCR and author of the book "A-Z of Quantitative PCR" which has been called "the bible of qPCR." Bustin pointed out that "the use of such arbitrary Cq cut-offs is not ideal, because they may be either too low (eliminating valid results) or too high (increasing false positive results)."[1363]

Remarkably, institutions such as the RKI cannot even provide data indicating the number of cycles (Cq value) at which the PCR tests used in practice are considered positive.[1364] Either they want to hide something or they are of the opinion that the Cq value has no relevance with regard to the significance of a positive PCR test result. Both of these positions would be simply absurd, if not scandalous.

However, as it happened the public only saw increasing numbers of "positive" tests. But these numbers were worthless, because (a) the Cq values used in the PCR-tests were not communicated, (b) most people testing "positive" were completely healthy, having no symptoms of disease and (c) in countries like Germany the number of sick, seriously ill and dying people had not increased (more about the worldwide mortality data later).

Moreover, there is another factor that can alter the result, before even starting with the actual PCR itself. When you are looking for presumed RNA viruses such as SARS-CoV-2, the RNA must be converted to complementary DNA (cDNA) with the enzyme Reverse Transcriptase (RT)—hence the "RT" at the beginning of "PCR" or "qPCR."

But this transformation process is "widely recognized as inefficient and variable," as Jessica Schwaber from the Centre for Commercialization of Regenerative Medicine in Toronto and two research colleagues pointed out in a 2019 paper. Stephen A. Bustin acknowledges problems with PCR in a comparable way. For example, he pointed to the problem that in the course of the conversion process (RNA to cDNA) the amount of DNA obtained with the same RNA base material can vary widely, even by a factor of 10—with the same high RNA starting base. This is a drastic difference.

Therefore the RT-PCR test can give a false negative result just because there was too little conversion of the sample's RNA to cDNA base material. In this scenario the Cq value that should have been adequate to make the PCR test positive (based on the amount of RNA) proves insufficient. This questions the validity of PCR tests in the other direction.

With regard to publications on RT-qPCR—and the so-called COVID-19 PCR tests = RT-qPCR tests!—Bustin also stated: "We demonstrate that elementary protocol errors, inappropriate data analysis and inadequate reporting continue to be rife and conclude that the majority of published RT-qPCR data are likely to represent technical noise." And "technical noise" ultimately means nothing else but—to put it in a nutshell—"whirled up crap."

To make things even worse, during the tests for virus detection, (from which the RNA is extracted and to which the PCR tests are "calibrated",) substances such as antibiotics are used which can demonstrably "stress" the in vitro cultures. This can lead to new nucleic acid sequences being expressed that were previously undetectable—and which are of course not viral. Nobel Prize winner Barbara McClintock spoke of these "shocks" (see Chapter 1, section "Viruses: Lethal Mini-Monsters?"). Consequently, it is quite possible that the RNA that the PCR tests "pick up" is actually one of the new non(!)-viral nucleic acid sequences created by test tube "shocks."[1365]

Therefore, it was not surprising that using PCR tests for SARS-CoV-2 led to totally confusing results.[1366] In February 2020, even Wang Chen, President of the Chinese Academy of Medical Sciences, stated in a TV interview that PCR tests are only "30 to 50 percent accurate."[1367] In fact, some people who had been labelled as having COVID-19 and who had fully recovered were retested by PCR. Result: First they were tested "negative" but then another test concluded they were "positive" again.

Another example of the total test result chaos: According to a news report, patients in China were not considered cured until they were symptom free, had clear lungs and had tested "negative" twice. In the Chinese province of Guangdong, the country's most populous province with 113 million inhabitants, the health authorities reported that 14 percent of patients who had made a complete recovery, later tested "positive" again.[1368] Many other similar examples of nonsensical results can be illustrated.[1369]

And to explain such results, it would certainly seem plausible that the RNA that the PCR test is calibrated to is not of viral origin. All the more if one considers that there was no concrete study showing that people with disease symptoms who tested "positive" could actually make someone else ill (i.e. not only PCR "positive"). There was also no study that clearly proved that a person who tested "positive" for SARS-CoV-2 could make another person "positive." The Robert Koch-Institute was also unable to name such a study.[1370]

Drosten PCR Study: Seriously Deficient and Full of Conflicts of Interest

On November 27, 2020, a team of 22 renowned scientists—including our author Stefano Scoglio as well as Ulrike Kämmerer, Professor of Virology and Cell Biology, and Michael Yeadon, pharmacologist and former chief scientist of the pharmaceutical giant Pfizer in the UK—published an in-depth analysis of the aforementioned Drosten/Corman et al. paper.[1371] This paper, which was published in *Eurosurveillance* on January 23, 2020, claimed to have established a solid diagnostic workflow and RT-qPCR protocol for the detection and diagnosis of SARS-CoV-2. This protocol was the first in the world to be "accepted" (not validated!) by the WHO and was said to have been used in an estimated 70 percent of all PCR test kits worldwide (as of early December 2020).[1372]

The importance of this protocol was therefore enormous. And hence the conclusion drawn by the 22 researchers is all the more alarming: "We provide compelling evidence of several scientific inadequacies, errors and flaw. We outline and explain in greater detail ten fatal problems in this paper. Considering the scientific and methodological blemishes presented here, we are confident that the editorial board of Eurosurveillance has no other choice but to retract the publication."

The authors exposed numerous conflicts of interest that were concealed by Drosten and his colleagues. As the analysis states: "We find severe conflicts of interest for at least four authors, in addition to the fact that two of the authors of the Corman-Drosten paper—Christian Drosten and Chantal Reusken—are members of the editorial board of *Eurosurveillance*. A conflict of interest was added on July 29, 2020—Olfert Landt is CEO of TIB-Molbiol, Marco Kaiser is senior researcher at GenExpress and serves as scientific advisor for TIB-Molbiol—that was not declared in the original version (and is still missing in the PubMed version); TIB-Molbiol is the company which was 'the first' to produce PCR kits (Light Mix) based on the protocol published in the Corman-Drosten manuscript, and according to their own words, they distributed these PCR-test kits before the publication was even submitted.

Further, Victor Corman and Christian Drosten failed to mention their second affiliation: the commercial test laboratory 'Labor Berlin.' Both are responsible for the virus diagnostics there and the company operates in the realm of real time PCR-testing."

Horror Scenes from Italy Burn a Groundless Virus Dogma into People's Minds

But the idea that no virus could be at work here was almost unimaginable for the majority of the mainstream media and politicians and for most of the virologists who were paraded in the spotlight. This is all the more unbelievable when one considers that the predictions being passed on from super-virologists to politicians and journalists were based on the weakest data imaginable. Renowned statisticians such as Gerd Bosbach and Frank Romeike, founder of the RiskNET competence centre, as well as Stanford epidemiologist John P. A. Ioannidis voiced strong concerns at an early stage that far too little was known about the new virus and about case and death rates to justify the measures taken by politicians. According to Ioannidis, no one would have any interest in this virus if it had not been specifically sought out.[1373]

So let's face it: the PCR tests and the data were demonstrably lousier than lousy right from the start. From the perspective of the representatives of the official narrative, apparently only one thing helped: incessantly spreading horror reports through the media, thus pushing their demands for even more draconian measures—even if they were based on false information. For example, the German Society for Epidemiology (DGEpi) warned on 19 March 2020 that because of corona there would be more than one million patients in Germany within a short time who would need intensive medical care. The *Frankfurter Allgemeine Zeitung*, immediately made itself the mouthpiece of the DGEpi and carried the headline "Researchers for tougher measures: Flatten the curve? That is no longer enough."

One only had to read past the headline to discover what they were suggesting: "Now containment is the motto. That means: Tough measures for a long time."[1374] Shortly afterwards, the DGEpi revised its published data considerably, which put things into perspective again. The original predictions had been made on the basis of assumptions which, let's say politely, were not really scientifically proven. Despite this, the media did not adjust or correct their reports. According to the statistician Gerd Bosbach, this was mainly due to the fact that the DGEpi spoke about "adjusted model parameters" instead of admitting in an understandable and simple way that a gross mistake had been made. In truth, Bosbach says, the entire DGEpi simulation model was "unclear" and its approach simply "catastrophic."

But from the woolly wording of the DGEpi correction, "no journalist would have been able to quickly recognize the error of the previous day. And so the threatening figure [of one million patients who will require intensive medical care] will continue to have an effect on some people," as Bosback stated. In fact, "the most important argument for the lockdown [in March 2020] was not to overload the number of intensive care beds in the hospitals, but this was never the case in Germany," as Stefan Aust, former editor-in-chief of *Der Spiegel* and publisher of the newspaper *Die Welt*, wrote on September 6 in an article with the headline "Because they [= the decision-makers] do NOT know what they are doing." Aust demanded: "The view of reality should be the yardstick for action. Not the fear and fogging of the facts."[1375]

But sense of reality seemed to be a foreign concept to most journalists. Instead, TV channels and social media platforms were spreading frightening images around the world—actively supported by the drastic warnings from virologists, which were recited mantra-like. And these images burned one message into most people's heads: Only one thing can be going on here—a life threatening virus.

As we have seen, this "scam" has worked very well previously with HIV/AIDS. At that time, we were shown pictures of emaciated world stars, of whom it was said that the HIV virus was responsible for their unfortunate physical condition and later for their death. The first was Hollywood superstar Rock Hudson, whose tragic fate "gave AIDS a face" all over the world, as the *Frankfurter Allgemeine Zeitung* put it[1376] (see epilogue after this chapter). Later on, the fates of world-famous personalities such as Freddie Mercury, front man of the rock band Queen, the tennis professional Arthur Ashe (see chapter 3) and many others were linked with HIV in the media.

And what Rock Hudson was for HIV/AIDS, Italy was for SARS-Cov-2/COVID-19. By mid-March 2020, media coverage was practically dominated by only one topic: that the corona-related death toll in Italy had skyrocketed. Of course, the reporting was always based on the narrative "SARS-CoV-2 = death"—and it was accompanied by dramatic pictures of coffins without end, queues of military vehicles etc. And why not be a little dramatic about it? The *Süddeutsche Zeitung*, for example, declared the whole country a "death zone" in their headline on 24 March 2020—and placed a moving picture of a funeral ceremony with a man wearing a face mask in front of a coffin underneath (see screenshot).

It becomes clear how unfounded it was to represent a virus as the only cause when one looks at the different worldwide mortality data for the first six months of 2020. We will go into this in more detail soon. At this point, it is sufficient to know that by mid-March the nationwide excess mortality in Italy was less than what it had been in early 2017 for example.

As in the case of HIV/AIDS, stories of personal tragedies had a particularly intense effect, as they tug at people's heartstrings. One example of this was a report by *Vatican News* on 24 March 2020: "The drama associated with the spread of the coronavirus has a new face. In the particularly affected Italian region around Bergamo, a sick priest has given up his respirator to save a younger patient. The 72-year-old priest died as a result"[1377] (see screenshot).

Those who had the 'SARS-CoV-2 = death' mantra more or less firmly anchored in their minds could hardly escape the effect of these images.

This applied also to neurologist Ulrich Dirnagl. He considered the claim of Stanford research-er Ioannidis (that without the mass application of PCR tests, nobody would be interested in SARS-CoV-2), to be „refuted" as reported in the *Süddeutsche Zeitung* on 24 March. He just considered Ioannidis' statement "with regard to Italy" to be refuted not because of any data showing significant excess mortality nationwide but due to the TV pictures from Italy. And the *Süddeutsche Zeitung* also brought a second gun into position against Ioannidis: Marc Lipsitch of the Harvard School of Public Health. But even his ammunition consisted of

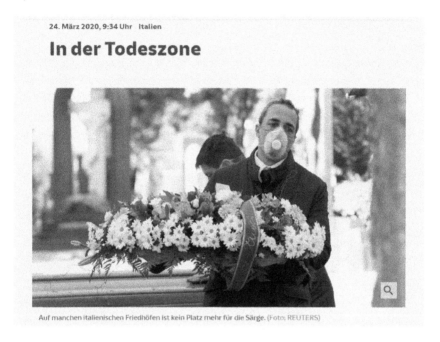

24. März 2020, 9:34 Uhr   Italien

In der Todeszone

Auf manchen italienischen Friedhöfen ist kein Platz mehr für die Särge. (Foto: REUTERS)

Article on sueddeutsche.de *on March 24, 2020. The headline Italy: In the death zone"*
implies that the whole of Italy was a "death zone," which was by far not the case!

blank rounds. Nevertheless, he was allowed to use the *Süddeutsche* to broadcast his prophecy of doom that the number of serious cases would "reach appalling proportions without control measures." Lipsitch was quoted as saying that this is particularly true "in Italy [where] the coffins of COVID-19 victims are gathered in churches." His conclusion: Whoever waits too long risks the collapse of the health system, and its functioning must be preserved in order to keep mortality rates low.[1378] Unfortunately, we do not know what evidence he based his statements on. And an evidence base certainly didn't exist at that time. There was no reliable information to prove that excess death figures had increased significantly overall or even in certain regions. "We would have to make sure that the media do not use the power of images to generate emotions that influence our judgement," said statistics professor Gerd Bosbach. "When pictures of coffins and death departments from Italy are shown, or pictures of absolutely empty shelves, their effects exceed even the stated facts. If we pick out only a small part of the whole with a magnifying glass, we lose the overview."[1379]

Also overlooked was what the Italian newspaper *Corriere della Sera* reported in January 2018: Italian intensive care units had already collapsed under the flu epidemic of 2017/2018, so that operations had to be postponed and nurses recalled from their holidays.[1380] The British *Telegraph* asked the question on 23 March: "Why have so many coronavirus patients died in Italy?" The newspaper then addressed three points in par-

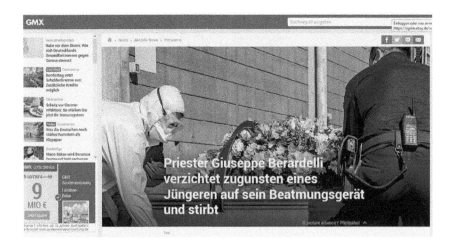

On March 25, 2020, gmx.net, like many other media outlets, reported on the moving act of Italian priest Giuseppe Berardelli giving up a ventilator to a younger patient—of course with the narrative of a killer virus being responsible.

ticular: The high death rate in the country is due to an ageing population, the health care system is overburdened and the way deaths are reported is distorted.[1381] One of the people quoted in this context was Walter Ricciardi, scientific advisor to the Italian Minister of Health, who said that "the way we count deaths in our country was very generous."

In fact, all people who died in hospital and had tested "positive" (with a PCR test), were automatically assumed to have died from the coronavirus. But a re-evaluation by the National Institute of Health revealed that 88 percent of the patients who died had at least one underlying illness, and many even had two or three.

Even a Bloomberg report from 18 March stated that "more than 99 per cent" of those who died and tested "positive" for corona were people who had underlying illnesses, according to a study by the national health authority. At the same time, the average age of the deceased was 79.5 years. And "all victims in Italy under 40 years of age were men with serious illnesses."[1382]

The palliative care physician Matthias Thöns commented on this on 11 April 2020: "In Italy, only three out of 2003 deaths had been patients without serious pre-existing conditions."[1383] Klaus Püschel, head of Hamburg Forensic Medicine, told the *Hamburger Abendblatt* four days later that the so-called COVID-19 fatalities he examined all had such serious pre-existing conditions that, "even if this sounds harsh, they would all have died in the course of this year."

In other words, many people would have died anyway, regardless of them testing "positive." Essentially, a reclassification has taken place, i.e. previously people died of heart failure, cancer, etc., but since the beginning of the "corona age," the seriously ill are tested—and when they test "positive" and die, their death is no longer classified as a heart or cancer death, but as a COVID-19 death. In the end, the president of the RKI also conceded this—unfortunately only on the request of a journalist.[1384]

Additionally, orthodox virologist Hendrik Streeck confirmed that deaths were being reclassified in the aforementioned interview with the *FAZ*: "It must also be taken into account that the SARS-CoV-2 deaths in Germany were exclusively among old people. In Heinsberg, for example, a 78-year-old man with pre-existing conditions died of heart failure, and that without any lung involvement from SARS-2. Since he was infected, he naturally appears in the Covid-19 statistics. But the question is whether he would not have died anyway, even without SARS-2."[1385]

The USA similarly reclassified mortality numbers to create misleading figures thus "confirming" the horror scenarios. The authorities began to recommend that all deceased people who tested "positive," and even suspected cases without a "positive" test result, be registered as "COVID-19 deaths," as the *New York Post* reported on 7 April in the article "Feds classifying all coronavirus patient deaths as 'COVID-19' deaths, regardless of cause."

A US physician and state senator from Minnesota declared that this was tantamount to manipulation. Furthermore, there were financial incentives for hospitals to declare patients as COVID-19 patients.[1386] In the same vein a doctor from the US state of Montana blew the whistle in her YouTube video "COVID-19 death certificates are being manipulated."

Good summaries of manipulated data were published very early, for example on April 5th, 2020 in the *OffGuardian* ("Covid19 Death Figures: 'A Substantial Over-Estimate': Bizarre guidelines from health authorities around the world are potentially including thousands of deceased patients who were never even tested") and on April 13th in the German online magazine *Rubikon* ("The Lethality Scam: So much for 'millions of deaths' worldwide. The numbers are manipulated and are estimated to be twenty times inflated").

COVID-19 Mortality Data Reveals:
Viral Cause Impossible, Drugs Key Factor

Any self-respecting scientist should always look at things from a "wide angle," especially in microbiology—a world that could hardly be more complex. There are some very good reasons, as we have explained, to regard the COVID-19 viral theory as unfounded and un-sound. At the same time, there is another factor that must be acknowledged as a possible cause: the use of drugs with severe side effects including potential death. Especially, if one considers that "our prescription drugs are the third leading cause of death after heart disease and cancer in the United States and Europe," as Peter C. Gøtzsche states.[1387]

As far as corona was concerned, politicians were given the "green light" for implementing their lockdown measures when virologists like Christian Drosten declared their prophecies of doom. On March 6, he stated that, "278,000 corona death victims are to be expected" in Germany. We have explained that such horror scenarios lacked any scientific foundation. The observational data also showed that in the first six months of 2020 there was no ex-cess mortality in numerous countries, including Germany—so a virus cannot be blamed as the cause of the increased mortality in countries such as Spain, France, England or the USA.

Instead, there is overwhelming evidence for the theory that in these latter countries it was primarily the mass and experimental administration of preparations such as hydroxychloroquine, Kaletra and azithromycin that caused countless people to die prematurely. On another note, in the middle of 2020 the Australian state of Victoria showed the world just how absurd the behavior of the decision makers could be – with orders such as the police being allowed to enter anyone's home without a warrant, an 8 o'clock curfew, and even a ban on weddings. Jeffrey A. Tucker, editorial director of the American Institute of Economic Research, commented: „Melbourne has become a living hell. Tacitus's line about the Roman empire comes to mind: ,Where they make a desert, they call it peace.'"

The mere fact that „in Australia since March, there have been 50 percent more deaths from suicide than official numbers show for Covid-19," as Tucker pointed out, should have given everyone plenty to think about. The lockdown in Australia was all the more absurd if you consider that „the per capita deaths are about 26 per million over a six months period," as David James, journalist from Down Under, stated in an *OffGuardian* article. With the best will in the world this cannot be called a virus pandemic.

Especially since, as James added: „the chief health officer in Victoria admitted that they were not testing for the virus, just assuming that if there were flu-like symptom it must be COVID-19; and deaths by flu in Australia, it should be added, are running unusually low."

Like Australia, many other countries did not record any excess mortality in the first six months of 2020 either. For example in Germany and Portugal the mortality rates for this period were even lower than some of the previous years. This was the conclusion of the previously mentioned analysis titled „For [the decision makers] know not what they do" by Stefan Aust, former editor-in-chief of Germany's best known news magazine *Der Spiegel*.
As Aust stated, the fact that Germany and other countries did not experience any excess mortality could not be considered the result of the governments' lockdown measures. A main reason: The majority of those who were declared corona deaths were elderly and came from the seriously ill in aged care facilities. So „their lives could not have been saved even with the strictest general social lockdown measures."

Indeed, some countries recorded noticeably more deaths in the first half of 2020 than in some previous years. This holds true especially for Italy, Spain, France, England, Belgium, the Netherlands and the USA. However, the hypothesis that only lockdowns could slow down a new, deadly corona virus was contradicted by the fact that these countries in particular pursued rigid lockdown policies. Meanwhile, Sweden which did not implement any lockdown, should have experienced an extremely high excess mortality, which it did not.

In addition, Belgium, for example, had eight times more deaths (per 100,000 inhabitants) than its neighbour Germany, Spain 22 times more than Poland, while Portugal, Spain's direct neighbour, did not experience any excess mortality. But in today's times how can a virus afflict countries so differently? – It couldn't have changed its very nature with each border crossing. This is why our author, Claus Köhnlein, MD, stated in a letter, published at the end of June in the German *Ärzteblatt*: „In view of the fact that very different mortality rates are reported in different European countries, it is reasonable to assume that a different aggressive therapy could be responsible for this."

This is also clearly supported by the fact that the largest part of the excess mortality in these countries took place during a very short period of time, within about two to three weeks around early/mid-April. As the Euromomo mortality statistics show, in Spain and the UK the charts had been relatively „boring" until around the end of March, but then the excess mortality suddenly shot up, only to drop drastically again around mid-April causing a "peak" around April – where the majority of the deaths were of old age. (see diagram 11 with the charts of Spain, Portugal, UK and Sweden).

In number terms this means that within a few weeks 60 to 70 thousand more deaths occurred in these European countries than is usual at this time of the year. And there were around 130,000 additional deaths in the US during the first six months of 2020 compared to the same period of the previous two years (the death rate in the USA for the first half of 2020 was 0.48 percent, in 2018 and 2019 it was 0.44 percent). The only difference between the European countries and the U.S. is that the „peak" in America's chart is a bit wider, i.e. it extends over more than two weeks in April, and the peak is on April 11, about two weeks later than that of Italy, where the worldwide death drama started (see diagram 12).

So it really makes it impossible to declare that it was a virus that killed many tens of thousands in a two week period outside of peak flu season. A respiratory virus simply does not behave this way. And even if such a super deadly virus existed, according to the lockdown proponents, it would have caused a staggering „peak" in Sweden's chart, a country that did not lock down at all. But Sweden's chart shows only a flat hump in mid April. Additionally, the death rate, i.e. the proportion of deaths per total number of inhabitants, for the first six months of 2020 was 0.48 percent which is within expected range and only slightly higher than in 2017 and 2018 (0.46 percent). On October 9, the Foundation for Economic Education (FEE) published the analysis „5 Charts That Show Sweden's Strategy Worked. The Lockdowns Failed." Conclusion: „We know better now. There ist no correlation between lockdown stringency and COVID-19 deaths, while their harms are indisputable."

Diagram 11   Excess Mortality (z-score) for Selected European Countries
                    (Dec. 2019 till Sept. 2020)

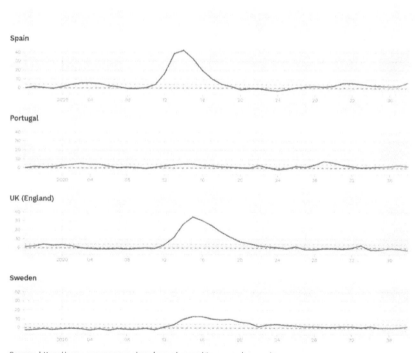

Source: https://www.euromomo.eu/graphs-and-maps/#z-scores-by-country

In Italy, there was also a "peak" in the chart in April, but (just like in Switzerland, as we shall see) the deaths were concentrated in certain regions like Bergamo. Even allowing for demographics a respiratory virus that is deadly in only certain regions of a country seems odd! A closer look at Germany's data also shows that the virus only thesis is not plausible.

The data from the Federal Statistical Office shows the weekly death rates (see diagram 13). This chart shows that in March 2019, about 86,500 people died. Yet, „in March 2018, i.e. in a year when the flu epidemic was particularly severe, the figure was 107,100. Even without a corona pandemic, the death toll can therefore fluctuate considerably, especially during the typical flu season," as it says on their website. Clearly there is no evidence of a corona virus death train looking at the 2020 curve, even with the best will in the world. The study „Excess mortality due to COVID-19 in Germany" by the University Duisburg-Essen, published in September 2020 in the *Journal of Infection*, even indicates that „during the first COVID-19 wave" ther was „under-mortality" with a „deficit of 4,926 deaths," when the increasing number of elderly is taken into account.

Nor do the figures for 2020 as a whole, which the Federal Statiscital Office in Germany presented on January 22, 2021, provide evidence for a raging virus. There were almost 41,000

Diagram 12   Weely Mortality Rates in the USA (June 2018 till August 2020)

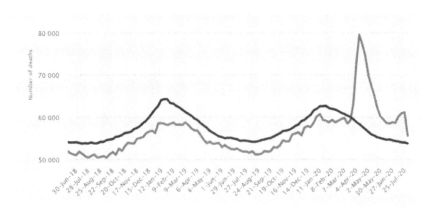

Source: statista.com

or 4 percent more deaths in 2020 than on average from 2016 to 2019, and almost 20,000 more deaths (+ 2.1%) than in 2018. But not only were about 1 Million more inhabitants in Germany in 2020 than in 2016, but far more than half of those who died came from the over-80 age group—and their share increased from 5.8 to 6.8 percent between 2016 and 2019, an increase of almost 20 percent. This, together with the aforementioned heat wave in the late summer 2020, which led to more than 9,000 more deaths than normal in Germany, already explains a significant part of the almost 41,000 deaths in 2020.

The rest is then "easily" explained by the wide-spread experimental and high-dose administration of potentially lethal drugs—drugs that have been used in worldwide trials and also outside of these trials, costing the lives of tens of thousands of "test" subjects. Over the course of time the „patient supply" dried up which is largely suggested by the rapid drop in the curves creating these „peaks" in April 2020.

By the way, the flat „peak" in the 2020 chart from Germany with an excess mortality of a few thousand in April (compared to 2019 and 2018) corresponds almost exactly with the increased experimental use of the malaria drug hydroxychloroquine in so-called COVID-19 patients (more on the crucial role of this drug later). As the German news

Diagram 13   Weekly death rates in Germany 2020

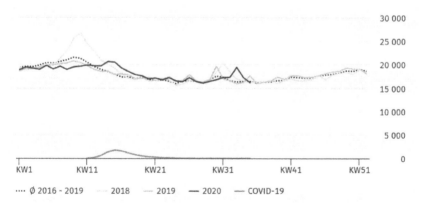

Source: German Federal Statistical Office

411

magazine *Spiegel* reported, according to an analysis from the German health insurer AOK the drug had found many supporters in Germany from March on. In this month the drug was prescribed to almost 10,000 more patients than in the previous month—mostly to patients who were very old, with serious health problems and for whom potentially toxic drugs were therefore particularly life-threatening. In April and May, the numbers of hydroxychloroquine prescriptions in Germany dropped again. In June, the figures were then below the average of the previous year.

In fact, it seems likely that the general COVID-19 panic, which was particularly striking in the second half of March, led to an increased experimental use of highly toxic drugs such as hydroxychloroquine and the antiviral preparation Kaletra (Lopinavir/Ritonavir) in Germany. However, the use of these drugs in countries such as Germany was obviously noticeably lower than in Belgium or Great Britain.

In this context it is noteworthy that on March 20, 2020 an interview by Margarita Bityutskikh from *Russia Today* with our author Claus Köhnlein was broadcasted on YouTube. In it he criticized the experimental use of highly toxic drugs. The interview had more than 900,000 views within a short time (a second *Russia Today* interview with him, posted on YouTube on September 18, with the title "Dr. Claus Köhnlein on 'fatal corona experiments' by the WHO" gained almost 1.4 million views within a short time). A few days later, the physician from Kiel received a call from a former doctoral student at the Charité's Institute for Social Medicine.

She asked Köhnlein if he was aware that his critical statements had torpedoed the application of the antiviral therapy in connection with COVID-19. His answer: If his interview statements had really contributed to the fact that significantly less medication was used, then he would have achieved exactly what he wanted to, because such drug therapy is always immunosuppressive and thus can be fatal, especially for already severely ill people.

In the mentioned letter to the journal *Ärzteblatt* Claus Köhnlein wrote: "It could be that we got off so well in Germany because we were therapeutically more reserved from the beginning and/or because we have learned from the bad experiences in countries such as Italy, Spain, France and England and hardly used any antiviral substances."[1388]

In the course of corona mega-panic, experiments with drugs with a plethora of side effects were started very early on worldwide, although their effect on COVID-19 patients had not been comprehensively investigated at all. For example, the *Pharmazeutische Zeitung* reported as early as 28th January 2020 that, although there are "no specific drugs against corona viruses ... certain HIV drugs are used experimentally"—seemingly with the motto: trial and error. It should be noted that "certain HIV drugs" can be potentially fatal (this is particularly true for old and frail people suffering from more severe diseases).

There were also reports in the media that "a spokeswoman for the US pharmaceutical company AbbVie has confirmed that the Chinese health authorities have requested the HIV drug Kaletra"[1389]—a combined preparation (Lopinavir and Ritonavir), which, like other antiviral drugs, can have "life-threatening" side effects.[1390]

The precipitant of the massive experimental use of medication was probably papers such as the single-case study, published in *The Lancet* on February 18, 2020. Perhaps if it had been assessed more critically it would have served as an early warning *against* the use of such drugs. It described a case of a 50-year-old man who presented with fever, chills, coughing, tiredness and shortness of breath who was classified as a "COVID-19" patient.

Thereupon he was treated with a total drug armada consisting of the antiviral drugs interferon alfa-2b, lopinavir and ritonavir, the antibiotics moxifloxacin and meropenem as well as high dose cortisone (methylprednisolone)—substances that can have severe side effects, including death, even when administered alone. Moreover, the autopsy revealed liver damage—and this the authors of the *Lancet* paper at least conceded may have been caused by the drugs. But the strong possibility that the patient actually died due to drug toxicity cannot be ignored.

And if such a man who was „in his best years" at the age of 50 with no apparent underlying illnesses other than severe flu symptoms, died after receiving such a „drug cocktail," then one can imagine how such highly toxic "treatments" could affect people classified as COVID-19 patients in their 70s or 80s with underlying illnesses including cancer.

But why did the attending physicians treat the 50-year-old this way? And why does this *Lancet* paper emphatically conclude that the patient "died from severe infection with severe acute respiratory syndrome coronavirus 2 (SARS-CoV-2)," i.e. from nothing other than a virus? The answer seems to be: monocausal virus tunnel vision, the deep-seated belief that only drugs can bring salvation to the ill and out of the fear, typical in today's medical system, that one could have left a remedy untried, which then often enough leads to more drug administration. All the more so during the panic of a "pandemic", as in this case.

Because the tragic 50-year-old was short of breath, he was given cortisone, a lymphocyte suppressant that slows down the inflammatory response. Many symptoms then subside and fever, for example, goes down. The patient feels temporarily better, he can breathe more easily again. However, there is a cost: the immune system is heavily suppressed, which can end up being fatal, as was possible in this case, especially if other potentially lethal medication is administered in addition. Nevertheless, the *Lancet* study concluded that the patient died only of a virus, and despite the drugs not because of the drugs. And this kind of study, published in a journal whose content is widely considered de facto law, served as a blueprint for the treatment of COVID-19 patients.

In fact, only a few weeks later, highly toxic drugs were used excessively, especially in all of the above-mentioned countries with excess mortality, both experimentally and off-label, meaning that the drugs were used outside of their regulatory approval. Even worse was that the drugs were mostly given to people who were old and already had serious illnesses, prior to testing „positive" for COVID-19.

The available data gives the impression that increased deaths migrated quickly like a huge wave from Italy via Spain and France to the UK and Belgium and then spilled over to the USA and Brazil.

In Italy, and especially in Lombardy, the „drug frenzy" started around March 17th, and was particularly rampant in nursing homes and clinics. For Italy, there was a telling death statistic from April 9, 2020, which showed that 84% of the deceased patients received antibiotics, especially azithromycin, 55% received antiviral drugs, 33% received corticosteroids and 18.6% a combination of all three.

With regards to azithromycin, in 2013 the U.S. Food and Drug Administration (FDA) issued a warning that its use may lead to a potentially fatal irregular heart rhythm. That antiviral drugs can be lethal has also been sufficiently shown. This includes the combination Lopinavir-Ritonavir, which was also given to the 50-year-old patient mentioned above.

As for corticosteroids, a study published in the *Journal of Infection* on April 10, 2020 concluded: "Patients with severe conditions are more likely to require corticosteroids. Corticosteroid use is associated with increased mortality in patients with coronavirus pneumonia." Despite the authors suggesting that "corticosteroid should be used with caution in the treatment of COVID-19", it really indicates that there was no evidence for corticosteroid use in this setting.

France Culture described how the great drug experiment was being done in practice in an article titled „Covid-19: in France, Italy, Spain, Germany, how doctors are tackling the disease," by quoting the neurologist Francesco Alberti, president of the Order of Physicians of the Province of Imperia (a subdivision of the Liguria region bordering France), who had returned to work due to the pandemic:

"We are doing a lot of experimentation and many trials, because the disease is very different and more or less serious depending on the patient. If there is only fever and it doesn't last more than 4 or 5 days, we prescribe paracetamol. Beyond that, we use antivirals to limit the progression of the disease: the most commonly used drugs are hydroxychloroquine, brand name Plaquenil, combined with an antibiotic, azithromycin, bearing in mind that hydroxychloroquine can cause heart rhythm problems. We also give other antivirals such as remdesivir and favipiravir. In case of immune system runaway, we are also experimenting with tocilizumab, an immunological drug usually prescribed for rheumatoid problems."

For now, we will discuss hydroxchloroquine, its potentially deadly effects and the devastating role it played as well as remdesivir later. As far as tocilizumab is concerned, it can also be deadly, by causing lethal allergic reactions. Since this immunosuppressive drug was launched in the US in 2010, more than 1,000 deaths have been reported to the FDA.

However, the actual number is likely to be much higher as the FDA's reporting system only covers a fraction of the adverse events that occur in patients.

Meanwhile Alberti continued: „There is no single therapeutic protocol. The drugs we use are ‚off label', i.e. we prescribe them outside their indications. The Ministry of Health and the Italian Drug Agency have authorized us to use these drugs, even if they were originally prescribed for other diseases."

And a quick word on ventilation. Jean-François Timsit, Head of the Department of Intensive Care Medicine and Resuscitation of Infectious Diseases at the Bichat Hospital in Paris, for his part said: „For the moment, the mortality rate is estimated at around 30 percent for patients who are in intensive care, with a variation depending on whether or not patients are intubated [for machine ventilation]. When patients are intubated, the death rate rises to 50 percent."

30 percent is already a very high figure, 50 percent all the more. In fact, intubations were increasingly used because it was initially feared that the significantly less invasive mask respiration would carry a higher risk of viral infection. However, it had already been observed that patients died more frequently as a result of invasive ventilation in relation to SARS in 2002/2003. This trend appeared to continue in the treatment of COVID-19 patients. A *Lancet* study in February 2020 drew a very bleak picture: only three out of 22 intubated patients survived.

On December 23, 2020, *focus.de* published the article "Too high mortality due to intubation—pulmonologist: 'Early ventilation is biggest mistake in the fight against corona.'" In it, pulmonologist Thomas Voshaar states that intubation causes the mortality of those labeled as COVID-19 victims to rise extremely. "Fifty percent of invasively ventilated COVID-19 patients die. This is a clear sign that we need to take a different approach in medicine," Voshaar appeals to colleagues. Unfortunatley, this appeal also went unheard.

The Hydroxychloroquine Overdose Tragedy

Hydroxychloroquine which had already been widely administered to patients in Italy, played a significant part in making countless people die prematurely. Hydroxychloroquine is far from harmless and, has many serious side effects including death by causing cardiac arrhythmias. This is especially so if it is given in higher doses, which is exactly what happened in the treatment of so-called COVID-19 patients, in Italy, Spain, France, England and the USA. Yale epidemiologist Harvey Risch, who is one of the best known researchers who saw a potential curative effect if the drug was administered in low doses, wrote by email: "I agree about hydroxychloroquine overdosing, both from a reduced function point of view and toxicity."

In Spain, the Agencia Española de Medicamentos y Productos Sanitarios (AEMPS)—the Agency of Medicines and Healthcare Products—started the extensive distribution of hydroxychloroquine and its somewhat more toxic variant chloroquine for COVID-19 in hospitals on March 16, 2020 through the application of Management of Medicines in Special Situations (MSE). As Miquel Barceló from the hospital Cerdanya around 150 km north of Barcelona and just south of the French border told *France Culture* at the beginning of April:

"There is a more or less reckless behavior in relation to this drug [hydroxychloroquine] … There are many patients in intensive care and many deaths compared to Occitania [directly opposite on the French site] … Faced with this drift of the disease, people say to themselves: we must do something. There is perhaps less reluctance to use this drug."

Just two days later (March 18), none other than Tedros Adhanom Ghebreyesus, Director-General of the WHO, proclaimed a major study-based drug offensive to combat COVID-19:

"Multiple small trials with different methodologies may not give us the clear, strong evidence we need about which treatments help to save lives. WHO and its partners are therefore organizing a study in many countries in which some of these untested treatments are compared with each other. This large, international study is designed to generate the robust data we need, to show which treatments are the most effective. We have called this study the SOLIDARITY trial."

And the focus of this SOLIDARITY trial was on the following already mentioned highly toxic drugs: remdesivir, lopinavir/ritonavir (Kaletra), Interferon-β in combination with Kaletra and hydroxychloroquine and chloroquine.

"However, the doses were not specified on WHO's list of the drugs to be trialed, nor were the actual doses specified, surprisingly, in WHO's consultation on chloroquine dosing, dated April 8," as Meryl Nass, a physician from Maine, pointed out in an article for the Alliance for Human Research Protection.

Instead, the introduction of the report of that meeting notes, "The chloroquine or hydroxychloroquine schedule selected for the trial includes two oral loading doses (250 mg per tablet CQ or 200 mg per tablet HCQ), then oral twice-daily maintenance doses for ten days. This meeting convened to discuss the appropriateness of the selected doses for the trial."

But according to Nass, this statement about "dosing seems to be deliberately vague or even misleading, as the actual dose used in the SOLIDARITY trial is 2,400 mg during the first 24 hours, and a cumulative dose of 9.2 grams [9,200 mg] over 10 days."

This extremely high dose is all the more strange when you consider the document from the WHO's March 13 informal consultation on the potential role of chloroquine. Incidentally, it showed that the Gates Foundation was among those involved in studying chloroquine's pharmacokinetics (of the 25 participants at this meeting, 5 were from the Gates Foundation). In this file it says "Higher doses would be considered for treatment, i.e., [a loading dose of] 10mg/kg base, followed by 5mg/kg twice daily for seven days." (A 250 mg chloroquine tablet contains 150 mg of "base" drug.)

If this had been followed a typical 70 kg person would receive 700 mg base, which equals 1,200 mg of chloroquine, as a loading dose. This is much lower than the dose of 2,400mg hydroxychloroquine used in the first 24 hours in the Solidarity trial when one considers that chloroquine and hydroxychloroquine are given in comparable doses.

Note that both, chloroquine and hydroxychloroquine, are very difficult for the body to break down: in fact, they have elimination half-lives of one to two months. Thus the doses can rapidly cumulate with potentially fatal effects, even more so in older people. In 1986, the German journal *Zeitschrift für Rechtsmedizin* published the article „Tod nach Gabe von 1250 mg Chloroquin bei Porphyria cutanea tarda" (Death after administration of 1250 mg [1.25 g] chloroquine in [the metabolic disease] Porphyria cutanea tarda). Other sources put the lethal dose at 2 to 3 g.

In 1979, the WHO hired a consultant named H. Weniger to explore the toxicity of chloroquine. He looked at 335 episodes of adult poisoning by chloroquine. On page 5 Weniger notes that a single dose of 1.5 to 2.0 g of chloroquine base [= 2.5 to 3.3 g chloroquine] may be fatal." It should be emphasized again that the dose of the highly comparable hydroxychloroquine used in the SOLIDARITY trial was 2.4 g in the first 24 hours alone and a total dose of 9.2g over 10 days.

According to Nass, "all experts agree on this: ' ... chloroquine has a small toxic to therapeutic margin,' according to Goldfrank's Toxicologic Emergencies. The drug is very safe when used correctly, but not a lot more can potentially kill. Prof. Nicholas White, a Wellcome Trust Principal Research Fellow and expert in malaria treatment, who attended both WHO consultations on the chloroquines, has confirmed this."

This is aggravated by the fact that the WHO report of its meeting on chloroquine dosing states, "Although the preponderance of opinion tilted towards a reasonable benefit risk profile for the intervention, there was some scepticism about what was considered a 'minimalistic safety data collection' currently included in the protocol." Nass' commentary: "The high dose regimen being used in the SOLIDARITY trials has no medical justification. The trial design, with its limited collection of safety data, may make it more difficult to identify toxic drug effects, compared to standard drug trials. This is entirely unethical."

Nevertheless, many countries around the globe joined the SOLIDARITY trial, among them Spain, France, Switzerland and Belgium — countries that had noticeable excess mortality (mostly limited to April).

At the end of March, 2020 none other than US President Donald Trump praised hydroxy-chloroquine as "a gift from God," which certainly gave the demand for the drug and the belief in its possible healing powers an extra boost. But as promising as the well-meaning name "SOLIDARITY" and Trump's proclamation sounded, the whole thing ended in disaster, due to the overdosing with hydroxychloroquine, which in many cases was given together with other toxic drugs.

How dangerous chloroquine could be, was demonstrated in Brazil. On April 13, the *Chicago Tribune* reported that a study in Brazil where "national guidelines recommend the use of chloroquine in coronavirus patients" was halted early for safety reasons after "coronavirus" patients taking a higher dose of chloroquine were found to have an increased risk of a potentially fatal heart arrhythmia. Patients in the trial were also given the antibiotic azithromycin, which carries similar risks.

"To me, this study conveys one useful piece of information, which is that chloroquine causes a dose-dependent increase in an abnormality in the electrocardiogram [which measures the heart's electrical activity] that could predispose people to sudden cardiac death," said Dr. David Juurlink, a physician and the head of the division of clinical pharmacology at the University of Toronto.

Roughly half the study participants were given a dose of 450 milligrams of chloroquine twice daily for five days, i.e. 4.5 g total, while the rest got a higher dose of 600 milligrams every 12 hours for 10 days, i.e. 12 g total. Within three days, researchers started noticing heart arrhythmias (abnormal heartbeats) in patients taking the higher dose. By the sixth day of treatment, 11 of them had died, leading to an immediate end to the high-dose segment of the trial.

In Switzerland, empirical evidence raised suspicions that a major cause of excess mortality was also due to drugs after 16 hospitals joined the SOLIDARITY study. In the alpine country a significant excess mortality was only evident in the Italian-speaking canton of Ticino and the French-speaking part of the country but not in the German-speaking region, as data from the Federal Statistical Office show. And the German speaking canton of Zurich with its 1,521,000 inhabitants had about the same number of deaths as Ticino, despite the latter's much smaller population (353'000 inhabitants). The idea that a respiratory virus alone could attack Switzerland's cantons in such different ways, is just completely irrational.

The cluster of deaths in certain places also occurred incredibly quickly. For example in the St. Antonius retirement and nursing home in Saas-Grund (in the Valais region which was participating in the SOLIDARITY trial). As Swiss television reported, the first „positive" test was on April 1, 2020, the first death on April 17, and shortly afterwards another 14 died, i.e. a total of almost a third of the home's residents passed away very rapidly.

"We had many inhabitants, who were relatively well on the way with the virus, and we had actually seven to eight days the feeling that the people were over the hump, and suddenly things went very badly," said the housemaster Patricia Pfammatter. „Within a few hours they were then partly no longer responsive, terminal, you could tell they were coming to an end."

„It appears that the SOLIDARITY trials are not testing the benefits of hydroxychloroquine on Covid-19, but rather testing whether patients tolerate toxic, non-therapeutic doses," as Meryl Nass criticized.

However, the SOLIDARITY studies weren't the only experimental trials. On March 22, IN-SERM, the French biomedical research agency, announced it was coordinating an add-on trial in Europe, named DISCOVERY, that would follow the WHO's example and include 3,200 patients from at least seven countries, including 800 from France. It was said the trial would test the same drugs, with the exception of chloroquine.

On April 8, *Newsweek* reported that the University Hospital in Nice (CHU), which had been selected for the DISCOVERY study on March 22, had to stop an experimental treatment with hydroxychloroquine. In an interview with the French daily newspaper *Nice-Matin*, Emile Ferrari, Head of Cardiology at the Pasteur Hospital, which is part of the CHU, stated that some patients should have discontinued treatment because of the risk of cardiac arrhythmia.

According to Ferrari, the cardiac risk is increased if the antibiotic azithromycin is given in addition to hydroxychloroquine. For some patients, who are treated with these medicines, the medicine is more harmful than the illness itself, stated Ferrari. "The new observations are quite significant, as the combination is currently being tested in numerous other COVID-19 studies," as the German journal *Deutsche Apotheker Zeitung* (German Pharmacists Newspaper) reported.

As far as France is concerned, massive drug experimentation had taken place there as well. On March 23 the newspaper *L'Express* reported that the High Council of Public Health (Haut Conseil de santé publique) "encourages doctors to include as many patients as possible in the various therapeutic trials underway in our country because it is the surest way to quickly determine whether a treatment is effective or not." And according to a list of different kinds of COVID-19 therapy projects first published on April 1, 2020 various drugs are mentioned, including remdesivir, Kaletra and hydroxychloroquine.

And as an official Belgian guideline document issued on June 8, 2020 shows, high doses of hydroxychloroquine were also used in the DISCOVERY trial in the EU.

But we are far from reaching the end of the study road! On April 3, the UK government announced, „almost 1,000 patients from 132 different hospitals [in the UK] have been already recruited in just 15 days and thousands more are expected to join the Randomized Evaluation of COVID-19 Therapy (RECOVERY) trial in the coming weeks, making it the largest randomized controlled trial of potential COVID-19 treatments in the world. The trial is testing a number of medicines. They include: Lopinavir-Ritonavir, [the anti-inflammatory drug] Dexamethasone, Hydroxychloroquine." The RECOVERY trial was also designed to test the already mentioned azithromycin and tocilizumab as well as REGN-COV2, described as „a combination of monoclonal antibodies directed against coronavirus."

The RECOVERY trial—funded in part by the Wellcome Trust and the Bill & Melinda Gates foundation—had proceeded at unprecedented speed, enrolling over 11,000 patients from 175 National Health Service hospitals in the UK within a relatively short period of time. But then, the hydroxychloroquine arm of the study was abruptly discontinued. The rationale was that the „data convincingly rule out any meaningful mortality benefit of hydroxychloroquine in patients hospitalized with COVID-19." But this was a euphemism that completely distorted reality, because a quarter (25.7 %) of the people treated with hydroxychloroquine had died.

In fact, this is not really surprising when you look at RECOVERY's hydroxychloroquine dosage which resembles that of the SOLIDARITY trial. As Martin Landray, professor of medicine at the University of Oxford and co-head oft he UK based RECOVERY trial said in an interview with the French online newspaper *France-Soir* on June 6, 2020 „it is 2400 mg in the first 24 hours and 800 mg from day 2 to day 10. It is a 10 day course of treatment in total." That makes a total of almost 10 g, with 2.4 g on the first day alone.

In addition, dosing failed to take into account weight, renal and hepatic function," as Meryl Nass pointed out. „The RECOVERY trial used 1.860 grams hydroxychloroquine base (equal to 2400 mg of hydroxychloroquine) in the first 24 hours for treatment of already very ill, hospitalized Covid-19 patients, a potentially lethal dose."

Landray was asked whether "there is any maximum dosage for hydroxychloroquine in the UK?," and Landray answered in all seriousness: „I would have to check but it is much larger than the 2,400mg, something like six or 10 times that." And then he was asked: „Are there any doses considered lethal for hydroxychloroquine in the UK by the Medicines and Healthcare products Regulatory Agency, MHRA?" Landray: „The treating doctors did not report that they thought any of the deaths were due to hydroxychloro-quine. We did not stop the [hydroxychloroquine] arm not because of safety but because it doesn't work. For a new disease such as COVID, there is no approved dosing proto-col. But the HCQ dosage used are not dissimilar to that used, as I said, in for example amoebic dysentery."

The chief investigator of the RECOVERY trial, Peter Horby, claimed that the *France Soir* misinterpreted Landray's comments, but *France Soir* could easily refute the criticism as they were simply quoting Landray.

Hence, Landray's statements can only be viewed as careless, if not irresponsible. The UK's maximum recommended daily dosage for hydroxychloroquine is 6.5mg per kg, i.e. approximately 500mg per day. Incredibly, the RECOVERY trial's hydroxychloroquine dosage of 2,400mg in the first 24 hours is even higher than what the L'autorisation de mise sur le marché (AMM) in France considers the overdose rate of 25mg/kg (e.g. 1,875mg per day for a 75kg patient), requiring immediate emergency hospital care. Furthermore, the RECOVERY dosage is well above that recommended by the World Medical Association (WMA) in France, as *France Soir* reported in its article „Recovery trial: Brexit and overdose" on June 8, 2020.

The RECOVERY and SOLIDARITY trials abruptly ended their hydroxychloroquine study arms on June 5 and June 17, respectively—coincidentally as people began noticing the excessive potentially lethal doses, especially on Twitter (hashtag #Recoverygate).

Another very strange thing was that on May 28, just before the hydroxychloroquine study was stopped, the RECOVERY Control Committee indicated that there was no problem with hydroxychloroquine and therefore recommended that recruitment should be continued without interruption until the next meeting, scheduled for June 11. They didn't seem to take into account a *Lancet* study that had appeared on May 22, which reviewed over 96,000 patient records. This revealed a much higher death rate in patients receiving hydroxychloroquine, while an even higher death rate was observed in subjects receiving hydroxychloroquine plus a macrolide such as azithromycin compared to the control group.

But the debacle just got worse. On May 29, the Indian Council of Medical Research had alerted the WHO about the incredibly high dose of hydroxychloroquine being used in the RECOVERY trial, being four times higher than that used in the Indian trials. And on June 4, the UK's Medicines and Healthcare products Regulatory Agency asked the RECOVERY team to look at the data for hydroxychloroquine. The French Minister of Health, by the way, had done the same on May 23, 2020. Only four days later, on May 27, the French government decided to stop using hydroxychloroquine after receiving an adverse report on its use by the National Agency for the Safety of Medicines and Health Products.

Then, on June 4, the *Lancet* retracted its comprehensive study that showed the high lethality of hydroxychloroquine (plus an antibiotic).

It begs the question: What was actually going on here? Officially, the *Lancet* study had been retracted after independent peer reviewers informed three study-authors that Surgisphere, a Chicago-based company providing and summarizing the raw hospital patient data, would not transfer the full dataset, client contracts, and the full ISO audit report for their analysis. But how realistic is it to assume that the authors of such an important study—among them cardiologist Mandeep Mehra of Harvard University said to be „one of the stars of the field" and „as straight an arrow as you can find"—compiled it without examining the raw data or the study had not gone through the peer review process when it was approved for publication?

This gives rise to the thought: Why was it „necessary" to withdraw this study? Imagine, what would have happened if this *Lancet* study had not been labeled as dubious and retracted. Then of course it would be apparent that there had been "a lot of collateral damage in terms of patients not surviving the treatment," as Roger Lord, a Research Fellow with The Prince Charles Hospital in Brisbane and lecturer in medical sciences at The Australian Catholic University pointed out. Indeed, this would have been the final proof that hydroxychloroquine administered in high doses is a potential „killer" and led to countless unnecessary deaths all over the world. And then, wouldn't it also have been much more difficult to justify the RECOVERY study's reckless use of hydroxychloroquine?

Or maybe it was smoke and mirrors: First, on May 22, hydroxychloroquine was demonized when the *Lancet* study was published in order to distract attention from other toxic drugs such as remdesivir. Then, on June 5, hydroxychloroquine was taken out of the line of fire by the retraction of the *Lancet* study as well as by the termination of the hydroxychloroquine arms in the RECOVERY and SOLIDARITY trials (June 5 and 17). They claimed this drug was not effective (instead of telling the truth that this drug had been administered in potentially fatal doses), which in turn caused so much confusion that the topic of "lethal drug effects" fell out of sight.

Another very important question is: when discussing the maximum dosage for hydroxychloroquine in the UK why on earth did co-chief investigator Landray state „I would have to check but it is much larger than the 2,400mg, something like six or 10 times …

the hydroxychloroquine dosage used are not dissimilar to that used, as I said, in for example amoebic dysentery"?

With regards to this, Christian Perronne, professor of infectious and tropical diseases, pointed out to *France Soir*:

„In 1975, when I did my medical internship at the Claude Bernard hospital, which was the temple of infectious diseases, I saw a lot of amoebiasis and chloroquine was no longer used to treat that disease. It is the first time that I learn [from Martin Landray] that we use hydroxychloroquine in amoebic dysentery, in super-toxic doses for humans. The classic treatment for colonic amoebiasis is the hydroxyquinoline combination of tiliquinol and tilbroquinol, the trade name of which is Intetrix."

This is why Perronne thinks „Landray confused hydroxychloroquine with hydroxyquinoline. This man, who calls himself a doctor, is incompetent and dangerous. This is scandalous."

The question remains, why did Landray tell *France Soir* hydroxychloroquine was not lethal and that they stopped the hydroxychloroquine „arm not because of safety but because it doesn't work"?

Perhaps because the mortality rate in the comparison group (randomized to standard care) in the RECOVERY trial was 23.6 percent and was therefore not much lower than in the subjects receiving hydroxychloroquine (25.7 percent). But there is something very odd here because 23.6% seems unusually high.

For example, in a study published in the *Journal of the American Medical Association* on May 11, 2020, on severe hospitalized patients comparing hydroxychloroquine plus azithromycin with hydroxychloroquine alone, with azithromycin alone and neither drug, the mortality rate for the latter was 12.7 percent. Another study published in the *New England Journal of Medicine* showed an intubation or mortality rate of 32.3 percent for the hydroxychloroquine group and 14.9 percent for the no hydroxychloroquine group.

The latter two studies focused on the New York state. That is to say, we have the simple result that twice as many patients died in the New York area when they received hydroxychloroquine. Unfortunately, they were observational studies and the authors applied statistical modelling to conclude that hydroxychloroquine was not associated with increased mortality, rather than looking at the raw data and suspecting drug toxicity as a factor.

These studies do provide very good information about which medicines were prescribed at that time in regions such as New York. And hydroxychloroquine, in particular, was also widely dispensed by general practitioners and other physicians. In practice, it appeared that patients who tested "positive" queued up in front of clinics for a pack of hydroxychloroquine. A pack that is quite capable of sending a person to the afterlife. And there were certainly some who thought that twice as much is twice as good.[1391]

With regards to the pharmacological frenzy, the US physician and molecular biologist Andrew Kaufman commented: "In order to put the people in the USA on the ventilators, since they were awake and alert, they had to use many drugs. They used paralytics—related to curare poison—, sedatives, and anesthesia. They also used prophylactic drugs on them, such as proton pump inhibitors, anti-clotting drugs, etc. This is, of course, in addition to antibiotics, antivirals/chemotherapy drugs, and others like hydroxychloroquine and corticosteroids. I wish we were in a position to do a chart review in the hot spots and see what really killed each individual."[1392]

Anyone who thought it couldn't get any worse, was mistaken. Another study was initiated, named REMAP, that targeted patients who were on ventilators, or in shock, i.e. near death—using the same hydroxychloroquine loading dose (2.4 g in the first 24 hours) as the RECOVERY and the SOLIDARITY trial and 6.4 g total within six days. But there were even more problems as physician Meryl Nass outlined at the time:

- As a participant, you have to be close to death to be included in the trial, according to the trial documents.

- You may receive hydroxychloroquine alone or in combination with two more drugs, lopinavir/ritonavir, which, as mentioned, may not only be fatal themselves. Yet lopinavir/ritonavir predisposes to QT prolongation, as does hydroxychloroquine (QT prolongation is a measure of delayed ventricular repolarisation, which means the heart muscle takes longer than normal to recharge between beats). And the drug label states, 'Avoid use in combination with QTc- or PR-interval prolonging drugs.'

- Patients who are in shock or on a ventilator may be unable to give their consent to enroll in a clinical trial. But the trial investigators have deemed that consent may not be required: 'For patients who are not competent to consent, either prospective agreement or entry via waiver of consent or some form of deferred consent can be applied, as required by an appropriate ethical review body.'

- For patients too sick to swallow a pill, the drug will be administered via a feeding tube. This could entail an extra procedure for patients."

The REMAP trials took place at 200 sites in 14 countries, among them Belgium, the Netherlands, Spain, the UK, and the USA—all countries with an excess mortality over a relatively short period of time.[1393]

Before starting such massive human experiments, one should have at least taken a look back in history to avoid making the same mistakes. As the aforementioned article in the *Pharmazeutische Zeitung* stated: "During the SARS pandemic in 2002/2003, patients were also treated with corticosteroids and the hepatitis C drug ribavirin. Initial reports had sounded promising, according to a review from 2007, but it turned out that the toxicity of ribavirin was too high ... The intake regimen and the dosage of corticosteroids were controversial ... [And] at that time the HIV drug Kaletra was also given to SARS patients on an experimental basis. It contains the two HIV protease inhibitors lopinavir and ritonavir."[1394]

The article refers to a WHO report,[1395] whose negative commentary regarding the use of the drugs in SARS patients is not surprising, since many of the medications used can be associated with the most severe side effects. Further, if one takes a closer look at the structures of the WHO, one might also wonder whether the conclusions about so-called SARS medications should have been even more damning. This idea seems justified, considering the WHO's close ties with Big Pharma.

Bill Gates, the Greed for World Control and the Insanity with the COVID-19 Vaccine

The WHO to a large extent is dependent on private foundations, especially the Bill & Melinda Gates Foundation. In the 2011 article "The power of money: A fundamental reform of the WHO is overdue," published in the journal *Dr. med. Mabuse* which opened with a photo of Bill Gates (see article clipping), it said: "Increasingly, private money or earmarked donations from individual states are deciding on the goals and strategies of the WHO. The extent of their influence was recently demonstrated by the way the WHO dealt with the 'swine flu.'"

On the advice of its Standing Committee on Immunization, the WHO declared the highest pandemic alert level for H1N1 (swine flu) in June 2009. "The worldwide vaccination campaign that it thus set in motion became a multi-billion dollar business for the pharmaceutical companies," wrote the author Thomas Gebauer, a psychologist and spokesman for the medico international foundation. „This was made possible, according to a Council of Europe study, partly because WHO had previously lowered the criteria for pandemic alerts." At the same time, health authorities around the world had entered into contractual purchase guarantees with vaccine manufacturers. The taxpayers and, as mentioned, those who were physically harmed by the recklessly approved vaccines were left to pay the cost.[1396]

In fact, until the beginning of May 2009 the WHO website stated under the question "What is a pandemic?" that it was "associated with an enormous number of deaths and illnesses." But all of a sudden the WHO deleted this text passage—and only a few weeks later, on June 11, the organization declared the highest pandemic alert level (phase 6) for "swine flu." At this time there were hardly any "swine flu" victims to report, even according to official numbers. The WHO had thus deceived the public, as even an internal report revealed. With this brazen elimination of the text passage in question, it had changed the very definition of the word "pandemic".

This also laid the foundation to declare COVID-19 a worldwide death epidemic, without a sound scientific basis. Even according to the authorities, corona claims only a fraction of deaths compared to cancer, heart disease, hunger or even particulate matter.[1397]

As far as Bill Gates is concerned it was revealed how little he seems to care about the welfare of people in a 2007 *Los Angeles Times* article entitled "Dark cloud over good works of Gates Foundation". According to the article, the multi-billionaire's foundation owned extensive shareholdings in companies that broke acceptable social responsibility standards as they destroyed the environment, discriminated against their employees and violated workers' rights.

In Nigeria, for example, the Gates Foundation supported a vaccination program against polio and measles. However, on the other hand it owned shares in an oil company of the Italian Eni group, which, like many companies in the Niger Delta, burnt off excess oil in huge gas flares that polluted the region.

This caused a veritable rain of 250 toxic substances to fall on people and the environment. Many children became ill as a result—and there is reason to believe that these children's immune systems were so weakened by the poisons that they developed exactly the diseases they were being vaccinated against.[1398] Three years later, the British physician David McCoy also criticized the Gates Foundation. He pointed out that the foundation was primarily a means of exercising power and influence, avoiding taxes and supporting large corpora-

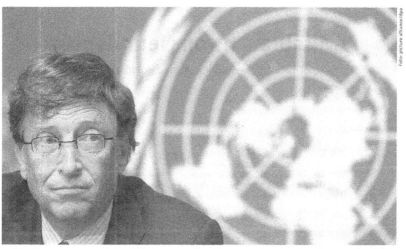

Die Macht des Geldes

Eine grundlegende Reform der WHO ist überfällig

Microsoft-Gründer
Bill Gates auf der Weltge-
sundheitsversammung in
Genf im Mai diesen Jahres:
Seine Stiftung ist
der zweitgrößte Finanzier
der WHO.

Thomas Gebauer

In 2011, the medical journal Dr. med. Mabuse *published the article "The power of money: A fundamental reform of the WHO is overdue"—due to the big influcence of major backers of the WHO, especially Bill Gates (shown in the photo).*

429

tions such as the pharmaceutical giants Novartis, Glaxo-Smith-Kline, Sanofi and Merck.[1399] According to McCoy, it is also apparent that the assets of the Gates Foundation are largely investments in companies such as Monsanto, Coca-Cola, McDonalds and Shell.[1400]

In April 2020, Robert F. Kennedy Jr. pointed out in his article "Gates' Globalist Vaccine Agenda: A Win-Win for Pharma and Mandatory Vaccination" that the multi-billionaire "is funding a private pharmaceutical company that produces vaccines and donating $50 million to 12 pharmaceutical companies to accelerate the development of a coronavirus vaccine. Gates has invested in Drosten's Charité as well as in media outlets such as *Spiegel*, *Zeit* and *Guardian* (see "Awarded Grants" at www.gatesfoundation.org).

Even though the Microsoft founder put on his spending pants in connection with the development of a COVID-19 vaccine, it seems less about the well-being of the people, and more about money. Co-incidentally, he was able to more than double his fortune between 2010 and 2020 – a timespan that Bill and his wife Melinda Gates called the "Decade of Vaccines" – from around 50 billion to 120 billion US dollars.

This was made possible above all by the investment company he founded: Cascade Investment. In 2020, a huge amount of their funds were in fellow multi-billionaire Warren Buffet's Berkshire Hathaway holding company, whose investments were well positioned in the pharmaceutical industry.

But money is not "the ultimate goal of Gates' activities," as the Corbett report stated in "Bill Gates' Plan to Vaccinate the World". "Money is only the tool he uses to buy what he really wants: control. Control not only of the health industry, but control of the world population itself."[1401]

In 2019, his activities caused the news platform *Modern Ghana* to headline: "Why The World Health Organization Treats Bill Gates Like A President."[1402] And in the *Politico* article "Meet the world's most powerful doctor: Bill Gates" (April 5, 2017), a Geneva-based NGO representative is quoted as saying that Gates "is treated liked a head of state, not only at the WHO, but also at the G20."

It was also the Gates Foundation that announced in mid-April 2020 that "There are seven billion people on the planet, we are going to need to vaccinate nearly every one", because this would be the only way to effectively counter the corona pandemic.[1403] In the search for a vaccine against COVID-19, the pharmaceutical companies started a real "race" at an early stage, as reported by *Der Spiegel* a month earlier. "Research on a new vaccine against Covid-19 is being conducted under high pressure. Therefore, common rules are now being softened in drug development."[1404]

And on March 19, Christian Drosten also exerted pressure by demanding: "We have to see where we can conjure up a vaccine."[1405]

According to the World Health Organization (WHO), near the end of 2020, no fewer than 48 possible vaccine candidates were being tested, with a further 164 candidates in preclinical development.[1406]

On December 1, the pharmaceutical giants then went on the PR offensive. The media announced, three vaccine candidates were close to possible approval in the EU and the USA - from the companies BioNTech/Pfizer, Moderna and AstraZeneca/University of Oxford. All three, it was claimed, showed high efficacy in final studies, while serious side effects did not occur. The next day it was reported that the British Medicines Agency (MHRA) had granted emergency approval for the corona vaccine of the Mainz-based pharmaceutical company BioNTech and its US partner Pfizer.[1407]

However, the vaccine studies were not lengthy enough to allow a realistic estimate of the long term effects.

"As in the narcolepsy cases following the swine flu vaccination in 2009, millions of healthy people would be exposed to an unacceptable risk if an emergency approval were planned, with the possibility of monitoring the late effects only afterwards," said Michael Yeadon and Wolfgang Wodarg in their petition submitted on December 1, 2020 to the European Medicine Agency (EMA) that is responsible for EU-wide drug approval. In this petition, they demanded the immediate suspension of all SARS-CoV-2 vaccine studies, in particular the BioNTech/Pfizer study.[1408]

Wolf-Dieter Ludwig, Chairman of the German Medical Commission, also criticized corona vaccinations and sharply attacked the miserable data situation relating to the scientific trials.[1409]

Despite the lack of adequate data, decision-makers were nevertheless prepared to take a huge risk and carry out population-wide trials with the vaccines. This was made clear by

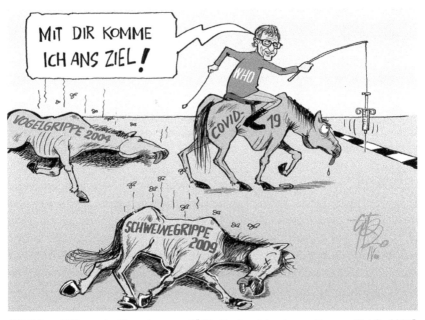

Bill Gates: „With you I will reach my goal!" (On the two lying horses it says: „Bird flu 2004" *and „Swine flu 2009").* © expresszeitung.com *Ausgabe 32, www.wiedenroth-karikatur.de*

Stephan Becker, Head of Virology at the University of Marburg in an interview with the ZDF's *heute* TV program on November 20, 2020, with regards to the corona vaccine from BioNTech and Pfizer:

ZDF news anchor: "Emergency approval—that sounds like quick, quick … Of course there is no time to test possible effects and side effects extensively. How much worry do you have about this?"

Becker: " … Now it's just a matter of watching the side effect profile very closely—after all, we want to vaccinate millions and billions of people."

ZDF: "But only while the whole thing is running, so to speak. So, we administer the vaccination and then, while it's running, we see if there could be any other side effects."

Becker: "Exactly, that's the point of such an emergency approval. It should then lead to a completely normal approval as soon as the sufficient safety data are available."

ZDF: "But now I have stumbled over a word you just said, namely 'as far as we know.' That is a very interesting point. So far we have press releases from the companies involved. They are naturally cheering. How much of all this is scientifically proven?"

Becker: "Yes, that is exactly what we as scientists are still missing a little bit at the moment: the exact knowledge of the study and what has come out of it. I hope that this will be there in the near future."

This is all the more serious when you consider the nature of RNA vaccines, which were not well developed. As Dr Joseph Mercola reported, "An October 20, 2020, article in the *Observer* lists the known side effects that have emerged in the various trials. Chills, fever, body aches and headache are the most commonplace, but at least two cases of transverse myelitis—inflammation of the spinal cord—have also occurred. A December 1, 2020, *CNBC* article, which looked at the frequency of adverse reactions, noted that 10% to 15% of participants in the Pfizer and Moderna trials reported 'significantly noticeable' side effects.

The article also admits they have no idea what, if any, long-term reactions there might be." Moreover, a participant in India's AstraZeneca trial started a lawsuit against the firm claiming the vaccine caused "serious neurological damage." Then there are concerns about COVID-19 mRNA vaccines causing long term genetic expression alterations at a cellular level.[1410]

Almost 4,000 COVID vaccine related adverse events, including 13 deaths, were reported in the U.S. to the Vaccine Adverse Event Reporting System (VAERS) in December alone (by mid-January 2021, there were already nearly 7,000 cases, including 55 deaths). This is all the more remarkable when you consider that fewer than 1 percent of adverse events are reported to VAERS, as the 2010 analysis "Electronic Support for Public—Health Vaccine Adverse Event Reporting System", conducted by the federal Agency for Healthcare Research an Quality (AHRQ), revealed.

The write-ups that accomapny VAERS reports showed that five or six of the 13 deaths occured on the same day as vaccination, and sometimes within 60 to 90 minutes of the injection. Furthermore, some of the deceased had actually experienced and recovered from COVID-19—raising the question about why they were vaccinated.

"The write-ups also illustrate the subtle pressure to attribute the cause of death to something other than COVID-19 vaccination," as Children's Health Defense writes in the article "Tip of the Iceberg? Thousands of COVID Vaccine Injuries and 13 U.S. Reported in December Alone." "For example, a grandchild who submitted a report wrote, 'My 85 year old grandmother died a few jours after receiving the Moderna COVID vaccine booster 1. While I don't expect that the events are related, the treating hospital did not acknowledge this and I wanted to be sure a report was made.'"

The 13 deaths communicated to VAERS did not inlcude any deaths in the state of New York. However, a disturbing news report from Syracuse.com showed that that a single nursing home in upstate New York vaccinated 193 residents beginning on December 22 and subsequently reported 24 deaths within a few weeks. Although the facitlity claimed the deaths occured due to a COVID-19 "outbreak," there had been no COVID-19 deaths in any nursing homes in the entire county "until the first three deaths ... were reported December 29."

The majority of the mass media simply ignored these concerns and instead acted like a PR agency of the vaccine manufacturers by hailing the Corona vaccination as a "serum of hope" (as the daily newspaper *Bild* on December 1, 2020). The magazine *Stern* crowned this media tragedy when it sold its readers the vaccination on December 23rd on the cover in all seriousness as an "act of love of neighbour." The complete cover was a painting on which one of the three kings from the Orient holds a vaccine vial, the label of which bears the name of the manufacturing company Biontech, in the direction of the baby Jesus and his mother Mary (see image).

Apart from the fact that *Stern* refused to take any notice of the data, which shows unambiguously that there is no evidence whatsoever for the usefulness of vaccinations, the question arises as to what the cover picture is supposed to tell us: That the virus is so dangerous that even the Son of God needs a Corona vaccination? Or is Jesus supposed to sell the vaccination to humanity as an act of Christian love? Either way, it is shameful for a journalistic medium to use the baby Jesus to promote a drug. More religious transfiguration is hardly possible.

Against this background, it is even more disturbing that those who voluntarily participated in the vaccine trials were not even informed in the consent process that the vaccine could make them more susceptible to a worsened disease course. This was the

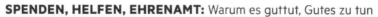

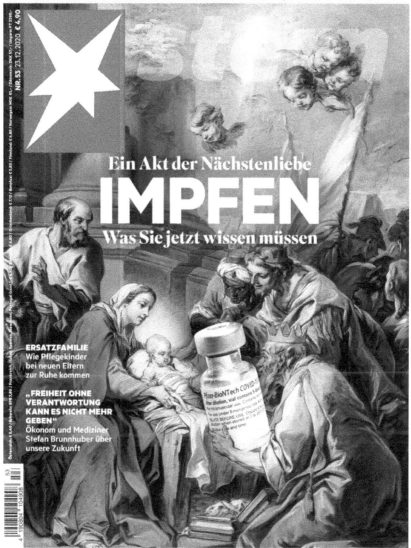

To elevate vaccination as an „act of charity" into religious spheres while also promoting a vaccine manufacturer (in this case BionTech), as Stern *magazine did on December 23, 2020, is just unworthy of a journalistic medium. Source: Screenshot from* stern.de conclusion of the study "Informed Consent Disclosure to Vaccine Trial Subjects of Risk of COVID-19 Vaccine Worsening Clinical Disease", published in the *International Journal of Clinical Practice* on Oct. 28[1411]

According to the study, this risk was so obscured in the clinical trial protocols and in the consent forms that an adequate understanding by patients is unlikely to have been possible. Quite simply they were not aware that the vaccine had the potential to worsen their health in this way.

At the same time, the paper pointed out that vaccines against other putative corona viruses—that of Severe Acute Respiratory Syndrome (SARS-CoV) and Middle Eastern Respiratory Syndrome (MERS-CoV) as well as the Respiratory Syncytial Virus (RSV)—have never been approved and the futile efforts to realize them raised serious concerns.

Incidentally, a "COVID-19" vaccine makes no sense not only from an ethical but also from a scientific point of view because:

1) There was and still is no direct evidence of the entity SARS-CoV-2—the virus targeted by the vaccines.
2) The SARS-CoV-2 PCR tests used to "diagnose" COVID-19 are meaningless.
3) There is no conclusive evidence whatsoever that vaccinations on the whole are generally useful. As shown in particular in Chapter 11 "10 Reasons against Measles Vaccination," the historical curves for so-called infectious diseases show that mass vaccinations were introduced after the severe complications and deaths associated with these diseases had already decreased to somewhat negligible levels.

Even authoritative institutions such as the RKI were unable to name one single study that clearly shows that vaccinated people have better health than unvaccinated people.

On the other hand, there are dozens of studies that clearly show the opposite (see also chapter 11 about measles): that unvaccinated people have significantly improved health outcomes compared to vaccinated people. On November 22, 2020 another study appeared in the *International Journal of Environmental Research and Public Health* that reinforced this theme by concluding that "indeed the overall results may indicate that the unvaccinated pediatric patients ... are healthier overall than the vaccinated."[1412]

The Mask Madness

The evidence is no less overwhelming that it makes no sense to require people of all ages to wear cloth face masks to avoid further expansion of a claimed virus pandemic. For example, in its August 2020 meta-analysis of data from 24 countries and 25 U.S. states, the renowned independent U.S. National Bureau of Economic Research (NBER) showed that mandatory measures such as mask-wearing do not have a relevant impact on the incidence of infection.[1413] Three months earlier, a study in *Emerging Infectious Diseases* concluded that, according to 14 randomized controlled trials, interventions such as hand washing and wearing face masks had no effect on the transmission of „laboratory-confirmed influenza."[1414]

This result is all the more remarkable when one considers that this paper appeared in a journal published by the U.S. Centers for Disease Control and Prevention (CDC)—an institution that is one of the world's most powerful proponents of the COVID-19 pandemic thesis, but at the same time, as described, is beset by glaring conflicts of interest. On this point Lawrence R. Huntoon, physician and editor-in-chief of the eminent *Journal of American Physicians and Surgeons*, wrote in his editorial „CDC: Bias and Disturbing Conflicts of Interest" (published in the Fall 2020 issue):

„The CDC openly admits that it is fudging the COVID-19 death figures. These statistics have been made to look really scary by adding speculative guesses to the official database. Those false numbers are sanctioned by the CDC. The CDC has a long history of bias and troubling conflicts of interest. This history calls into question the scientific validity of recommendations made by the CDC. As evidenced by the CDC's ‚fudging' of COVID-19 death numbers during the current pandemic, political and/or philosophical biases continue"

As of December 28, 2020 , the website „Ärzte klären auf" (doctors clarify), published by the Hanover infectiologist Thomas Ly, lists (with the heading „Body of evidence in the matter of cloth face masks: Sense or Nonsense? Protection or danger?") a total of 48 studies published between the years 1981 and 2020 in which „the data do not support the wearing of mouth-nose coverings. This is especially true with regard to children!"[1415]

One of those 48 studies is the Danish analysis published in November 2020 in the world-renowned journal *Annals of Internal Medicine*, which concluded: „The trial found no statistically significant benefit of wearing a face mask."[1416] Shortly before, U.S. researcher Yinon Weiss updated his charts on cloth face masks mandates in various countries and U.S. states—and they also showed that mask mandates have made no difference or may even have been counterproductive.[1417] The aforementioned website „Ärzte klären auf" showed a graph with data going until December 4, 2020, which also refutes the effectiveness of the mask obligation.

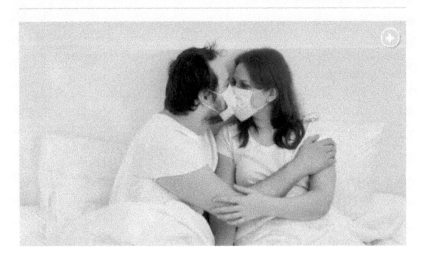

Theresa Tam, Canada's 3rd chief public health officer, advised in Sepember 2020 to skip kissing and wearing a mask while having sex to protect yourself from contracting the coronavirus. To this, one can only state that whoever proposes such a thing in all seriousness must be completely removed from what constitutes a fulfilled life, let alone sexuality, or foolish—or both. All the more so as the SARS-CoV-2=COVID-19 hypothesis is unsubstantiated and hence mask mandates without meaning. Source: Screenshot from nypost.com

This graph also shows that the number of „positive" PCR test results shot up sharply in mid-October 2020 – and this despite the fact that it was precisely at this time in Germany that the regulations on wearing a cloths face masks in many schools and public places had been tightened. This also clearly speaks against the meaningfulness of the introduction of a masks obligation – and for the fact that simply more tests were carried out and thus more „positive" results were obtained.

In fact, the number of tests in Germany already rose significantly in the course of March 2020, from just under 130,000 to around 350,000 per week. By mid-October, the number of weekly tests had already reached 1.2 million, and within a short period of time this figure had risen to more than 1.6 million.[1418] (in other countries, such as Great Britain, the situation was similar[1419]). It is true that the „positive rate" – i.e. the percentage of „positive" tests out of the total number of tests – also increased from mid-October. However, apart from the fact that the metric „positive rate" is based on speculation, the increase of this „positive rate" was not due to an increasingly „raging" virus, but merely to the fact that the laboratories were totally overloaded and, in addition, even lousier tests had been introduced.

For example, in early November, the RKI reported that „overall, the backlog of PCR samples has increased almost fivefold since calendar week 42 [= October 12-18]. There were 69 laboratories reporting a total backlog of 98,931 samples to be processed."[1420] And it was not only due to this overload that the quality of testing decreased noticeably and the number of false „positive" tests increased accordingly. Also, in October 2020, the national testing strategy was expanded to include, among other things, rapid antigen tests – so-called point of care tests (POCT).[1421] And these POCT are associated with a rate of false „positive" results that is even significantly higher than that of PCR tests.

There was an 11 percent increase in deaths in Germany in November as a whole compared to the 2016-20 average, as the Federal Statistical Office wrote.[1422] But this is not surprising and does not mean that a virus killed more people, either. As the *Frankfurter Allgemeine Zeitung* wrote on December 30, 2020, citing the Federal Statistical Office, „the above-average death rate in November 2020 was almost exclusively due to an increase in deaths in the age group of people aged 80 and older."[1423] And the group „of people over 80 [in 2020] is no less than 11 percent larger than the average from 2016 to 2019," as Friedrich Breyer, professor of economics at the University of Konstanz and member of the Scientific Advisory Board of the German Federal Ministry of Economics, noted.[1424] This alone practically dissolves the alleged excess mortality in the second half of November.

Incidentally, the general panic is drastically increased when a strong rise in „positive" test results is reported (as of the end of October, there was an increase of more than 100,000 „positive" results per week!). This in turn, tends to result in more potentially lethal drugs and invasive ventilations being used, or even increased isolation of elderly people in nursing homes, which can also quickly become fatal. This conclusion is also supported by the fact that, according to the Federal Statistical Office, the total number of deaths in the first half of October was still „within the range of the average of previous years." This means that the death figures did not rise noticeably until mid-October and thus were only climbing exactly parallel to the drastic expansion of testing (with 1.18 million weekly tests in the second week of October to 1.63 million in the fourth week of October[1425]).

Franz Knieps, head of the association of company health insurance funds in Germany and for many years in close contact with Chancellor Angela Merkel, even told the *Redaktionsnetzwerk Deutschland* in mid-January 2021 that "if you would not test anymore, corona would have disappeared."

On October 23, 2020, even the *Norddeutscher Rundfunk* (*Northern German Broadcasting*, a public radio and television broadcaster, based in Hamburg) — normally „fully in line" with politics and RKI as well as hoard of Christian Drosten's Corona podcast — published the article „Is the number of corona cases rising because more testing is being done? Three times as many tests as in spring and at the same time rising numbers of new infections: Is there a connection?" In this piece it says:

„The short answer to that is: you don't know. 'Of course, if I test three times more, I will find more people infected,' says Dirk Brockmann. As a professor at the Institute of Biology at Humboldt University in Berlin, he deals with statistical modeling of epidemics and also conducts research at the Robert Koch Institute (RKI). However, no one can reliably say at present how strong this effect will be. This is a statement that is shared in principle by all the scientists with whom NDR spoke for this research. One researcher even referred to the question of how high the number of unreported cases is as a 'million-dollar quest.'"
Politics and the RKI are also poking around in the fog on this central point — but instead of admitting this publicly, they simply claimed, without having any solid evidence, that it

was certain that the world, including Germany, was affected by a worldwide deadly pandemic that could only be effectively combated by measures such as imposing compulsory cloth face masks on young children during face-to-face learning at schools.

And even if one does not want to let go of the belief that a super-lethal coronavirus is circulating, it is fact that the simple cloth face masks cannot hold back these viruses at all. This is because the size of the particles called SARS-CoV-2 is said to be around 125 nanometers (0.125 microns), whereas the size of the „pores" of simple cotton masks is 0.3 microns. Thus, what has been termed SARS-CoV-2 flies through conventional fabric MNBs as through an open window. Yet even the WHO stated that „there is insufficient evidence" that the so-called SARS-CoV-2 virus is transmitted through the air, as *Nature* reported.[1426]

On the December 9, 2020, even someone like Hamburg's school senator Ties Rabe criticized in the TV talkshow *Markus Lanz* that the top decision-makers of the corona measures, „in truth [lack] the power to look into the detail"—and as for that detail, he wondered: „The different infection rates in the states—where do they actually come from? Where does they come from? You've asked it yourself several times. And I'm a bit upset that we can't get this crucial question for governance in Germany clarified. I'd like to know what the— I don't know—the North Frisians are doing right and what others [like the Bavarians] are doing wrong … My reproach is that we don't know what the problem is."[1427]

In fact, it is possible to know what the cause is, but this would require a departure from the viral tunnel vision, which many decision-makers were and are unwilling to do—with the tragic consequence that even well-known figures such as the magician Roy Horn have been sold therapies whose benefits have never been demonstrated and of which only the lethal potential has been proven, as the last possible sheet anchor.

The Death of Magician Roy Horn—and the Dubious Approval of Remdesivir by Dr. "Baron of Lies" Anthony Fauci

Roy Horn, the legendary magician (of Siegfried & Roy), passed away on May 8, 2020 at the age of 75 years in Las Vegas. He was the first megastar worldwide who was said to have died from COVID-19 and thus from the so-called coronavirus SARS-CoV-2. However, again there is no evidence to support this story. In fact, Roy Horn, born in Nordenham close to the German city Bremen, was in such poor health that it seems downright absurd to ignore non-viral factors as the cause of his sad demise. Horn, as German daily newspaper *Bild* reported (see screenshot), was diagnosed with advanced skin cancer in December 2016. "Chemotherapy and radiation should help, but they weakened him furthermore," as

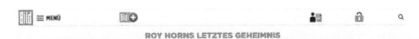

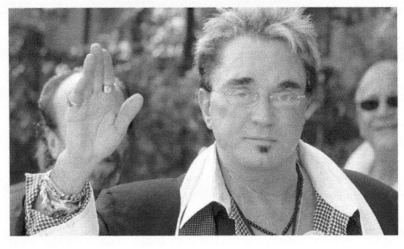

On the 11th of May 2020, the German daily newspaper Bild *reported that the legendary magician Roy Horn had died on 8 May 2020 in Las Vegas at the age of 75 after being treated with the highly toxic drug remdesivir: "Roy Horn's last secret: He has been fighting skin cancer for four years." Source: Screenshot from* bild.de

bunte.de wrote. "He had to take strong medication every day. A friend: 'Before dinner, Roy took in the many pills like smarties.' Not only did he fight cancer, but also the pains he has suffered from since the tiger attack almost 17 years ago."

On top of that, after he had tested "positive" for COVID-19, he received Gilead Sciences' drug remdesivir, which had been fast-tracked in the US and approved for emergency use only on the 2nd of May. This medication inhibits cell reproduction in the body and can undoubtedly lead to fatal outcomes in an unwell older person. This justifies the conclusion that the already terminally ill and heavily medicated Horn died tragically, not in spite of, but because of the administration of remdesivir.

In connection with the drug remdesivir the most serious side effects reported include multi-organ dysfunction, septic shock (usually fatal blood poisoning) and respiratory failure. Additionally, in experiments with so-called Ebola patients it was found that the drug elevates liver enzyme values, which can be a sign of liver damage.

Even after Horn had been given Remdesivir, it had not received full approval from the American Food and Drug Administration (FDA) for use in COVID-19, Ebola or any other disease. And the European Medicines Agency (EMA) was just lagging behind the FDA, again not with a full approval, but only in recommending it for use when it came to "hardship cases" ("compassionate use").
The fact that remdesivir was presented as the great rescue for COVID-19 patients can only be described as a scandal—especially when you look at the fraudulent way in which the drug was approved for "emergency use."

In late April 2020, Anthony Fauci, director of the US Department of Health's National Institute of Allergy and Infectious Diseases (NIAID) since 1984 and probably the mightiest ringmaster in the international virus circus (see also chapter 3 about HIV/AIDS and especially the fraudulent approval of the first "AIDS drug" AZT), claimed a study had found that remdesivir would reduce recovery time and reduce mortality.

But an article from the Alliance for Human Research and Protection (AHRP)—"Fauci's Promotional Hype Catapults Gilead's remdesivir"—brought up a sensitive subject:

That "Fauci has a vested interest in remdesivir. He sponsored the clinical trial whose detailed results have not been peer-reviewed. What's more, he declared the tenuous results to be 'highly significant,' and pronounced remdesivir to be the new 'standard of care.' Dr. Fauci made the promotional pronouncement while sitting on a couch in the White House, without providing a detailed news release; without a briefing at a medical meeting or in a scientific journal—as is the norm and practice, to allow scientists and researchers to review the data. When he was asked about a recently published remdesivir Chinese study, in *The Lancet* (April 29th , 2020); a trial that was stopped because of serious adverse events in 16 (12%) of the patients compared to four (5%) of patients in the placebo group, Dr. Fauci dismissed the study as 'not adequate.'"

Fauci warns of 'a bad fall and a bad winter' as Kushner claims victory over pandemic

A second wave of coronavirus infections is 'inevitable' if the the country opens too early, Fauci warns.

By Jeff Parrott | Apr 29, 2020, 2:09pm MDT

   SHARE

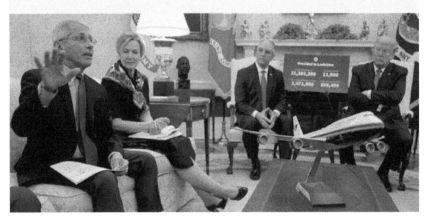

Anthony Fauci, director of the National Institute of Allergy and Infectious Diseases (NIAID) and the "tsar" of US virology since 1984, made the promotional pronouncement regarding remdesivir while sitting on a couch in the Oval Office of the White House (far left in the picture with a raised hand)—and violated fundamental scientific and ethical rules. Fauci speaks as White House Coronavirus response coordinator Deborah Birx, Louisiana Gov. John Bel Edwards and President Donald Trump listen during a meeting on the Coronavirus on the 29th of April, 2020. Source: Screenshot from deseret.com

But while the Chinese study that Fauci denigrated, was a randomized, double-blind, placebo-controlled, multi-center peer-reviewed, published study in a premier journal, *The Lancet*, with all data available, the NIAID-Gilead study results have not been published in peer-reviewed literature—nor have details of the findings been disclosed.

"However, they were publicly promoted by the head of the federal agency that conducted the study, from the White House," as the AHRP underlined. "What better free advertisement?"

What Fauci also failed to disclose to the public in his promotional pronouncement was that the primary outcomes of the study were changed on April 16, 2020. Changes in the primary outcome are posted on clinicaltrials.gov. Previously there was an 8-point scale, which also included deceased patients, but subsequently there was only a 3-point scale. This then left deceased patients out of the equation and instead only measured the time until recovery or being released from hospital. "Changing primary outcomes after a study has commenced is considered dubious and suspicious," as the AHRP pointed out.

In addition, due to an allegedly shorter recovery time in the Remdesivir group, patients in the placebo group were later also given Remdesivir. Thus the study falls apart completely on its design alone and this was violently criticized by several experts.Moreover, *Reuters News* reported that highly respected prominent leaders in the medical community—such as Steven Nissen, MD, the chief academic officer at the Cleveland Clinic and Eric Topol, MD, director and founder of the Scripps Research Translational Institute in California— were unimpressed by remdesivir's tentative, modest benefit at best.

Referring to the *Lancet* report, Topol stated: "That's the only thing I'll hang my hat on, and that was negative." As for the NIAID modest results, Dr. Topol was unimpressed: "It was expected to be a whopping effect. It clearly does not have that."
The change in primary outcome measures raised serious red flags for scientists; but was largely ignored by the mainstream media which mostly repeated Fauci's promotional script. Steve Nissen told *The Washington Post*: "I think that they thought they weren't going to win, and they wanted to change it to something they could win on. I prefer the original outcome. It's harder. It's a more meaningful endpoint. Getting out of the hospital early is useful, but it's not a game-changer."[1428]

By the way, Fauci not only acted as "Dr. "Baron of Lies" with remdesivir in 2020, but did so almost continuously as head of the NIAID since he took office there in 1984. Under Fauci's aegis, Robert Gallo was able to promote his unfounded HIV/AIDS thesis to the world as the eternal truth. The "virus tsar" also succeeded in the mid-1980s in spreading the alleged "HIV test" worldwide, although it cannot detect the so-called "HIV virus" at all (see Chapter 3). And in 1987, Fauci presided over the fraudulent approval of the first AIDS drug AZT (see section "AZT Study 1987: A Giant Botch-up" in Chapter 3).

In the decades that followed, Fauci continued to spread one untruth after another. With the bird flu, he predicted "two to seven million deaths" worldwide, and in the end, according to official figures, only 100 deaths were counted (see Chapter 7).

With the swine flu vaccine, he claimed that it was only "very, very, very rarely" associated with severe side effects, although the data for such statements was not even available and later it became apparent that there were many side-effects including severe neurological complications (see chapter 8).

And with regards to HIV/AIDS the recommendation of "pre-exposure prophylaxis," PrEP for short, in which even people who are "HIV-negative" take medication.

But when we asked Fauci to back up his claims, he refused to comment on whether there is any solid scientific evidence for PrEP. Hillary Hoffman from the communications department of NIAID merely let us know: "Dr. Fauci respectfully declines to respond to the questions that you emailed."[1429]

Fauci's pattern of not wanting to answer critical questions pervades his entire career. For example in 1987, *NBC News* reporter Perri Peltz wanted to confront the virus tsar with criticisms about the AZT approval study—but Fauci characteristically refused (see section "AZT Study 1987: A Giant Botch-up" in Chapter 3).

"Welcome to the club, Perri!", wrote John Lauritsen in his book "The AIDS War: Propaganda, Profiteering and Genocide from the Medical-Industrial Complex." According to Lauritsen, Fauci also "refused to speak to the BBC, Canadian Broadcasting Corporation Radio, Channel 4 (London) television, Italian television, *The New Scientist*, and Jack Anderson" about the fraudulent 1987 AZT trial.

Two years before that, on October 2 1985, Rock Hudson, who gave HIV/AIDS "a face," died during Fauci's term in office. And just like Roy Horn in 2020, world-famous stars in the early days of the "AIDS era" were experimented on with potentially lethal drugs. The first really famous victim was Hudson, who was treated with agents such as HPA-23, a drug, for which ...

... no scientifically controlled studies had been carried out.
... there was no proof of efficacy with regards to Hudson's illness.
... the liver-damaging and potentially lethal effects alone were sufficiently documented.
... the highly toxic effects were especially dangerous for patients that already had underlying health problems.

Sounds a lot like COVID-19, except that there are 35 years in between.

Epilog

Rock Hudson Gave „AIDS" a Face – and His Fallacious Story the Virus Hunters Godlike Status

> „We would have to ensure that the media do not use the power of images to
> create emotions that influence our judgment."[1430]
> Gerd Bosbach
> Professor of Statistics and Empirical Economic and Social Research

On the 23rd of April 1984, the US microbiologist Robert Gallo and the then US Secretary of Health and Human Services Margret Heckler claimed towards the world in front of running cameras: „The probable cause of AIDS has been found: a variant of a known human cancer virus." The word „probable" was practically unnoticed, not least because the two also used phrases like „Today's discovery represents the triumph of science over a dreaded disease" (see chapter 3, subchapter „23 April 1984: Gallo's TV Appearance Carves the Virus Dogma in Stone").

But the whole thing was still relatively theoretical. So for people to really realize, even really feel, that a deadly virus is „raging", more is needed. It needs stories of fates, of dramas that touch us deeply.

With Corona, these were particularly the dramatic TV pictures from Italy, which went around the world in mid-March and showed military vehicles that carried away numerous coffins. And in the case of HIV/AIDS, it was the Hollywood world star Rock Hudson who depicts a kind of „big bang" here. Hudson was one of the first to undergo an „HIV antibody test". This happened on June 5, 1984, just a few weeks after Gallo's TV appearance on stage.

The test was not even officially licensed at that time, as this was only done nine months later by the US FDA.[1431] Moreover, the first HIV antibody test, developed in 1985, was designed to screen blood products, not to diagnose AIDS, as it says in the study „Human Immunodeficiency Virus Diagnostic Testing: 30 Years of Evolution", published 2016 in the journal *Clinical and Vaccine Immunity*. Nevertheless, Gallo and Heckler were not afraid to send the completely unfounded message around the globe: „We now have a blood test for AIDS. With a blood test, we can identify AIDS victims with essentially 100 percent certainty."[1432]

So it happened that the 1.96-metre tall image of American manhood received a „positive" test report.[1433] [1434] [1435] Hudson did not make this public for a long time, but about a year later, on the 25th of July 1985, he finally passed on the news to the world public that he had AIDS.

And the fact that Hudson was the first Hollywood star to be officially considered an AIDS patient and who died only a few months after his „AIDS-Outing" finally brought the AIDS phenomenon out of the gay community and conveyed the message that a real epidemic was underway.

According to the motto: if AIDS can affect someone like Hudson, it can affect anyone, men and women alike. Or as the German news magazine *Spiegel* put it in August 1985: „At the latest since the long death and public confession of AIDS by the film idol Rock Hudson, once the epitome of radiant health and (heterosexual) love, the mood has changed. 'Danger for us all—a new epidemic plague,' discovered the Munich tabloid *Quick*. 'No one is safe from Aids anymore,' was a title of the US magazine *Life* ... 'Aids—now the women are dying' (*Bild am Sonntag*)."[1436]

But especially the medical history of Hudson shows on a closer inspection that it is, there is no other way to put it, a lie to claim that AIDS can affect anyone—just as it is wrong to assume that a so-called „HIV test" would reliably indicate that a deadly HI Virus is haunting the body of the person concerned (see chapter 3).

Hudson was at least bisexual—and in any case homosexually active throughout his entire acting career.[1437] And apparently even the Hollywood personage indulged in a fast-lane lifestyle typical of many gays, which is characterized by the excessive consumption of highly toxic drugs and medication and which can cause precisely the symptoms that occur in seriously ill AIDS patients.

For example, one of Hudson's lovers, the writer Armistead Maupin, reported how Hudson lovingly presented him with the sex drug Poppers, which is extremely popular

among gays, from a leather case with „RH" engraved on it.[1438]
But especially Poppers can be very liver-damaging and even carcinogenic (see chapter 3, subchapters „The Early 1980s: Poppers and AIDS Drugs" and „How the 'Fast-Lane Lifestyle' Topic Went Out of Sight"). Therefore, it is not surprising that Hudson is reported to have been diagnosed with the cancer Kaposi's sarcoma in 1984.[1439] In addition he has drunk and smoked heavily over decades. Even after a quadruple heart bypass surgery in 1981, he still took a pack of cigarettes every day—even though his doctors warned him that if he didn't stop, he would soon be in dire need.[1440] [1441]

And so it came about that Hudson becamethe star guest of the first episode of Doris Day's „Best Friends" show on July 16th , 1985—and that his long-time acting colleague was visibly shocked by the frail appearance of the 59-year-old, whom she and the world had known as the model of a handsome man.[1442] Shortly afterwards, on July 21st, 1985, he collapsed in a Paris hotel and on the same day asked his spokesman to announce that he had „inoperable liver cancer", as the *New York Times* also reported.[1443] [1444]

But liver cancer, unlike HIV/AIDS, does not have the potential to create headlines that the masses are craving. In contrast to the HIV=AIDS narrative, liver cancer does not touch the most secret of human intimacy. In 1987, the *Spiegel* journalist Wilhelm Bittorf wrote the following in a personal experience report on HIV/AIDS: „Even the worst environmental damage is further away than an infection in the erogenous zone. And if the Pershing missiles in Baden-Württemberg only affected the sex lives of Germans, they would be long gone by now."[1445]

And so it was that on the 25th of July 1985 Hudson had it announced from Paris that he was „dying of AIDS"—and it became a story the world had hardly seen before. At the end of his stay in the French capital, he was even flown out of his hotel by helicopter, lying motionless on a stretcher, in front of running cameras of course, and loaded into a chartered Boeing 747. In addition to himself, there were only two doctors, two assistants, a nurse and four of his confidants.[1446] Hudson is said to have spent a few hundred thousand dollars on this transport action to make it possible for him to „die in his own bed" in Los Angeles.

As a result, „HIV testing" experienced a real boost, and an AIDS industry was boosted, generating hundreds of billions of dollars each year. Elizabeth Taylor also benefited enormously.

451

The Hollywood icon reportedly called Hudson shortly after his collapse to thank him for his announcement that he was dying of AIDS, believing it would „save millions of lives." A few weeks later, in September 1985, Taylor co-organized the „Commitment for Life" gala dinner in Los Angeles to raise money for AIDS sufferers. Originally, only 200 tickets were sold for this event, but after Hudson's „AIDS confession" more than 2500 tickets were sold—and even the then US President Ronald Reagan felt compelled to send a greeting telegram saying that it was of „highest priority" for the US government to stop the spread of AIDS.

In the following years, Taylor was even able to raise funds of several hundred million for AIDS research. But although the Hollywood diva is said to have been a close friend of Hudson since their film „Giant" in 1956, it is reported that she paid him only one visit to his bed in the last months of his life, the day before his death.[1447]

But why had Hudson set off for Paris in the summer of 1984? The reason was that his „HIV test" turned out „positive"—and he had the opportunity to receive a drug from doctors in the capital of France, which he was led to believe was a kind of last resort before an AIDS death. This drug was called HPA-23, which the Pasteur Institute in France provided for experimental purposes. One of the inventors was Luc Montagnier.

But as melodious as the names Pasteur Institute and Montagnier may be to some, the administration of HPA-23 to Hudson (and many other desperate people) can only be described as highly irresponsible. The liver-destroying effect of this drug alone was suf-ficiently documented, but there was no proof of its effectiveness in the context of AIDS.

William A. Haseltine of Harvard Medical School, for example, stated that the reports on the success of HPA-23 in France were of „the crummiest kind of anecdotal stories"—and they didn't "do the scientifically controlled trials" for HPA-23, although these are neces-sary to provide the evidence about a drug's safety and efficacy. According to Haseltine, it was „really a crime", as had been done here.[1448]

Other physicians took the same line and emphasized that HPA-23, due to its high toxicity, was especially dangerous for patients who were already ailing.[1449] And Rock Hudson, when he started taking HPA-23, was a man who was severely ill. Yet virtually no one in the major media asked if there was any solid evidence of the efficacy of HPA-23 in treat-ing AIDS—or why patients, rather than chasing after such a lousy drug, should not tackle their underlying health problems.

Apparently, journalists and their recipients had fallen victim to the fallacy at the time that it can only be good if a famous actor like Hudson receives this drug, but the average citizen does not. In addition, even then the public interest in tabloid stories spiced with sex was huge. And so the general attention was only directed to find out if Rock Hudson would have infected his acting colleague Linda Evans with HIV after he kissed her in the

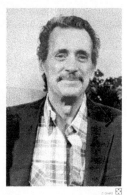

ROCK HUDSON

Er gab Aids ein Gesicht

VON PETER-PHILIPP SCHMITT · AKTUALISIERT AM 10.09.2010 · 20:19

In 2010, the German daily newspaper Frankfurter Allgemeine Zeitung *(FAZ) published the article „Rock Hudson: He gave AIDS a face" on the occasion of the 25th anniversary of the Hollywood legend's death and hit the nail on the head with it. Indeed, it was the world-famous actor who gave HIV/AIDS a face in 1985. Unfortunately, the FAZ article failed to tell its readers how scientifically untenable the message was that Hudson had died of HIV, and in what fatal way this gave the worldwide virus hunters unimagined power.* Source: Screenshot from faz.net

series „Denver-Clan".

Even the self-proclaimed assault gun for democracy, the news magazine the *Spiegel*, readily took up the subject in 1985, in its article on „Hollywood stars' fear of AIDS": „Linda Evans, who was carelessly kissed by the AIDS-infected Rock Hudson in the 'Denver Clan', is scared out of her sleep night after night. She screams for help on the phone, because her nightmares make her believe all stages of the disease. Burt Reynolds must reaffirm over and over again that he is neither gay nor has AIDS."[1450]

This smug reporting was diametrically opposed to the harsh reality for Rock Hudson, who had started taking HPA-23 in August 1984.[1451] And shortly afterwards he developed

453

severe itching, rashes and Vincent's disease, a painful, ulcerative gum disease. During the winter months of 1984, he was also confronted with loose teeth and a weeping rash called contagious impetigo.

The thesis that these severe reactions are due to HPA-23 is also supported by a study published in 1988 in the journal *Animicrobial Agents and Chemotherapy*, in which AIDS patients were administered HPA-23 over a period of just eight weeks. The result: the patients showed exactly the same severe symptoms that Hudson had to struggle with. At the same time, the study showed that the drug had no clinical benefit for the patients.[1452]

It is therefore not surprising that Hudson's appearance had already changed considerably by the end of 1984 — after only a few months of HPA-23 medication — and had lost a lot of weight in the process. Hudson claimed in this connection that he was merely suffering from anorexia (loss of appetite) — but even the magazine *People*, which was already riding the AIDS panic wave at the time, considered this to be an „unbelievable" explanation.[1453] It seems plausible, however, that Hudson's already weakened liver was once again severely affected by HPA-23 — and that he therefore had hardly any appetite left, which often happens with liver damage.

The preparation, which is rich in side effects, brought Hudson, who was already very badly „hit" in terms of health, close to physical knockout after a short time. It is not difficult to imagine how serious the consequences must have been for Hudson's already severely battered body that HPA-23 was used on him over a period of about a year.[1454]

In late July 1985, Hudson finally turned his back on Paris and flew back to the USA because his doctors in Paris assessed that he was too weak to continue taking HPA-23[1455] — whereby his French medical practitioners unspokenly admitted that the toxic effects of the drug were extremely severe. Nevertheless, Hudson is likely to have continued to be administered HPA-23 or similar preparations in the USA, which were also severely damaging to the liver.[1456]

Summarizing, Rock Hudson has been drinking and smoking chain for decades, which in itself is very damaging to the liver and the body as a whole. In addition to that is the intake of lifestyle drugs like poppers, which also have a highly toxic effect on organs such as the liver. Due to this wasting lifestyle Hudson was already a seriously ill man in his mid/late 50s, which was also reflected in his heart surgery at the age of 56. In this very unstable physical stage, the Hollywood legend received drugs such as HPA-23, which has liver-destroying effects, over the twelve (or even more) months before his death. And once the liver is gone, death is inevitably not far away.

Therefore it can only be concluded that the highly toxic medication played the crucial part in Hudson's death on the 2nd of October 1985.

Even if the medical establishment particularly or exclusively recommends vaccines and antiviral medicines in the fight against alleged viral diseases, "the determinants of health lie in large part outside the medical system," as Thomas McKeown, professor of social medicine, writes in his work "The Meaning of Medicine." The only effective way to combat so-called influenza, SARS, HIV or COVID-19 (baselessly connected to viruses), while also safeguarding our hearts, lungs, livers and brains, is to strengthen our immune systems.

The idea that only the blessings of modern high-tech industry can make us healthy (again) is as pervasive as it is false. If this were true, then there wouldn't be so many sick people — and affluent societies are primarily affected by chronic diseases like allergies, diabetes, heart disease, osteoporosis and cancer. In contrast, diseases like cancer are virtually unknown in wild animals, even in elephants, which have approximately the same life expectancy as humans, or in whales, which can live for more than 200 years.

The idea that artificial products could replace nature and maintain or even manufacture health is merely due to a Cartesian worldview (tracing back to René Descartes, 1596-1650), in which the "modern" individual's thoughts are ensnared. Ultimately, this viewpoint reduces living beings to machines that can be fueled artificially, with pills thrown in from time to time, and, if necessary, rigged with substitute replacement parts.

"And so we carry over principles that have been successfully applied to inanimate nature to living beings," writes McKeown. "This model would long have been rejected if it seriously contradicted experience"— if humanity, then, finally realized it had come to a false conclusion. We mistakenly believe that the "retreat of infectious diseases — the main reason for improvements in public health — is substantially due to advances in medical science," as McKeown points out. In truth, the "vast improvement to public health [only] profited a little from the contributions of science and technology. Instead, the advances can be traced to simple but momentous everyday discoveries": For instance, increases in food production through conservation of soil fertility, or hygiene improvements. Reports on certain primitive peoples also show that one can live very healthily without the blessings of the pharmaceutical industry. In his diary, the Frenchman Jean de Léry admiringly recounts the "wild Americans" with whom he lived in the mid-16th century, in what is now Brazil:

"They are a great deal healthier than us [Europeans] and suffer less from diseases. It is very rare to see lame, one-eyed, or deformed people among them. Not few of these people attain an age of one hundred to 120 years, and only a few have white or even grey hair." Léry is praised by specialists for the objective style of his descriptions. The famous ethnologist Claude Lévi-Strauss even paid him the compliment of the modern scholar in his book „Tristes Tropiques."

Besides Léry, all of the 16th century's other travelers were downright amazed at the vivid beauty and stable health of the native men and women, who cultivated a totally simple lifestyle and ate natural foods (so unlike ours today which, thanks to over-industrialized chemical farming often taste like cardboard and are deprived of important nutrients). Léry gushed poetically about the pineapples grown in the wilderness, whose strong strawberry scent "one could already smell from afar" and which "melt in your mouth and are naturally so sweet that they cannot be bettered by any of the jams we usually have in Europe." And so the people of the Renaissance ultimately observed with amazement that their own antique ideal had found its realization overseas in these native men.

One might wonder: If everything that many politicians, researchers and journalists sell us as truth is false, how could all the mistakes go undiscovered for so long? Shouldn't the conclusions outlined in this book have gone off like a bomb a long time ago?

The primary reason this has not happened is that it's too simple for many people to imagine. Intelligent researchers have chosen to overlook it for decades. It is too shocking for us to believe that we've been lied to by the very people charged with safeguarding our health. Above all, none of them are interested in these simple pursuits:

- Dctors would have to go on a totally different path in order to achieve fame and honor (or abandon such a goal altogether and change their definition of success).

- Medical statisticians would be sawing off the very branch on which they perch.
- Pharmaceutical companies would have to completely overhaul their bottom line-obsessed industry and actually invest resources in developing effective medications instead of ones that do nothing, harm or even kill.
- Ultimately, the only individuals who would profit from this would be patients. But first, they have to educate themselves and take back control of their own bodies.

And with this book, we hope we can make a contribution to this pursuit—for a better, more peaceful and healthier future for our beloved planet and all its habitants.

„We should all start to live before we get too old.
Fear is stupid, so are regrets."

Marilyn Monroe

———————————

„*For the New Year.*—I still live, I still think: I must still have to live, because I still have to think. *Sum, ergo cogito: cogito, ergo sum* ... I want to learn more and more to perceive the necessary characters in things as the beautiful—I shall thus be one of those who beautify things."

Friedrich Nietzsche
„The Joyous Science," aphorism 276

Literature

Beginning of the Book and Introduction

[1] Kass, Edward H., Infectious Diseases and Social Change, *The Journal of Infectious Diseases*, January 1971, pp. 110-114

[2] Golub, Edward, The Limits of Medicine: How Science Shapes Our Hope for the Cure, The University of Chicago Press, 1997, pp. 3-4

[3] Smith, Lewis, £1m scientific "gospel" of Newton's greatest rival, *Times*, 9 February 2006

[4] Hunter, Michael, The Royal Society and Its Fellows, 1660-1700: The Morphology of an Early Scientific Institution, British Society for the History of Science, 1982

[5] Robert Boyle (1627-1691), University of Dayton, see www.udayton.edu/~hume/Boyle/boyle.htm

[6] Starr, Paul, The Social Transformation of American Medicine. The rise of a sovereign profession and the making of a vast industry, Basic Books, 1982, p. 3

[7] Ibid., pp. 6-7

[8] McCarthy, Michael, Lies, Damn lies, and scientific research (Rezension des Buches The Great Betrayal: Fraud in Science von Horace Judson, Harcourt, 2004), *Lancet*, 6 November 2004, p. 1657

[9] Golub, Edward, The Limits of Medicine: How Science Shapes Our Hope for the Cure, The University of Chicago Press, 1997, p. 178

[10] McKeown, Thomas, Die Bedeutung der Medizin, Suhrkamp, 1979, p. 214

[11] Moss, Ralph, Fragwürdige Chemotherapie. Entscheidungshilfen für die Krebstherapie, Haug, 1997, p. 39-43

[12] Manipulating a Journal article, *New York Times*, Editorial, 11 December 2005, Sektion 4, p. 11

[13] Engelbrecht, Torsten, Ungesunde Verhältnisse. Wie die PharMayndustrie die Medien beeinflusst, *Journalist*, November 2005, pp. 40-42

[14] Lieberman, Trudy, Bitter Pills, *Columbia Journalism Review*, July/August 2005

[15] Engelbrecht, Torsten, Spitze des Eisbergs: Warum Journalisten auch den angesehenen Wissenschaftszeitschriften nicht blindlings vertrauen sollten, *Message*, 3/2005, pp. 70-71

[16] Smith, Richard, Medical Journals Are an Extension of the Marketing Arm of Pharmaceutical Companies, *Plos Medicine*, May 2005, p. e138

[17] Krimsky, Sheldon, Science in the Private Interest. Has The Lure Of Profits Corrupted Biomedical Research?, Rowman & Littlefield, 2004, pp. 163-176

[18] Chargaff, Erwin, Das Feuer des Heraklit, Luchterhand, 1989, p. 224

[19] Krugman, Paul, Drugs, Devices and Doctors, *New York Times*, 16 December 2005

[20] Judson, Horace, The Great Betrayal. Fraud in Science, Harcourt, 2004, p. 9

[21] Sharav, Vera, Scientific Fraud & Corruption on Both sides of Atlantic: Merck/Proctor & Gamble, press release, Alliance for Human Research Protection, 11 December 2005

[22] Taylor, Rosie, Cash Interest taint drug advice, *Nature*, 20 October 2005, pp. 1070-1071

[23] Abramson, John, The Effect of Conflict of Interest on Biomedical Research and Clinical Practice Guidelines: Can We Trust the Evidence in Evidence-Based Medicine?, *The Journal of the American Board of Family Practice*, September 2005, pp. 414-418

24   Ioannidis, John, Why most published research findings are false, *Plos Medicine*, August 2005, p. e124

25   Charlton, Bruce, The need for a new specialist professional research system of "pure" medical science, *Plos Medicine*, 13 July 2005, p. e285

26   Engelbrecht, Torsten, „Die Industrie macht Druck," Interview with Marcia Angell, former editor in chief of the *New England Journal of Medicine*, on editorial autonomy, fraud in science and the purpose of peer reviewing, *Message*, 3/2005, pp. 66-69

27   Martinson, Brian, Scientists behaving badly, *Nature*, 9 June 2005, pp. 737-738

28   Engelbrecht, Torsten, Gaunereien und Betrug sind auch in der Wissenschaft verbreitet (review of the book „The Great Betrayal: Fraud in Science" from Horace Judson, Harcourt, 2004), *Neue Zürcher Zeitung am Sonntag*, 9 January 2005, p. 69

29   Washburn, Jennifer, University, Inc: The Corporate Corruption of Higher Education, Basic Books, 2005

30   Krimsky, Sheldon, Science in the Private Interest. Has The Lure Of Profits Corrupted Biomedical Research?, Rowman & Littlefield, 2004

31   Moynihan, Ray, Who pays for the pizza? Redefining the relationships between doctors and drug companies, *British Medical Journal*, 31 May 2003, pp. 1189-1192

32   Gøtzsche, Peter C., Our prescription drugs kill us in large numbers, *Polskie Archiwum Medycyny Wewnetrznej*, epub 30 October 2014

33   Global Corruption Report 2006. Special Focus: Corruption and Health, Transparency International, February 2006, see http://www.transparency.org/publications/gcr

34   Judson, Horace, The Great Betrayal. Fraud in Science, Harcourt, 2004, p. 41

35   McCarthy, Michael, Lies, Damn lies, and scientific research (Rezension des Buches The Great Betrayal: Fraud in Science von Horace Judson, Harcourt, 2004), *Lancet*, 6 November 2004, p. 1658

36   Miller, Donald, On Evidence, Medical and Legal, Journal of American Physicians and Surgeons, Fall 2005, p. 70

37   See de.wikipedia.org/wiki/William_Osler

38   Miller, Donald, On Evidence, Medical and Legal, Journal of American Physicians and Surgeons, Fall 2005, p. 70

39   Weihe, Wolfgang, Klinische Studien und Statistik: Von der Wahrscheinlichkeit des Irrtums, *Deutsches Ärzteblatt*, 26 March 2004, p. C683

40   Judson, Horace, The Great Betrayal. Fraud in Science, Harcourt, 2004, p. 39

41   Prange, Astrid, Hoffnung kostet 140 Dollar, *Rheinischer Merkur*, 48/2005, p. 14

42   Solomon, John, NIH Medical Safety Officer Reinstated. Government Reinstates Safety Officer Who Alleged Misconduct in AIDS Research, Associated Press, 24 December 2005

43   Engelbrecht, Torsten, AIDS-Krimi. WHO spielt Nebenwirkungen herunter, *Freitag*, 11 February 2005, p. 18

44   Klon-Star Hwang hat Studie gefälscht, *Spiegel Online*, 23 December 2005

45   Klonskandal: Kritik an der Sensationsgier der Forscher, *Spiegel Online*, 24 December 2005

46   McKeown, Thomas, Die Bedeutung der Medizin, Suhrkamp, 1979, p. 237

47   Tracey, Michael, Mere Smoke of Opinion; AIDS and the making of the public mind, *Continuum*, Summer/Fall 2001

48   Krugman, Paul, Drugs, Devices and Doctors, *New York Times*, 16 December 2005

49   Duesberg, Peter, Inventing the AIDS Virus, Regnery Publishing, 1996, p. 129

50   Burnet, Sir MacFarlane, Genes, Dreams and Realities, Medical and Technical Publishing, 1971, pp. 217, 219

51   Epstein, Samuel, Losing the „War against Cancer": A Need for Public Policy Reforms, *International Journal of Health Services and Molecular Biology*, 4 February 1992, pp. 455-469

[52] Engelbrecht Torsten, Aneuploidie. Paradigmenwechsel in der Krebstherapie, *Co'Med*, August 2005, pp. 30-35

[53] Duesberg, Peter, Multistep Carcinogenesis—A Chain Reaction of Aneuploidizations, *Cell Cycle*, May/June 2003, p. 204

[54] Miklos, George, The Human Cancer Genome Project—one more misstep in the war on cancer, *Nature Biotechnology*, May 2005, pp. 535-537

[55] Engelbrecht, Torsten, Schuss auf den Matrosen, interview with US molecular biologist Peter Duesberg on anti-smoking campaigns, gene-mutations, aneuploidy, and the failure of the established cancer research, *Freitag*, 27 April 2005, p. 18

[56] Deutschen Institut für Ernährungsforschung Potsdam-Rehbrücke (DIFE), World Cancer Research Fund, American Institute for Cancer Research, Krebsprävention durch Ernährung, 1999, see www.dife.de/de/publikationen/krebsbrosch99k.pdf

[57] Epstein, Samuel, US National cancer Institute. Misguided policies, funding lucrative drug treatments, caving in to corporate interests, see www.preventcancer.com/losing/nci/why_prevent.htm

[58] Epstein, Samuel, Cancer-Gate: How to Win the Losing Cancer War, Baywood Publishing, 2005, p. 114

[59] Engelbrecht, Torsten, Schuss auf den Matrosen, interview with US molecular biologist Peter Duesberg on anti-smoking campaigns, gene-mutations, aneuploidy, and the failure of the established cancer research, *Freitag*, 27 April 2005, p. 18

[60] Critser, Greg, Generation Rx: How Prescription Drugs Alter Our Bodies, Houghton Mifflin, 2005

[61] Sharav, Vera, Selling Sickness: Pharma Industry Turning Us All into Patients, press release, Alliance for Human Research Protection, 12 September 2005

[62] Engelbrecht, Torsten, Risiken und Todesfälle eingeschlossen. Killer Nummer eins: In den USA sterben jährlich 800.000 Patienten durch fehlerhaftes ärztliches Handeln, schätzen Experten. Dennoch fehlt es nach wie vor an einem gezielten Fehlermanagement, *Freitag*, 3 December 2004, p. 18

[63] Gøtzsche, Peter C., Our prescription drugs kill us in large numbers, *Polskie Archiwum Medycyny Wewnetrznej*, epub 30 October 2014

[64] Angell, Marcia, The Truth About the Drug Companies. How They Deceive Us And What To Do About It, Random House, 2004, p. 120

[65] Lacasse, Jeffrey, Serotonin and Depression: A Disconnect between the Advertisements and the Scientific Literature, *Plos Medicine*, December 2005, p. e392

[66] Sharav, Vera, Eli Lilly finances World Health Org (WHO) promoting psychotropic drugs. The Credibility of the World Health Organisation is in doubt since its financial ties to Eli Lilly and Johnson and Johnson, press release, Alliance for Human Research Protection (AHRP), 20 August 2005

[67] Dobson, Roger; Lenzer, Jeanne, US regulator suppresses vital data on prescription drugs on sale in Britain, *Independent*, 12 June 2005

[68] Lenzer, Jeanne, NIH Secretes, *The New Republic*, 30 October 2006

[69] Lenzer, Jeanne, Conflicts of Interest are common at FDA, *British Medical Journal*, 29 April 2006, p. 991

[70] Lurie, Peter, Financial conflict of interest disclosure and voting patterns at Food and Drug Administration Drug Advisory Committee meetings, *Journal of the American Medical Association*, 26 April 2006, pp. 1921-1928

[71] Sharav, Vera, Disease Mongering Conference/Plos Special Issue, press release, Alliance of Human Research Protection (AHRP), 10 April 2006

[72] House of Commons Health Committee, The Influence of the Pharmaceutical Industry, Forth Report of Ses-

sion2004-05, Volume 1, 22 March 2005

[73] Angell, Marcia, The Truth About the Drug Companies. How They Deceive Us And What To Do About It, Random House, 2004, p. 133

[74] Ibid., p. 126

[75] Epstein, Steven, Impure Science—AIDS, Activism and the Politics of Knowledge, University of California Press, 1996, pp. 57-58

[76] Marcuse, Herbert, Der eindimensionale Mensch, Luchterhand, 1988, pp. 29-32

[77] Golub, Edward, The Limits of Medicine: How Science Shapes Our Hope for the Cure, The University of Chicago Press, 1997, p. 160

[78] Ibid., p. 176

[79] Epstein, Steven, Impure Science—AIDS, Activism and the Politics of Knowledge, University of California Press, 1996, p. 57

[80] Golub, Edward, The Limits of Medicine: How Science Shapes Our Hope for the Cure, The University of Chicago Press, 1997, p. 160

[81] Dubos, René, Mirage of Health: Utopias, Progress, and Biological Change, Harper&Brothers, 1959, p. 86

[82] Michael Specter, The Vaccine, The New Yorker, 3 February 2003, p. 59

[83] Roach, Mary, Germs, Germs Everywhere. Are You Woried? Get Over It, New York Times, 9 November 2004

[84] Review of the book „Leben auf dem Menschen" (by Jörg Blech, Rowohlt 2000), Spektrum der Wissenschaft, 11/2000

[85] Kruis, Wolfgang, Informationen über eine Therapiestudie: Rezidivprophylaxe bei Patienten mit Colitis ulcerosa durch Mutaflor im Vergleich zu Mesalazin, Der Bauchredner, 3/1996, pp. 64-68

[86] Bjorksten, Bengt, Effects of intestinal microflora and the environment on the development of asthma and allergy, Springer Seminars in Immunopathology, 25 February 2004, pp. 257-70

[87] Knight, David, Gut flora in health and disease, Lancet, 24 May 2003, p. 1831

[88] Tannock, Gerald, Medical Importance of the Normal Microflora, Kluwer Academic Publishers, 1999

[89] Langosch, Angelika, Einfluss der Ernährung insbesondere der Rohkost auf die Darmflora und Infektabwehr, Institut für Medizinische Balneologie und Klimatologie der Universität München, 1984 (Dissertation)

[90] Golub, Edward, The Limits of Medicine: How Science Shapes Our Hope for the Cure, The University of Chicago Press, 1997, p. xiii

[91] Ibid., pp. 3-5

[92] Duesberg, Peter, Inventing the AIDS Virus, Regnery Publishing, 1996, p. 457

[93] Katzenellenbogen, Jonathan, Third of Africans Undernourished, Business Day (Johannesburg), 20 August 2004

[94] Duesberg, Peter, The African AIDS Epidemic: New and Contagious—or—Old under a New Name?, Report to Thabo Mbeki's AIDS Panel, 22 June 2000

[95] Engelbrecht, Torsten; Crowe, David, Avian Flu Virus H5N1: No Proof for Existence, Pathogenicity, or Pandemic Potential; Non-'H5N1' Causation Omitted, Medical Hypotheses, 4/2006; pp. 855-857

[96] Schwägerl, Christian, „Die Gefahr wird unterschätzt", Interview with Reinhard Kurth, Frankfurter Allgemeine Zeitung, 18 August, 2005

[97] Köhnlein, Claus, Zur Epidemiologie moderner Test-Seuchen, Fachhochschule Dortmund, 6 December, 2003

[98] Köhnlein, Claus, Hepatitis C—the epidemic that never was?, British Medical Journal (online), 7 March 2002, see bmj.bmjjournals.com/cgi/eletters/324/7335/450

[99] Duesberg, Peter, Rasnick, David, AIDS in Africa, *British Medical Journal* (online), 1 March, 2003

[100] World Health Organisation, Summary of probable SARS cases with onset of illness from 1 November to 31 July 2003, see www.who.int/csr/sars/country/table2003_09_23/en

[101] Mullis, Kary, Dancing Naked in the Mind Field, Vintage Books, 1998, p. 180

[102] Johnson, Judith, AIDS funding for federal government programs: FY1981-FY2006, CRS Report for Congress, Congressional Research Service, The Library of Congress, 23 March 2005

[103] Engelbrecht, Torsten, Therapien ohne Beweiskraft, *Freitag*, 12 March, 2004, p. 18

[104] Sharav, Vera, 38 Senators With $13.4 Million in Pharma Stock Approved Sweeheart Deal; Rumsfeld's Growing $$ Stake in Tamiflu (*Fortune*), press release, Alliance for Human Research Protection, 23 December 2005

[105] Abramson, John, The Effect of Conflict of Interest on Biomedical Research and Clinical Practice Guidelines: Can We Trust the Evidence in Evidence-Based Medicine?, *The Journal of the American Board of Family Practice*, September 2005, p. 417

Chapter 1
Medicine Presents a Distorted Picture of Microbes

[106] French Wikipedia article about "Antoine Béchamp"

[107] Verner, Robinson, Rational Bacteriology, chapter 1: Bacteria In General, H. Wolff, 1953

[108] Nicholson Jeremy, The challenges of modeling mammalian biocomplexity, *Nature Biotechnology*, 6 October 2004, p. 1270

[109] Noelle-Neumann, Elisabeth, Die Schweigespirale: Öffentliche Meinung – unsere soziale Haut, Langen Müller, 2001, p. 211

[110] The Humane Society of the United States, Facts about the Canadian Seal Hunt, 2005, see www.hsus.org

[111] Engelbrecht, Torsten, Dying To Entertain Us: A harrowing insight into the hugely profitable and brutal world of captive dolphins, *The Ecologist*, October 2004, pp. 53-57

[112] Myers, Ransom, Rapid worldwide depletion of predatory fish communities, *Nature*, 15 May 2003, pp. 280-283

[113] Dubos, René, Mirage of Health: Utopias, Progress, and Biological Change, Harper&Brothers, 1959, p. 71

[114] Golub, Edward, The Limits of Medicine: How Science Shapes Our Hope for the Cure, The University of Chicago Press, 1997, p. xiii

[115] Noelle-Neumann, Elisabeth, Die Schweigespirale: Öffentliche Meinung – unsere soziale Haut, Langen Müller, 2001, p. 210

[116] Chargaff, Erwin, Das Feuer des Heraklit, Luchterhand, 1989, p. 229

[117] Epstein, Steven, Impure Science – AIDS, Activism and the Politics of Knowledge, University of California Press, 1996, p. 57

[118] Chargaff, Erwin, Das Feuer des Heraklit, Luchterhand, 1989, Luchterhand, 1989, p. 229

[119] Ibid., p. 209

[120] Ibid., pp. 232-233

[121] Super Size Me: Wer dauerhaft super size isst, endet beim XXL-Gewicht, *medizin.de*, 29 July 2004

[122] Martindale, Diane, Burgers on the brain: Can you really get addicted to fast food? The evidence is piling up, and the lawyers are rubbing their hands, *New Scientist*, 1 February 2003

[123] Dronda, Fernando, CD4 cell recovery during successful antiretroviral therapy in naive HIV-infected patients:

the role of intravenous drug use, *AIDS*, 5 November 2004, pp. 2210-2212

[124] Fast Food macht süchtig wie Heroin: *New Scientist* Studie warnt vor Burgers, Pommes und Co, *naturkost.de*, 3 February 2003

[125] A high with your fries: Even if fast food is not as addictive as tobacco it still merits a health warning, *New Scientist*, 1 February 2003

[126] Engelbrecht, Torsten, Krank durch tierisches Eiweiß: Eiweißspeicherkrankheiten – die unterschätzte Gefahr, *Bio*, December 2004, pp. 32-34

[127] Campbell, Colin, The China Study: The Most Comprehensive Study of Nutrition Ever Conducted and the Startling Implications for Diet, Weight Loss and Long-Term Health, BenBella Books, 2005

[128] Wendt, Lothar, Gesund werden durch Abbau von Eiweißüberschüssen. Wissenschaftliche Einführung in neueste Forschungsergebnisse der Eiweißspeicherkrankheiten, Schnitzer, 1987

[129] Jede Hand hilft! Prominente unterstützen den Weltkindertag bei McDonald's, *news-ticker.org*, 10 November 2005

[130] McDonald's-Website

[131] DJV lehnt Reding-Vorschläge zum Product Placement ab, press release, Deutscher Journalisten-Verbandes (DJV), 13 December 2005

[132] Stiftung Warentest, Die Andere Medizin: „Alternative" Heilmethoden für Sie bewertet, Stiftung Warentest, 2005

[133] Personal e-mail communication with Stiftung Warentest, 22 December 2005

[134] Abbott, Alison, Gut reaction, *Nature*, 22 January 2004, p. 284

[135] Tannock, Gerald, New Perceptions of the Gut Microbiota: Implications for Future Research, *Gastroenterology Clinics*, September 2005, p. 363

[136] Fast Food macht süchtig wie Heroin: *New Scientist* Studie warnt vor Burgers, Pommes und Co, *naturkost.de*, 3 February 2003

[137] Langosch, Angelika, Einfluss der Ernährung insbesondere der Rohkost auf die Darmflora und Infektabwehr, Institute for Medical Balneology and Climatology at the University of Munich, 1984 (dissertation), p. 89

[138] Canibe, Nuria, An overview of the effect of organic acids on gut flora and gut health, Danish Institute of Agricultural Sciences, Research Centre Foulum, 2002

[139] Haysche Trennkost ist als langfristige Ernährungsform nicht zu empfehlen, Deutsche Gesellschaft für Ernährung, 21 April 1998

[140] Tunsky, Gary, The Battle For Health Is Over pH, Crusador, 2004

[141] Lloyd, Tuhina, Lifestyle factors and the development of bone mass and bone strength in young women, Journal of Pediatrics, June 2004, pp. 776-82

[142] Tylavsky, Frances, Fruit and vegetable intakes are an independent predictor of bone size in early pubertal children, *American Journal of Clinical Nutrition*, February 2004, pp. 311-317

[143] Sellmeyer, Deborah, A High Ratio of Dietary Animal to Vegetable Protein Increases the Rate of Bone Loss and the Risk of Fracture in Postmenopausal Women, *American Journal of Clinical Nutrition*, March 2001, pp. 118-122

[144] Campenhausen, Jutta, Sauer macht gebrechlich: Neuen Forschungen zufolge ist nicht Kalziummangel die Ursache für Knochenschwund, sondern ein ernährungsbedingte Übersäuerung des Körpers, *Stern* 49/1999, pp. 256-257

[145] Die richtige Ernährung kann einer Osteoporose vorbeugen und sie günstig beeinflussen, brochure „Osteplus" from Merckle Arzneimittel

[146] Kruis, Wolfgang, Informationen über eine Therapiestudie: Rezidivprophylaxe bei Patienten mit Colitis ulcerosa

durch Mutaflor im Vergleich zu Mesalazin, *Der Bauchredner*, 3/1996, p. 64

[147] Personal interview with Francisco Guarner, 26 January 2006

[148] Eckburg, Paul, Diversity of the human intestinal microbial flora, *Science*, 1 June 2005, pp. 1635-1638

[149] Prados, Andrew, Milestones in gut microbiome science in 2019, www.gutmicrobiotaforhealth.com, 26 December 2019

[150] Blech, Jörg, Leben auf dem Menschen: Die Geschichte unserer Besiedler, Rowohlt, 2000, p. 47

[151] Abbott, Alison, Gut reaction, *Nature*, 22 January 2004, p. 285

[152] Guarner, Francisco, Gut flora in health and disease, *Lancet*, 8 February 2003, pp. 512-519

[153] E-Mail to te EU, 7 February 2006; no response

[154] E-Mail to the DIFE, 7 February 2006; no response

[155] Abbott, Alison, Gut reaction, *Nature*, 22 January 2004, p. 284

[156] Probiotics for Human Health. European Commission, Research, see http://europa.eu.int/comm/research/quality-of-life/wonderslife/project05_en.html

[157] Epstein, Samuel, The Stop Cancer Before It Starts Campaign, February 2003, p. 4, see www.preventcancer.com/press/pdfs/Stop_Cancer_Book.pdf

[158] Hinsliff, Gaby, Drugs firms "creating ills for every pill": Expensive new medicines are oversold when cheaper therapies or prevention would work better, say MPs, *The Observer*, 3 April 2005

[159] Abramson, John, Overdosed America, The Broken Promise of American Medicine: How The Pharmaceutical Companies Are Corrupting Science, Misleading Doctors, And Threatening Your Health, Harper Perennial, 2005, pp. 169-186

[160] Greg Ciola, Health Maverick Turns Medical Science Upside Down, Interview mit dem Mediziner Gary Tunsky, Healthliesexposed.com, 23 December 2005, see www.healthliesexposed.com/articles/article_2005_12_23_3950.shtml

[161] Blech, Jörg, Leben auf dem Menschen: Die Geschichte unserer Besiedler, Rowohlt, 2000, p. 204

[162] Dubos, René, Mirage of Health: Utopias, Progress, and Biological Change, Harper&Brothers, 1959, p. 64

[163] Jenuwein, Hans, Tropische Nutzpflanzen für Wintergarten und Terrasse, Ulmer, 1992, p. 22

[164] Langbein, Kurt; Ehgartner, Bert, Das Medizinkartell: Die sieben Todsünden der Gesundheitsindustrie, Piper, 2003, p. 37

[165] Burkart, Thomas, Pro- und Eukaryontenzellen, in: Mikrobiologie/Infektiologie (Grundlagen), Thema 02, Institut für Infektionskrankheiten der Universität Bern; see www.ifik.unibe.ch/uploads/education/02_pro_und_eukaryontenzellen.pdf

[166] Loibner, Johann, Bakterien, die Gesundheitserreger; see www.aegis.at

[167] Alfred-Nissle-Gesellschaft, Darmflora und chronische entzündliche Darmerkrankungen: Colitis ulcerosa, Morbus Crohn, Hagen, 2002

[168] Blech, Jörg, Leben auf dem Menschen: Die Geschichte unserer Besiedler, Rowohlt, 2000, p. 201

[169] Nicholson, Jeremy, The challenges of modeling mammalian biocomplexity, *Nature Biotechnology*, 6 October 2004, p. 1270

[170] Personal Interview, E-Mail from Jeremy Nicholson, 23 January 2005

[171] Dubos, René, Mirage of Health: Utopias, Progress, and Biological Change, Harper&Brothers, 1959, p. 70

[172] Ibid., p. 69

[173] Ibid., p. 74

[174] Ibid., p. 71

[175] Null, Gary; Dean, Caroly, Death by Medicine, December 2003, mercola.com/2003/nov/26/death_by_medicine.htm

[176] Null, Gary M. et al., Death by Medicine, Praktikos Books, 2010

[177] Dubos, René, Mirage of Health: Utopias, Progress, and Biological Change, Harper & Brothers, 1959, p. 64

[178] Lazarou, Jason, Incidence of adverse drug reactions in hospitalized patients: a meta-analysis of prospective studies, *The Journal of the American Medical Association*, 15 April 1998, pp. 1200-1205

[179] Suh Dong-Churl, Clinical and economic impact of adverse drug reactions in hospitalized patients, *The Annals of Pharmacotherapy*, December 2000, pp. 1373-1379

[180] US Food and Drug Administration, Antibiotic Resistance; see www.fda.gov/oc/opacom/hottopics/anti_resist.html

[181] Lönnroth, Anna, Eindämmung der mikrobiellen Resistenz, *FTE info — Magazin für die europäische Forschung*, published by the European Commission, May 2003, pp. 32-34

[182] Grayston, Thomas, Azithromycin for the Secondary Prevention of Coronary Events, *New England Journal of Medicine*, 21 April 2005, pp. 1637-1645

[183] Dubos, René, Mirage of Health: Utopias, Progress, and Biological Change, Harper & Brothers, 1959, p. 75

[184] Dubos, René, Mirage of Health: Utopias, Progress, and Biological Change, Harper & Brothers, 1959, pp. 75, 90-91

[185] Maggots eat away need for wound surgery, *ABC News Online*, 13 May 2005

[186] Website of the Institute Pasteur de Lille, see www.pasteur-lille.fr/fr/accueil/Nature_medicaments.htm

[187] Golub, Edward, The Limits of Medicine: How Science Shapes Our Hope for the Cure, The University of Chicago Press, 1997, p. 166

[188] Ibid., pp. 160-173

[189] Ibid., p. 169

[190] Brandt, Allan, No Magic Bullet: A Social History Of Venereal Disease In The United States Since 1880, Oxford University Press, 1985, p. 161

[191] Strahm, Barbara, Vom Bioterror zum Thema gemacht. Jenseits von Hysterie und Panikmache: Ein sachlicher Blick in die Geschichte der Pockenerkrankung und Pockenimpfung, *Die Tagespost*, 22 February 2003

[192] Dubos, René, Mirage of Health: Utopias, Progress, and Biological Change, Harper & Brothers, 1959, p. 90

[193] Robert Koch Institut fordert dringende Vorbereitung auf Pocken-Impfungen, *WELT.de*, 13 January 2003

[194] Miller, Neil, Vaccines: Are They Really Safe & Effective?, New Atlantean Press, 2005, p. 74

[195] Shelton, Herbert, Vaccine and Serum Evils, Health Research, 1966, p. 23

[196] Miller, Neil, Vaccines: Are They Really Safe & Effective?, New Atlantean Press, 2005, pp. 75-76

[197] Ibid., pp. 76-77

[198] Ibid., p. 80

[199] Buchwald, Gerhard, Impfen. Das Geschäft mit der Angst, Knaur, 1997, pp. 24-27

[200] Karberg, Sascha, Mit den spitzen Waffen eines Virus, *Financial Times Deutschland*, 3 May 2005

[201] Engelbrecht, Torsten; Crowe, David, Avian Flu Virus H5N1: No Proof for Existence, Pathogenicity, or Pandemic Potential; Non-"H5N1" Causation Omitted, *Medical Hypotheses*, 4/2006; pp. 855-857

[202] Houghton, Michael (Mit-Entdecker des HC-Virus): „*Where is the hepatitis C virus? Has anybody seen it?*", At the 8th International HCV Congress in Paris in 2001

[203] Papadopulos-Eleopulos, Eleni; Turner, Valendar, A critique of the Montagnier evidence for the HIV/AIDS hypothesis, *Medical Hypotheses*, 4/2004, pp. 597-601

[204] de Harven, Etienne, Problems with isolating HIV, Vortrag auf einem Symposium des EU-Parlaments in Brüssel

am 8 December 2003, see: www.altheal.org/texts/isolhiv.htm

[205] Personal e-mail communication

[206] Papadopulos-Eleopulos, Eleni; Turner, Valendar, Is a Positive Western Blot Proof of HIV Infection?, *Nature Biotechnology*, June 1993, pp. 696-707

[207] Brown, Terence, The Polymerase Chain Reaction, in: Genomes, chapter 4.3., Bios Scientific Publishers, 2002

[208] See page 76 under http://www.tig.org.za/Parenzee_prosecution_transcripts/Gallo_complete.pdf

[209] Einblick in den Bauplan des Menschen—Seite 2, Nationales Genomforschungsnetz, see www.ngfn.de/17_489.htm

[210] Kremer, Heinrich, Die stille Revolution der Krebs- und AIDS-Medizin, Ehlers, p. 173

[211] Buzás, Edit I. et al., Antibiotic-induced release of small extracellular vesicles (exosomes) with surface-associated DNA, *Scientific Reports*, 15 August 2017

[212] Grolle, Johann, Siege, aber kein Sieg, *Der Spiegel*, 29/1995

[213] Papadopulos-Eleopulos, Eleni; Turner, Valendar, Oxidative Stress, HIV and AIDS, *Research in Immunology*, February 1992, pp. 145-148

[214] Meyerhans, Andreas, Temporal fluctuations in HIV quasispecies in vivo are not reflected by sequential HIV isolations, *Cell*, 8 September 1989, pp. 901-10

[215] Burnet, Sir MacFarlane, Genes, Dreams and Realities, Medical and Technical Publishing, 1971, pp. 217-218

[216] Geison, Gerald, The Private Science of Louis Pasteur, Princeton University Press, 1995

[217] Judson, Horace, The Great Betrayal. Fraud in Science, Harcourt, 2004, pp. 69-71

[218] Georgescu, Vlad, Lebensmittelverpackungen: Weichmacher könnte Hirngewebe schädigen, *Spiegel Online*, 13 December 2005

[219] McClintock, Barbara, The Significance of Responses of The Genome to Challenge, Nobel speech, 8 December 1983

[220] Scobey, Ralph, Is Human Poliomyelitis Caused By An Exogenous Virus?, *Archives of Pediatrics*, April 1954, Vol. 71, pp. 111-123

[221] Kremer, Heinrich, Die stille Revolution der Krebs- und AIDS-Medizin, Ehlers, pp. 11-99, 169-208

[222] Papadopulos-Eleopulos, Eleni; Turner, Valendar, Reappraisal of AIDS: Is the Oxidation caused by the risk factors the primary cause?, *Medical Hypotheses*, March 1988, pp. 151-162

[223] Barbara McClintock, Wikipedia-Website, see en.wikipedia.org/wiki/Barbara_McClintock

[224] McClintock, Barbara, Letter from Barbara McClintock to J. R. S. Fincham, 16 May 1973, see profiles.nlm.nih.gov/LL/B/B/G/C/_/lbbgc.pdf

[225] Duesberg, Peter, Inventing the AIDS Virus, Regnery Publishing, 1996, pp. 238-239

[226] Rice, George, The structure of a thermophilic archaeal virus shows a double-stranded DNA viral capsid type that spans all doMayns of life, *Proceedings of the National Academy of Sciences*, 18 May 2004, pp. 7716-7720

[227] Sogin, Mitchell, Microbial diversity in the deep sea and the underexplored "rare biosphere," Proceedings of the National Academy of Sciences U S A., 8 August 2006, pp. 12115-12120

[228] Ocean Microbe Census Discovers Diverse World of Rare Bacteria, news release from the Marine Biological Laboratory, 31 July 2006, pp. 1-2

[229] Drehscheibe für Viren, Meldung des Wissenschaftlicher Informationsdienst des Europäischen Instituts für Lebensmittel- und Ernährungswissenschaften (EU.L.E.) e.V., 2/2000

[230] Nickels, Stefan, Feindliche Übernahme, *Financial Times Deutschland*, 3 January 2006

[231] Verner, Robinson, Rational Bacteriology, chapter 18: The Bacteriophage, H. Wolff, 1953

[232] Postgate, John, Microbiology and me in 1952, *Microbiology Today*, February 2003, p. 5

233 van Helvoort, Ton, When Did Virology Start? Despite discoveries of nearly a century ago, the unifying concept underpinning this discipline dates more recently to the 1950s, *American Society for Microbiology News*, 3/1996, p. 144

234 Verner, Robinson, Rational Bacteriology, chapter 18: The Bacteriophage, H. Wolff, 1953

235 van Helvoort, Ton, When Did Virology Start? Despite discoveries of nearly a century ago, the unifying concept underpinning this discipline dates more recently to the 1950s, *American Society for Microbiology News*, 3/1996, p. 145

Chapter 2
The Microbe Hunters Seize Power

236 Handel, Ted, Thomas Edison Home & Laboratory (Ft. Meyers, Fl.), Besuchsbericht, New Mexico Institute of Mining and Technology, see infohost.nmt.edu/~bridge/032298.html

237 Judson, Horace, The Great Betrayal. Fraud in Science, Harcourt, 2004, p. 68

238 Enserink, Martin, Virology. Old guard urges virologists to go back to basics, *Science*, 6 July 2001, p. 24

239 Judson, Horace, The Great Betrayal. Fraud in Science, Harcourt, 2004, p. 65

240 McCarthy, Michael, Lies, Damn lies, and scientific research (Rezension des Buches The Great Betrayal: Fraud in Science von Horace Judson, Harcourt, 2004), *Lancet*, 6 November 2004, p. 1657

241 Verner, Robinson, Rational Bacteriology, chapter 56: Four False Dogmas Of Pasteur, H. Wolff, 1953

242 Moschocwitz, Eli, Bulletin of the History of Medicine, Charles Pfizer, 1958, pp. 17-32

243 Langbein, Kurt; Ehgartner, Bert, Das Medizinkartell: Die sieben Todsünden der Gesundheitsindustrie, Piper, 2003, p. 27

244 de Kruif, Paul, Mikrobenjäger, 1941, Institut Orell Füssli, p. 94

245 Verner, Robinson, Rational Bacteriology, chapter 39: The Biont Cycle, H. Wolff, 1953

246 Wostmann, Bernard, Development of cecal distention in germ-free baby rats, *American Journal of Physiology*, December 1959, pp. 1345-1346

247 Verner, Robinson, Rational Bacteriology, chapter 39: The Biont Cycle, H. Wolff, 1953

248 O'Brien, Catheryn, The Mouse, Part 1, *ANZCCART News* insert, Winter 1993, p. 1

249 Wostmann, Bernard, Qualitative adequacy of a chemically defined liquid diet for reproducing germfree mice, *Journal of Nutrition*, May 1970, p. 498-508

250 National Research Council, Nutrient Requirements of Laboratory Animals, fourth revised edition, National Academy Press, 1995, p. 4

251 Wostmann, Bernard, Nutrition and metabolism of the germfree mammal, *World Review of Nutrition and Dietetics*, 1975, Vol. 22, pp. 40-92

252 Wostmann, Bernard, Development of cecal distention in germ-free baby rats, *American Journal of Physiology*, December 1959, pp. 1345-1346

253 Recessive Hairlessness: The "True Hairless" Rat, The Rat & Mouse Club of America, April 2003, see www.rmca.org/Articles/truehairless.htm

254 Snyder Sachs, Jessica, Are Anitbiotics Killing Us?, *Discover*, 10 October 2005

255 Langbein, Kurt; Ehgartner, Bert, Das Medizinkartell: Die sieben Todsünden der Gesundheitsindustrie, Piper, 2003, pp. 21-33

256   Geison, Gerald, The Private Science of Louis Pasteur, Princeton University Press, 1995

257   Langbein, Kurt; Ehgartner, Bert, Das Medizinkartell: Die sieben Todsünden der Gesundheitsindustrie, Piper, 2003, S. 22

258   Judson, Horace, The Great Betrayal. Fraud in Science, Harcourt, 2004, pp. 68-71

259   Ibid., p. 65

260   Geison, Gerald, The Private Science of Louis Pasteur, Princeton University Press, 1995

261   Judson, Horace, The Great Betrayal. Fraud in Science, Harcourt, 2004, p. 30

262   Ibid., p. 20

263   Ibid., p. 27

264   Engelbrecht, Torsten, „Die Industrie macht Druck," interview with Marcia Angell, former editor in chief of the New England Journal of Medicine, on editorial autonomy, fraud in science and the purpose of peer reviewing, Message, 3/2005, p. 69

265   Martinson, Brian, Scientists behaving badly, Nature, 9 June 2005, pp. 737-738

266   Judson, Horace, The Great Betrayal. Fraud in Science, Harcourt, 2004, p. 39

267   Ioannidis, John P. A., Why Most Published Research Findings Are False, PLoS Medicine, August 30, 2005

268   McCarthy, Michael, Lies, Damn lies, and scientific research (Rezension des Buches The Great Betrayal: Fraud in Science von Horace Judson, Harcourt, 2004), Lancet, 6 November 2004, p. 1658

269   Judson, Horace, The Great Betrayal. Fraud in Science, Harcourt, 2004, pp. 244-286

270   Engelbrecht, Torsten, „Die Industrie macht Druck," interview with Marcia Angell, former editor in chief of the New England Journal of Medicine, on editorial autonomy, fraud in science and the purpose of peer reviewing, Message, 3/2005, pp. 68-69

271   Judson, Horace, The Great Betrayal. Fraud in Science, Harcourt, 2004, p. 276

272   Smith, Richard, The Future of Peer Review, 1999, in: Godlee, Fiona; Jefferson, Tom, Peer Review in Health Sciences, BMJ Books, 2003

273   McCarthy, Michael, Lies, Damn lies, and scientific research (Rezension des Buches The Great Betrayal: Fraud in Science von Horace Judson, Harcourt, 2004), Lancet, 6 November 2004, pp. 1657-1658

274   Judson, Horace, The Great Betrayal. Fraud in Science, Harcourt, 2004, pp. 43-154, 191-243

275   Stollorz, Volker, Der große Irrtum des Doktor Koch, Frankfurter Allgemeine Sonntagszeitung, 25 September 2005

276   Gradmann, Cristoph, Krankheit im Labor. Robert Koch und die medizinische Bakteriologie, Wallstein, 2005, pp. 134-135

277   Daniel, Thomas, Captain of Death. The Story of Tuberculosis, Rochester, 1997, p. 76

278   Langbein, Kurt; Ehgartner, Bert, Das Medizinkartell: Die sieben Todsünden der Gesundheitsindustrie, Piper, 2003, p. 67

279   Porter, Roy, The Greatest Benefit to Mankind: a Medical History of Humanity, W. W. Norton & Company, 1997, p. 441

280   Langbein, Kurt; Ehgartner, Bert, Das Medizinkartell: Die sieben Todsünden der Gesundheitsindustrie, Piper, 2003, p. 68

281   Stollorz, Volker, Der große Irrtum des Doktor Koch, Frankfurter Allgemeine Sonntagszeitung, 25 September 2005

282   Langbein, Kurt; Ehgartner, Bert, Das Medizinkartell: Die sieben Todsünden der Gesundheitsindustrie, Piper, 2003, p. 68

283   Stollorz, Volker, Der große Irrtum des Doktor Koch, Frankfurter Allgemeine Sonntagszeitung, 25 September 2005

284   Langbein, Kurt; Ehgartner, Bert, Das Medizinkartell: Die sieben Todsünden der Gesundheitsindustrie, Piper,

2003, pp. 69-70

[285] Williams, Robert, Toward the Conquest of Beriberi, Harvard University Press, 1961, p. 18

[286] Golub, Edward, The Limits of Medicine: How Science Shapes Our Hope for the Cure, The University of Chicago Press, 1997, pp. 37-40

[287] Ibid., pp. 150-151

[288] Ibid., pp. 37-40

[289] Ibid., p. 103

[290] Langbein, Kurt; Ehgartner, Bert, Das Medizinkartell: Die sieben Todsünden der Gesundheitsindustrie, Piper, 2003, p. 51

[291] Golub, Edward, The Limits of Medicine: How Science Shapes Our Hope for the Cure, The University of Chicago Press, 1997, p. 97

[292] Ibid., p. 100

[293] Ibid., p. 99

[294] Ibid., p. 103

[295] Ibid., p. 109

[296] Keller, Evelyn, Barbara McClintock. Die Entdeckerin der springenden Gene, Birkhäuser, 1995, pp. 202-203

[297] Burnet, Sir Frank Macfarlane, Genes, Dreams and Realities, Medical and Technical Publishing, 1971, p. 145

[298] Furger, Sonja, Mit Rohkost gegen die Degeneration. Vor 100 Jahren: Max Bircher-Benner gründet das Sanatorium „Lebendige Kraft", Schweizerische Ärztezeitung, 5/2004, pp. 236-238

[299] McClintock, Barbara, The Significance of Responses of The Genome to Challenge, Nobelpreisrede, 8 December 1983

[300] Cannon, Walter, The Wisdom of the Body, Norton, 1932

[301] Zajicek, Gershom, Wisdom of the body, Medical Hypotheses, May 1999, pp. 447-449

[302] Doughty, Howard, The Limits of Medicine, Rezension des Buches The Limits of Medicine von Edward Golub (The University of Chicago Press, 1997), The Innovation Journal

[303] Duesberg, Peter, Inventing the AIDS Virus, Regnery Publishing, 1996, pp. 137-141

[304] Ibid., p. 134

[305] Ibid., pp. 137-145

[306] Ibid., pp. 137-138

[307] Etheridge, Elizabeth, Sentinel for Health: History of the Centers for Disease Control, University of California Press, 1992, p. 334

[308] Tracey, Michael, Mere Smoke of Opinion; AIDS and the making of the public mind, Continuum, Summer/Fall 2001

[309] Duesberg, Peter, Inventing the AIDS Virus, Regnery Publishing, 1996, p. 138

[310] Lemonick, Michael, Return to the Hot Zone, Time International, 22 May 1995, p. 56-57

[311] Signs that Ebola Virus Is Fading Away, San Francisco Chronicle, 24 May 1995, p. A6

[312] Sandler, Benjamin, Vollwerternährung schützt vor Viruserkrankungen: Das Drama unserer Gesundheitspolitik am Beispiel Kinderlähmung, emu-Verlag, 1986

[313] Miller, Neil, Vaccines: Are They Really Safe & Effective?, New Atlantean Press, 2005, p. 14

[314] McCloskey, Bertram, The relation of prophylactic inoculations to the onset of poliomyletis, Lancet, 18 April 1950, pp. 659-663

[315] Geffen DH, The incidence of paralysis occurring in London children within four weeks after immunization, Medical Officer, 1950, pp. 137–40

[316] Martin JK, Local paralysis in children after injections, *Archives of Disease in Childhood*, 1950, pp. 1-14

[317] Roberts, Janine, Polio: the virus and the vaccine, *The Ecologist*, May 2004, p. 36

[318] West, Jim, Pesticides and Polio: A Critique of the Scientific Literature, The Weston A. Price Foundation

[319] Scobey, Ralph, The Poison Cause of Poliomyelitis And Obstructions To Its Investigation. Statement prepared for the Select Committee to Investigate the Use of Chemicals in Food Products, United States House of Representatives, Washington, D.C., *Archives Of Pediatrics*, April 1952, Vol. 69, pp. 172-173

[320] Roberts, Janine, Polio: the virus and the vaccine, *The Ecologist*, May 2004, p. 36

[321] Ibid., pp. 36-37

[322] Chronological History of the Development of Insecticides and Control Equipment from 1854 through 1954, Clemson University Pesticide Information Program, see entweb.clemson.edu/pesticid/history.htm

[323] Lovett, Robert, The Occurrence Of Infantile Paralysis In Massachusetts In 1908, Reported For The Massachusetts State Board Of Health, *Boston Medical And Surgical Journal*, 22 July 1909, p. 112

[324] Roberts, Janine, Polio: the virus and the vaccine, *The Ecologist*, May 2004, p. 36

[325] Landsteiner, Karl; Popper, Erwin, Übertragung der Poliomyelitis acuta auf Affen, *Zeitschrift für Immunitätsforschung und experimentelle Therapie*, number 4, 1909, pp. 377-390

[326] Landsteiner, Karl; Popper, Erwin, *Wiener Klinische Wochnschrift*, Vol. 21, 1908, p. 1830

[327] Milestones in Poliomyelitis Eradication, World Health Organization Europe, 12 August 2003, see www.euro.who.int/document/pol/eeurotime2003.pdf

[328] Ibid., p. 37

[329] Zell, Roland, Medizinische Virologie. Picornavirusinfektionen, lecture at the Medical Faculty of the University of Jena, see www.med.uni-jena.de/virologie/zell/lehre/Vorlesung_3-Picornavirusinfektionen.pdf

[330] Dimercaprol (BAL), Krause & Pachernegg, see www.kup.at/db/antidota/dimercaprol.html

[331] Scobey, Ralph, The Poison Cause of Poliomyelitis And Obstructions To Its Investigation. Statement prepared for the Select Committee to Investigate the Use of Chemicals in Food Products, United States House of Representatives, Washington, D.C., *Archives Of Pediatrics*, April 1952, Vol. 69, pp. 172-193

[332] Eskwith, Irwin, Empirical Administration of BAL In One Case of Poliomyelitis, *American Journal of Diseases of Diseases of Children*, May 1951, pp. 684-686

[333] Ibid., p. 37

[334] Eggers, Hans, Milestones in Early Poliomyelitis Research (1840 to 1949), *Journal of Virology*, June 1999, pp. 4533-4535

[335] Landsteiner, Karl; Popper, Erwin, Übertragung der Poliomyelitis acuta auf Affen, *Zeitschrift für Immunitätsforschung und experimentelle Therapie*, number 4, 1909

[336] Flexner, Simon; Lewis, Paul, The transmission of acute poliomyelitis to monkeys, *Journal of the American Medical Association*, 13 November 1909, p. 1639

[337] Comroe, Julius, How to Succeed in Failing without Really Trying, *American Review of Respiratory Disease*, 1976, Vol. 14, p. 630

[338] Scobey, Ralph, The Poison Cause of Poliomyelitis And Obstructions To Its Investigation. Statement prepared for the Select Committee to Investigate the Use of Chemicals in Food Products, United States House of Representatives, Washington, D.C., *Archives of Pediatrics*, April 1952, pp. 172-193

[339] Flexner, Simon; Lewis, Paul, The transmission of acute poliomyelitis to monkeys, *Journal of the American Medical Association*, 13 November 1909, p. 1639

[340] Landsteiner, Karl; Popper, Erwin, Übertragung der Poliomyelitis acuta auf Affen, *Zeitschrift für Immunitätsforschung und experimentelle Therapie*, number 4 1909, pp. 377-390

[341] Scobey, Ralph, The Poison Cause of Poliomyelitis And Obstructions To Its Investigation. Statement prepared for the Select Committee to Investigate the Use of Chemicals in Food Products, United States House of Representatives, Washington, D.C., *Archives of Pediatrics,* April 1952, Vol. 69, pp. 172-193

[342] Scobey, Ralph, Is The Public Health Law Responsible For The Poliomyelitis Mystery?, *Archives of Pediatrics,* May 1951, Vol. 68, pp. 220-232

[343] Ostrom, Neenyh, Will The Poliovirus Eradication Program Rid the World of Childhood Paralysis?, Chronic Illnet, 20 April 2001, see http://www.chronicillnet.org/articles/paralyticpolio.html

[344] Roberts, Janine, Polio: the virus and the vaccine, *The Ecologist*, May 2004, p. 38

[345] Scobey, Ralph, The Poison Cause of Poliomyelitis And Obstructions To Its Investigation. Statement prepared for the Select Committee to Investigate the Use of Chemicals in Food Products, United States House of Representatives, Washington, D.C., *Archives of Pediatrics,* April 1952, Vol. 69, pp. 172-193

[346] Organisationen fordern mehr Impfungen gegen Polio, *Ärzte Zeitung* (online), 28 October 2005

[347] Roberts, Janine, Polio: the virus and the vaccine, *The Ecologist*, May 2004, p. 39

[348] Spice, Byron, Developing a medical milestone: the Salk polio vaccine: The Salk vaccine: 50 years later, *Pittsburgh Post-Gazette* (online), 3 April 2005

[349] Bayly, Beddow, The Story of the Salk Anti-poliomyelitis Vaccine, Animal Defence and Anti-Vivisection Society, 1956, chapters: Many Monkeys needed in Vaccine Production, Ban on Export by Indian Government?, see www.whale.to/vaccine/bayly.html#HUMAN-TISSUE%20VIRUS

[350] Scobey, Ralph, The Poison Cause of Poliomyelitis And Obstructions To Its Investigation. Statement prepared for the Select Committee to Investigate the Use of Chemicals in Food Products, United States House of Representatives, Washington, D.C., *Archives of Pediatrics,* April 1952, Vol. 69, p. 187

[351] Roberts, Janine, Polio: the virus and the vaccine, *The Ecologist*, May 2004, p. 39

[352] Ibid., p. 42

[353] Bayly, Beddow, The Story of the Salk Anti-poliomyelitis Vaccine, Animal Defence and Anti-Vivisection Society, 1956, capter "Claims for the Salk Vaccine"

[354] Ibid., chapter: The Salk Vaccine Disaster

[355] Roberts, Janine, Polio: the virus and the vaccine, *The Ecologist*, May 2004, p. 42

[356] Bayly, Beddow, The Story of the Salk Anti-poliomyelitis Vaccine, Animal Defence and Anti-Vivisection Society, 1956, chapter: The Salk Vaccine Disaster

[357] Officer Profiles: Neal Nathanson, Website der Centers for Disease Control and Prevention (CDC

[358] Bayly, Beddow, The Story of the Salk Anti-poliomyelitis Vaccine, Animal Defence and Anti-Vivisection Society, 1956, chapter: The Salk Vaccine Disaster

[359] Miller, Neil, Vaccines: Are They Really Safe & Effective?, New Atlantean Press, 2005, p. 14

[360] Biskind, Morton, Statement on clinical intoxication from DDT and other new insecticides, *Journal of Insurance Medicine*, March-May 1951, pp. 5-12

[361] Biskind, Morton, Public Health Aspects of the New Insecticides, *American Journal of Digestive Diseases*, November 1953, Vol. 20, p. 334

[362] Sabin, Albert, The Epidemiology of Poliomyelitis. Problems at Home and Among Armed Forces Abroad, *Journal of the American Medical Association*, 28 June 1947, pp. 754-755

363   Dichlordiphenyltrichlorethan (DDT), Wikipedia-Website, see de.wikipedia.org/wiki/DDT

364   Russell, Edmund, The Strange Career of DDT: Experts, Federal Capacity, and Environmentalism in World War II, *Technology and Culture*, Vol. 40, Nummer 4, October 1999, pp. 770-796

365   Biskind, Morton, Public Health Aspects of the New Insecticides, *American Journal of Digestive Diseases, November 1953, Vol. 20, pp. 331-341*

366   Biskind, Morton; Bieber, Irving, DDT poisoning: a new syndrome with neuropsychiatric manifestations; *American Journal Of Psychotherapy*; April 1949, p. 261

367   Dichlordiphenyltrichlorethan (DDT), Wikipedia-Website, see de.wikipedia.org/wiki/DDT

368   Zimmerman, Oswald; Lavine, Irvin DDT. Killer of Killers, Dover, N.H., Industrial Research Service, 1946

369   Dichlordiphenyltrichlorethan (DDT), Wikipedia-Website, see de.wikipedia.org/wiki/DDT

370   West, Jim, Pesticides and Polio, *Townsend Letter for Doctors and Patients*, June 2000, pp. 68-75, see www.geocities.com/harpub/overview.htm?20056

371   Biskind, Morton, Public Health Aspects of the New Insecticides, *American Journal of Digestive Diseases, November 1953, Vol. 20, pp. 331-341*

372   Dresden, Daniel, *Physiological Investigations Into The Action Of DDT*, G.W. Van Der Wiel & Co., Arnhem, 1949

373   Harrison, Tinsley, Harrison's Principles of Internal Medicine, McGraw-Hill, 1983, p. 1130

374   Biskind, Morton, Public Health Aspects of the New Insecticides, *American Journal of Digestive Diseases, November 1953, Vol. 20, p. 334*

375   Biskind, Morton, Public Health Aspects of the New Insecticides, *American Journal of Digestive Diseases, November 1953, Vol. 20, p. 332*

376   Biskind, Morton; Bieber, Irving, DDT poisoning: a new syndrome with neuropsychiatric manifestations; *American Journal Of Psychotherapy*; April 1949, p. 261

377   Biskind, Morton, Public Health Aspects of the New Insecticides, *American Journal of Digestive Diseases, November 1953, Vol. 20, p. 332*

378   Roberts, Janine, Polio: the virus and the vaccine, *The Ecologist*, May 2004, p. 39

379   Busse, Franziska, Als erstes Land der Welt verbietet Schweden den Einsatz von DDT. Vor 35 Jahren, *DeutschlandRadio Berlin*, 27 March 2005

380   Roberts, Janine, Polio: the virus and the vaccine, *The Ecologist*, May 2004, p. 39

381   West, Jim, Pesticides and Polio: A Critique of the Scientific Literature, The Weston A. Price Foundation

382   West, Jim, Pesticides and Polio, see http://www.geocities.com/harpub/overview.htm?20056

383   Worse Than Insects? *TIME*, 11 April 1949, see http://scitech.quickfound.net/environment/insecticides_news_index.html

384   Carson, Rachel, Silent Spring, Houghton Mifflin, 1962

385   Daniel, Pete, Toxic Drift. Pesticides And Health In The Post-World War II South, Louisiana State University Press, 2005, p. 82

386   Daniel, Pete, Toxic Drift. Pesticides And Health In The Post-World War II South, Louisiana State University Press, 2005, pp. 2, 16, 20-21, 33

387   Ibid., p. 81

388   Cottam, Clarence, The Handbook of Texas Online, see www.tsha.utexas.edu/handbook/online/articles/CC/fcoav_print.html

389   Daniel, Pete, Toxic Drift. Pesticides And Health In The Post-World War II South, Louisiana State University Press,

2005, p. 34

[390] Ibid., p. 79

[391] Ibid., p. 72

[392] Ibid., p. 82

[393] Scobey, Ralph, The Poison Cause of Poliomyelitis And Obstructions To Its Investigation. Statement prepared for the Select Committee to Investigate the Use of Chemicals in Food Products, United States House of Representatives, Washington, D.C., *Archives Of Pediatrics,* April 1952, Vol. 69, pp. 172-173

[394] de Harven, Etienne, The Recollections of an Electron Microscopist, *Reappraising AIDS,* November/December 1998

[395] Duesberg, Peter, Inventing the AIDS Virus, Regnery Publishing, 1996, p. 96

[396] Engelbrecht, Torsten, Schuss auf den Matrosen, interview with US molecular biologist and cancer expert Peter Duesberg on anti-smoking campaigns, gene-mutations, aneuploidy, and the failure of the established cancer research, *Freitag,* 27 April 2005, p. 18

[397] de Harven, Etienne, The Recollections of an Electron Microscopist, *Reappraising AIDS,* November/December 1998

[398] Duesberg, Peter, The Enigma of Slow Viruses, review of the book "Facts and Artefactcs. Archives of Virology" from Pawel Liberski (published at Springer), *Lancet,* 18 September 1993, p. 720

[399] Duesberg, Peter, Inventing the AIDS Virus, Regnery Publishing, 1996, p. 99

[400] Duesberg, Peter, Human immunodeficiency virus and acquired immunodeficiency syndrome: correlation but not causation, *Proceedings of the National Academy of Sciences U S A,* February 1989 Feb, pp. 755-764

[401] Gajdusek, Carleton, Unconventional Viruses and the Origin and Disappearance of Kuru, Nobelpreisrede, 13 December 1976, see p. 316 at nobelprize.org/medicine/laureates/1976/gajdusek-lecture.pdf

[402] Köhnlein, Claus, AIDS, Hepatitis C, BSE: Infectious or Intoxication Diseases?, *Continuum,* Fall 2001

[403] Duesberg, Peter, Inventing the AIDS Virus, Regnery Publishing, 1996, p. 77

[404] Kolata, Gina, Anthropologists Suggest Cannibalism Is A Myth, *Science,* 20 June 1986, pp. 1497-1500

[405] Scholz, Roland, Überlegungen zur Genese der bovinen spongiformen Encephalopathie (BSE), Biolab-Website, see http://www.biolab-muenchen.de/index.html?rightframe=http://www.biolab-muenchen.de/bse/scholz01.htm

[406] Ibid.

[407] See www.bigfootsurplus.com/bigfoot_tracker/03-0010.php

[408] Hartlaub, Peter, Sasquatch: Kitsch of death, *San Francisco Examiner,* 7 August 2000

[409] Stöcker, Christian, Kryptozoologie. Auf großem Fuß im Regenwald, *Spiegel Online,* 29 December 2005

[410] Papadopulos-Eleopulos, Eleni; Turner, Valendar, A Brief History of Retroviruses, *Continuum,* Winter 1997/1998, p. 27

[411] Beard, J. W., Physical methods for the analysis of cells, *Annals of the New York Academy of Sciences,* 16 December 1957, pp. 530-544

[412] Papadopulos-Eleopulos, Eleni; Turner, Valendar, A Brief History of Retroviruses, *Continuum,* Winter 1997/1998, p. 28

[413] Sinoussi, Françoise; Cherman, Jean Claude. Purification and partial differentiation of the particles of murine sarcoma virus (M. MSV) according to their sedimentation rates in sucrose density gradients, *Spectra* 1973, Vol. 4, pp. 237-243

[414] Papadopulos-Eleopulos, Eleni; Turner, Valendar, A Brief History of Retroviruses, *Continuum,* Winter 1997/1998, p. 29

[415] Personal interview, 1 February 2006

[416] de Harven, Etienne, Of Mice And Men; Viral Etiology Of Human Cancer: A historical perspective, *Continuum,* Summer/Fall 2001

[417] On 12 July, 2005, we requested supporting studies from the German Robert Koch-Institute (RKI) for the claims that (1) various viruses (SARS, Hepatitis C, HIV, Ebola, smallpox, polio) as well as the BSE-causing agent have been purified, fully characterized, and photographed by electron microscopy, that (2) these agents are transmissible and pathogenic to humans, and that (3) other possible causes for observed diseases (e.g., nutrition, pesticides, stress) can be ruled out. On 29 November, 2005, we also requested the same supporting studies from the German Friedrich-Loeffler-Institut (FLI) in relation to so-called H5N1—but we haven't received any study yet delivering the clear-cut proofs for these claims, neither from the RKI nor from the FLI

[418] Goodman, Jordan; Walsh, Vivien ,The Story of Taxol: Nature and Politics in the Pursuit of an Anti-Cancer Drug, Cambridge University Press, 2001

[419] de Harven, Etienne, The Recollections of an Electron Microscopist, *Reappraising AIDS*, November/December 1998

[420] Oberling, Charles, Krebs: das Rätsel seiner Entstehung, Rowohlt, 1959

[421] de Harven, Etienne, Remarks on Viruses, Leukemia and Electron Microscopy, in: Methodological approaches to the study of leukemias; a symposium held at the Wistar Institute of Anatomy and Biology, 5 and 6 April 1965, Defendi, Vittorio, The Wistar Institute Symposium Monograph, September 1965, pp. 147-156

[422] Weihe, Wolfgang, Klinische Studien und Statistik: Von der Wahrscheinlichkeit des Irrtums, *Deutsches Ärzteblatt*, 26 March 2004, p. C681

[423] Begley, Sharon, New Journals Bet. 'Negative Results' Save Time, Money, *Wall Street Journal*, 15 September 2006; p. B1

[424] Sharav, Vera, Negative Research Results—Mostly Concealed in Journals, press release, Alliance for Human Research Protection (AHRP), 26 Novembe 2006

[425] Bernhard, W.; Leplus, R., Fine structure of the normal and malignant human lymph node, Pergamon Press, 1965

[426] Bernhard, W.; Leplus, R., Fine structure of the normal and malignant human lymph node, Pergamon Press, 1964

[427] de Harven, Etienne, The Recollections of an Electron Microscopist, *Reappraising AIDS*, November/December 1998

[428] de Harven, Etienne, Structure of virus particles partially purified from the blood of leukemic mice, *Virology*, May 1964, pp. 119-124

[429] de Harven, Etienne, Structure of critical point dried oncornaviruses, *Virology*, October 1973, pp. 535-540

[430] de Harven, Etienne, The Recollections of an Electron Microscopist, *Reappraising AIDS*, November/December 1998

[431] Duesberg, Peter, Inventing the AIDS Virus, Regnery Publishing, 1996, pp. 121-122

[432] de Harven, Etienne, Of Mice And Men; Viral Etiology Of Human Cancer: A historical perspective, *Continuum*, Summer/Fall 2001

[433] Wade, Nicholas, Scientists and the Press: Cancer Scare Story That Wasn't, *Science*, Volume 1974, 1971, Vol. 174, pp. 679-680

[434] Temin, Howard, RNA-dependent DNA polymerase in virions of Rous sarcoma virus, *Nature*, 27 June 1970, pp. 1211-1213

[435] Baltimore, David, Viral RNA-dependent DNA polymerase, *Nature*, 27 June 1970, pp. 1209-1211

[436] The Nobel Prize in Physiology or Medicine 1975, Nobelprize.org, see nobelprize.org/medicine/laureates/1975/

[437] Epstein, Steven, Impure Science—AIDS, Activism and the Politics of Knowledge, University of California Press, 1996, p. 67

[438] The Australian Perth Group commenting the paper written by Robert Gallo and Luc Montagnier "The discovery of HIV as the cause of AIDS" (*New England Journal of Medicine*, 11 December 2003, pp. 2283-2285): „... all the HIV experts including Gallo and Montagnier have proven the presence of the enzyme indirectly, that is, by transcription of the synthetic template-primer An.dT," see www.theperthgroup.com/REJECTED/GalloMontagNEJM.html

439   de Harven, Etienne, The Recollections of an Electron Microscopist, *Reappraising AIDS*, November/December 1998

440   Montagnier, Luc; Barré-Sinoussi, Françoise; Cherman, Jean Claude, Isolation of a T-lymphotropic retrovirus from a patient at risk for acquired immune deficiency syndrome (AIDS), *Science*, 20 May. 1983, pp. 868-71

441   Temin, Howard; Baltimore, David, RNA-directed DNA synthesis and RNA tumor viruses, *Advances in Virus Research*, 1972; Vol. 17, pp. 129-186

442   Sinoussi, Françoise; Chermann, Jjean Claude, Purification and partial differentiation of the particles of murine sarcoma virus (M. MSV) according to their sedimentation rates in sucrose density gradients, *Spectra* 1973, pp. 237-243

443   Enserink, Martin, Virology. Old guard urges virologists to go back to basics, *Science*, 6 July 2001, p. 24

444   H. pylori nicht der einzige Magenbewohner? — Hinweis auf weitere exotische Bakterien, *Deutsches Ärzteblatt* (online), 9 January 2006

445   Bik, Elisabeth, Molecular analysis of the bacterial microbiota in the human stomach, *Proceedings of the National Academy of Sciences*, 17 January 2006, pp. 732-737

446   Moss, Ralph, Fragwürdige Chemotherapie, . Entscheidungshilfen für die Krebsbehandlung, Haug, 1997, pp. 36-38

447   Miklos, George, The Human Cancer Genome Project — one more misstep in the war on cancer, *Nature Biotechnology*, May 2005, pp. 535-537

448   Epstein, Samuel, Losing the "War Against Cancer": A Need for Public Policy Reforms, *International Journal of Health Services and Molecular Biology*, 4 February 1992, pp. 455-469

449   Moss, Ralph, Fragwürdige Chemotherapie, . Entscheidungshilfen für die Krebsbehandlung, Haug, 1997, p. 35

450   Engelbrecht, Torsten, Aneuploidie. Paradigmenwechsel in der Krebstherapie, *Co'Med*, 8/2005, pp. 30-35

451   Miklos, George, Iconoclast to the Max, review of the book „Oncogenes, Aneuploidy and AIDS" von Harvey Bialy (published by North Atlantic), *Nature Biotechnology*, July 2004, pp. 815-816

452   Halter, Hans, „Wir müssen den steinigen Weg gehen," *Der Spiegel*, 18/1986

453   Wecht, Cyril, The Swine Flu Immunization Program: Scientific Venture or Political Folly?, *Legal Medicine Annual*, 1978, pp. 227-244

454   Duesberg, Peter, Inventing the AIDS Virus, Regnery Publishing, 1996, pp. 141-143

455   Red Cross Knew of AIDS Blood Threat, *San Francisco Chronicle*, 16 May 1994

456   Mullis, Kary, Dancing Naked in the Mind Field, Vintage Books, 1998, p. 177

457   Duesberg, Peter, Inventing the AIDS Virus, Regnery Publishing, 1996, p. 124

458   Mullis, Kary, Dancing Naked in the Mind Field, Vintage Books, 1998, p. 177

Chapter 3
AIDS: From Spare Tire to Multibillion-Dollar Business

459   Mullis, Kary, Dancing Naked in the Mind Field, Vintage Books, 1998, pp. 171-174

460   Grolle, Johann, Siege, aber kein Sieg, *Der Spiegel*, 29/1995

461   Smith, Richard, Milton and Galileo would back the *BMJ* on free speech, *Nature*, 22 January 2004; p. 287

462   Kruse, Kuno; Schwarz, Birgit, Die Apokalypse wird abgesagt, *Die Zeit*, 15 June 1990

463   AIDS: Die Bombe ist gelegt, *Der Spiegel*, 45/1984

464   AIDS: eine neue Krankheit erschüttert Deutschland, *Bild der Wissenschaft*, 12/1985

465   Morganthau, Tom, AIDS: Grim Prospects, *Newsweek*, 10 November, 1986, pp. 20-21

[466] HIV/AIDS in Deutschland: Eckdaten (at the end of 2005), Website of the Robert Koch-Institute

[467] Suspension of Disbelief??, Health Education AIDS Liaison (HEAL), Toronto, see http://healtoronto.com/aids-drop.html

[468] Marcus, Ulrich, Glück gehabt? Zwei Jahrzehnte AIDS in Deutschland, Blackwell, 2000, S. 10

[469] Lang, Serge, Challenges; Springer, New York, 1998, p. 610

[470] Fiala, Christian, Lieben wir gefährlich? Ein Arzt auf der Suche nach Fakten und Hintergründen von AIDS, Deuticke, 1997, p. 202

[471] Keou, François-Xavier, World Health Organization clinical case definition for AIDS in Africa: an analysis of evaluations, *East African Medical Journal*, October 1992, pp. 550-553

[472] Lang, Serge, Challenges; Springer, New York, 1998, pp. 610-611

[473] de Harven, Etienne, Of Mice And Men; Viral Etiology Of Human Cancer: A historical perspective, *Continuum*, Summer/Fall 2001

[474] Mbeki, Thabo, A synthesis report of the deliberations by the panel of experts invited by the President of the Republic of South Africa, chapter 2.2.1.: Visualisation and Isolation of the Virus, March 2001, see www.polity.org.za/html/govdocs/reports/aids/chapter2.htm#2.2.1

[475] Tahi, Djamel, Did Luc Montagnier Discover HIV?, Interview mit Luc Montagnier, *Continuum*, Winter 1997/1998, pp. 31-35

[476] de Harven, Etienne, Problems with isolating HIV, European Parliament in Brussels, 8 December 2003, see: www.altheal.org/texts/isolhiv.htm

[477] Papadopulos-Eleopulos, Eleni; Turner, Valendar, A critique of the Montagnier evidence fort he HIV/AIDS hypothesis, *Medical Hypotheses*, 4/2004, pp. 597-601

[478] Structure of most deadly virus in the world revealed, press release, University of Oxford, 23 January 2006

[479] Briggs, John, The Mechanism of HIV-1 Core Assembly: Insights from Three Dimensional Reconstructions of Authentic Virions, *Structure*, January 2006, p. 16

[480] Ibid., pp. 15-20

[481] Structure of most deadly virus in the world revealed, press release, University of Oxford, 23 January 2006

[482] Briggs, John, The Mechanism of HIV-1 Core Assembly: Insights from Three Dimensional Reconstructions of Authentic Virions, *Structure*, January 2006, p. 19

[483] Metzler, Natasha, Generic AZT Hits the United States, *Pharmexec.com*, 10 October 2005

[484] Hodgkinson, Neville, How Giant Drug Firm Funds The AIDS Lobby, *Sunday Times* (London), 30 May 1993

[485] Briggs, John, The Mechanism of HIV-1 Core Assembly: Insights from Three Dimensional Reconstructions of Authentic Virions, *Structure*, January 2006, p. 16

[486] Ibid.

[487] Ibid.

[488] Personal interview with Val Turner, 3 February 2006

[489] Personal interview with Stepehn Fuller; 10 February 2006

[490] Gallo, Robert; Fauci Anthony, The human retroviruses, in: Fauci, Anthony, Harrison's Principles of Internal Medicine, McGraw-Hill, 1994, pp. 808-814

[491] Papadoupulos-Eleopulos, Eleni; Turner, Valendar, The request reMayns the same and is still pure and simple, *British Medical Journal* (online), 12 June 2003, see http://www.rethinking.org/bmj/response_33236.html

[492] HIV structure and Genome, Wikipedia-Website, see http://en.wikipedia.org/wiki/HIV_structure_and_genome

[493] Briggs, John, The Mechanism of HIV-1 Core Assembly: Insights from Three Dimensional Reconstructions of Authentic Virions, *Structure*, January 2006, p. 16

[494] Welker, Reinhold, Biochemical and Structural Analysis of Isolated Mature Cores of Human Immunodeficiency Virus Type 1, *Journal of Virology*, February 2000, pp. 1168-1177

[495] Bess, Julyan, Microvesicles are a source of contaminating cellular proteins found in purified HIV-1 preparations, *Virology*, 31 March 1997, pp. 134-144

[496] Gluschankof, Pablo, Cell membrane vesicles are a major contaminant of gradient-enriched human immunodeficiency virus type-1 preparations, *Virology*, 31 March 1997, pp. 125-133

[497] Hackenbroch, Veronika, „Der Optimismus ist verflogen." Der Virologe, AIDS-Forscher und Leiter des Berliner Robert Koch Instituts, Reinhard Kurth, über die ersten HIV-Impfstoff-Tests in Deutschland, *Der Spiegel*, 9/2004, p. 153

[498] Tahi, Djamel, AIDS—die großen Zweifel, Arte Television, 14 March 1996, see www.torstenengelbrecht.com/de/artikel_medien.html

[499] Papadopulos-Eleopulos, Eleni; Turner, Valendar, A critique of the Montagnier evidence for the HIV/AIDS hypothesis, *Medical Hypotheses*, 4/2004, p. 584

[500] Barré-Sinoussi, Françoise; Cherman, Jean Claude, Isolation of new lymphotropic retrovirus from two siblings with haemophilia B, one with AIDS, *Lancet*, 7 April 1984; pp. 753-757

[501] Macilwain, Colin, AAAS criticized over AIDS sceptics' meeting, *Nature*, 26 May 1994, p. 265

[502] Lang, Serge, Challenges; Springer, New York, 1998, p. 609

[503] Berger, Michael; Mühlhauser, Ingrid, Surrogatmarker: Trugschlüsse, *Deutsches Ärzteblatt*, 6 December 1996, pp. A3280-A3283

[504] ELISA Test-kit from Abbot Laboratories

[505] Papadopulos-Eleopulos, Eleni; Turner, Valendar, Is a Positive Western Blot Proof of HIV Infection?, *Nature Biotechnology*, June 1993, pp. 696-707

[506] Glücksspiel AIDS-Test, *Die Woche*, 5 August 1993, see AIDS-info.net/micha/hiv/AIDS/diewoche1.html

[507] Papadopulos-Eleopulos, Eleni; Turner, Valendar, The Isolation of HIV—Has It Really Been Achieved? The Case Against, *Continuum*, September/October 1996, Supplement, pp. 1-24

[508] Glücksspiel AIDS-Test, *Die Woche*, 5 August 1993, see AIDS-info.net/micha/hiv/AIDS/diewoche1.html

[509] Essex, Max; Kashala, Oscar, Infection with human immonodificiency virus type 1 (hiv-1) and human t-cell lymphotropic viruses among leprosy patients and contacts: correlation between hiv-1 cross-reactivity and antibodies to lipoarabinomanna; *Journal of Infectious Diseases*, February 1994, pp. 296-304

[510] Johnson, Christine, Whose Antibodies are they anyway?, *Continuum*, September/October 1996, pp. 4-5

[511] Hodgkinson, Neville, HIV diagnosis: a ludicrous case of circular reasoning, *The Business online*, 16 May 2004

[512] Duesberg, Peter; Koehnlein, Claus; Rasnick, David, The Chemical Bases of the Various AIDS Epidemics: Recreational Drugs, Anti-viral Chemotherapy and Malnutrition, *Journal of Biosciences*, June 2003, p. 390

[513] Hackenbroch, Veronika, „Der Optimismus ist verflogen." Der Virologe, AIDS-Forscher und Leiter des Berliner Robert Koch Instituts, Reinhard Kurth, über die ersten HIV-Impfstoff-Tests in Deutschland, *Der Spiegel*, 9/2004, p. 153

[514] Papadopulos-Eleopulos, Eleni; Turner, Valendar, HIV antibody tests and viral load—more unanswered questions and a further plea for clarification, *Current Medical Research and Opinion*, 3/1998, pp. 185-186

[515] Rich, Josiah, Misdiagnosis of HIV infection by HIV-1 plasma viral load testing: a case series, *Annals of Internal Medicine*, 5 January 1999, pp. 37-39

[516] Rodriguez, Benigno, Predictive value of plasma HIV RNA level on rate of CD4 T-cell decline in untreated HIV

infection, *Journal of the American Medical Association*, 27 September 2006, pp. 1498-1506

[517] Papadopulos-Eleopulos, Eleni; Turner, Valendar, A critical analysis of the HIV-T4-cell-AIDS hypothesis, *Genetica*, 1-3/1995; pp. 5-24

[518] Epstein, Steven, Impure Science – AIDS, Activism and the Politics of Knowledge, University of California Press, 1996, pp. 75, 109

[519] Concorde Coordinating Committee, Concorde: MRCC/ANRS randomised double-blind controlled trial of imme-diate and deferred zidovudine in symptom-free HIV-infection, *Lancet*, 9 April 1994, 343: 871-881

[520] Fleming, Thomas; DeMets, David, Surrogate end points in clinical trials: are we being misled?, *Annals of Inter-nal Medicine*, 1 October 1996, pp. 605-613

[521] Williams, Brian, HIV infection, antiretroviral therapy, and CD4+ cell count distributions in African populations, *Journal of Infectious Diseases*, 15 November 2006, pp. 1450-1458

[522] Chargaff, Erwin, Das Feuer des Heraklit, Luchterhand, 1989, p. 232

[523] Lichtblau, Eric, Settlement in Marketing of a Drug for AIDS, *New York Times*, 18 October 2005

[524] Duesberg, Peter; Koehnlein, Claus; Rasnick, David, The Chemical Bases of the Various AIDS Epidemics: Recre-ational Drugs, Anti-viral Chemotherapy and Malnutrition, *Journal of Biosciences*, June 2003, pp. 383-412

[525] Duesberg, Peter, Inventing the AIDS Virus, Regnery Publishing, 1996, p. 419

[526] Connor, Thomas, Methylenedioxymethamphetamine Suppresses Production of the Proinflammatory Cytokine Tumor Necrosis Factor-α Independent of a β-Adrenoceptor-Mediated Increase in Interleukin-10, *Journal of Pharmacology And Experimental Therapeutics*, January 2005, pp. 134-143

[527] Dronda, Fernando, CD4 cell recovery during successful antiretroviral therapy in naive HIV-infected patients: the role of intravenous drug use, *AIDS*, 5 November 2004, pp. 2210-2212

[528] Connor, Thomas, Methylenedioxymethamphetamine (MDMA, 'Ecstasy'): a stressor on the immune system, *Im-munology*, April 2004, pp. 357-367

[529] Duesberg, Peter; Koehnlein, Claus; Rasnick, David, The Chemical Bases of the Various AIDS Epidemics: Recre-ational Drugs, Anti-viral Chemotherapy and Malnutrition, *Journal of Biosciences*, June 2003, pp. 387-388

[530] Jaffe, Harold, National case-control study of Kaposi's sarcoma and Pneumocystis carinii pneumonia in homo-sexual men, Part 1. Epidemiologic results, *Annals of Internal Medicine*, August 1983, pp. 145-151

[531] What are the medical consequences of inhalant abuse?, Website des National Institute on Drug Abuse (NIDA), see www.drugabuse.gov/ResearchReports/Inhalants/Inhalants4.html

[532] Papadopulos-Eleopulos, Eleni; A Mitotic Theory, *Journal of Theoretical Biology*, 21 June 1982, pp. 741-57

[533] Harrison, Tinsley, Harrison's Principles of Internal Medicine, McGraw-Hill, 1983, p. 1206

[534] Papadopulos-Eleopulos, Eleni; Turner, Valendar, Oxidative Stress, HIV and AIDS, *Research in Immunology*, Febru-ary 1992, pp. 145-148

[535] Weiss, Robin, Induction of avian tumor viruses in normal cells by physical and chemical carcinogens, *Virology*, December 1971, pp. 920-38

[536] Duesberg, Peter, Inventing the AIDS Virus, Regnery Publishing, 1996, p. 149

[537] Ibid., pp. 146-148

[538] Tracey, Michael, Mere Smoke of Opinion; AIDS and the making of the public mind, *Continuum*, Summer/Fall 2001

[539] Shilts, Randy, And the Band Played on, Penguin Books, 1987, p. 67

[540] Gottlieb, Michael, Pneumocystis Pneumonia – Los Angeles, *Morbidity and Mortality Weekly Report*, 5 June 1981, pp. 250-252

[541] Duesberg, Peter, Inventing the AIDS Virus, Regnery Publishing, 1996, p. 148

[542] Haverkos, Harry; Dougherty, John, Health Hazards of Nitrite Inhalants, Research Monograph Series 83, National Institute on Drug Abuse, 1988, p. 1, see www.drugabuse.gov/pdf/monographs/83.pdf

[543] Ibid., p. 5

[544] Duesberg, Peter, Inventing the AIDS Virus, Regnery Publishing, 1996, pp. 260-261

[545] Labataille, Lorette, Amyl nitrite employed in homosexual relations, Medical Aspects of Human Sexuality, 1975; Vol. 9, p. 122

[546] Haverkos, Harry; Dougherty, John, Health Hazards of Nitrite Inhalants, Research Monograph Series 83, National Institute on Drug Abuse, 1988, pp. 5, 87, see www.drugabuse.gov/pdf/monographs/83.pdf

[547] Lauritsen, John, NIDA Meeting Calls For Research Into The Poppers-Kaposi's Sarcoma Connection, New York Native 13 June 1994

[548] Duesberg, Peter, Inventing the AIDS Virus, Regnery Publishing, 1996, p. 377

[549] Poppers advertising, see www.liquidaromas.com/ads.html

[550] Lauritsen, John, The AIDS War. Propaganda, Profeteering and Genocide from the Medical-Industrial Complex, Asklepios, 1993, pp. 108-110

[551] Haverkos, Harry; Dougherty, John, Health Hazards of Nitrite Inhalants, Research Monograph Series 83, National Institute on Drug Abuse, 1988, p. 6, see www.drugabuse.gov/pdf/monographs/83.pdf

[552] Ibid., pp. 6, 11

[553] What are the medical consequences of inhalant abuse?, Website des National Institute on Drug Abuse (NIDA), see www.drugabuse.gov/ResearchReports/Inhalants/Inhalants4.html

[554] Haverkos, Harry; Dougherty, John, Health Hazards of Nitrite Inhalants, Research Monograph Series 83, National Institute on Drug Abuse, 1988, pp. 2-4, see www.drugabuse.gov/pdf/monographs/83.pdf

[555] Lauritsen, John, The AIDS War. Propaganda, Profeteering and Genocide from the Medical-Industrial Complex, Asklepios, 1993, p. 109

[556] Haverkos, Harry; Dougherty, John, Health Hazards of Nitrite Inhalants, Research Monograph Series 83, National Institute on Drug Abuse, 1988, pp. 2-4, see www.drugabuse.gov/pdf/monographs/83.pdf

[557] Haley, Thomas, Review of the physiological effects of amyl, butyl and isobutyl nitrites, Clinical Toxicology, May 1980, pp. 317-329

[558] Masur, Henry, An outbreak of community-acquired Pneumocystis carinii pneumonia: initial manifestation of cellular immune dysfunction, New England Journal of Medicine, 10 December 1981, pp. 1431-1438

[559] Siegal, Frederick, Severe acquired immunodeficiency in male homosexuals, manifested by chronic perianal ulcerative herpes simplex lesions, New England Journal of Medicine, 10 December 1981, pp. 1439-1444

[560] Durack, David, Opportunistic infections and Kaposi's sarcoma in homosexual men, New England Journal of Medicine, 10 December 1981, pp. 1465-1467

[561] Adams, Jad, AIDS: The HIV Myth, St. Martin's Press, 1989, p. 129

[562] Shilts, Randy, And the Band Played on, Penguin Books, 1987, p. 81

[563] Current Trends Update on Acquired Immune Deficiency Syndrome (AIDS) — United States, Morbidity and Mortality Weekly Report, 24 September 1982, pp. 507-508

[564] Lauritsen, John, The AIDS War; Propaganda, Profeteering and Genocide from the Medical-Industrial Complex, Asklepios, 1993, pp. 11-14

[565] Epstein, Steven, Impure Science — AIDS, Activism and the Politics of Knowledge, University of California Press,

1996, pp. 49-50

566 Shilts, Randy, And the Band Played on, Penguin Books, 1987, p. 121

567 Epstein, Steven, Impure Science – AIDS, Activism and the Politics of Knowledge, University of California Press, 1996, p. 55

568 Halter, Hans, Eine Epidemie, die erst beginnt, *Der Spiegel*, 23/1983

569 Duesberg, Peter; Koehnlein, Claus; Rasnick, David, The Chemical Bases of the Various AIDS Epidemics: Recreational Drugs, Anti-viral Chemotherapy and Malnutrition, *Journal of Biosciences*, June 2003, pp. 392-401

570 Duesberg, Peter, Inventing the AIDS Virus, Regnery Publishing, 1996, pp. 377-381

571 Lauritsen, John, Prickly Poppers. An AIDS activist wonders how a flammable drug become so popular among gay men, *Xtra!*, 23 March 2000

572 Lauritsen, John, NIDA Meeting Calls For Research Into The Poppers-Kaposi's Sarcoma Connection, *New York Native* 13 June 1994

573 Lauritsen, John, The AIDS War. Propaganda, Profeteering and Genocide from the Medical-Industrial Complex, Asklepios, 1993, p. 110

574 see www.allaboutpoppers.com

575 see www.bearcityweb.com

576 Epstein, Steven, Impure Science – AIDS, Activism and the Politics of Knowledge, University of California Press, 1996, p. 23

577 Shilts, Randy, And the Band Played on, Penguin Books, 1987, p. 83

578 Etheridge, Elizabeth, Sentinel for Health: History of the Centers for Disease Control, University of California Press, 1992, p. 326

579 Tracey, Michael, Mere Smoke of Opinion; AIDS and the making of the public mind, *Continuum*, Summer/Fall 2001

580 Haverkos, Harry, Disease Manifestation among Homosexual Men with Acquired Immunodeficiency Syndrome: A Possible Role of Nitrites in Kaposi's Sarcoma, *Sexually Transmitted Diseases*, October-December 1985, pp. 203-208

581 Krieger, Terry; Caceres, Cesar; The unnoticed Link in AIDS cases, *Wall Street Journal*, 24 October 1985

582 Tom Bethell, AIDS and Poppers, *Spin*, November 1994

583 Engelbrecht, Torsten, Sex, Blut und Tod, „HIV verursacht AIDS." An der Verfestigung dieses Theorems lässt sich zeigen, wie der Wissenschafts-Journalismus folgenreiche Widersprüche ausblendet und Zweifel wegdrückt, *Message*, 1/2005, pp. 39-40

584 Halter, Hans, Eine Epidemie, die erst beginnt, *Der Spiegel*, 23/1983

585 Engelbrecht, Torsten, Sex, Blut und Tod, „HIV verursacht AIDS." An der Verfestigung dieses Theorems lässt sich zeigen, wie der Wissenschafts-Journalismus folgenreiche Widersprüche ausblendet und Zweifel wegdrückt, *Message*, 1/2005, p. 40

586 Shilts, Randy, And the Band Played on, Penguin Books, 1987, p. 81

587 Köhnlein, Claus, Das neue "Super-AIDS". Hysterie mit neuen Untertönen: Die Meinstream-Medien entdecken ganz nebenbei die „Co-Faktoren," *Eigentümlich Frei*, March 2005, p. 14

588 McMillan, Dennis, SF Responds To Media Hysteria About "Super-HIV", *San Francisco Bay Times*, 24 February 2005

589 Graham, Judith, Meth use adds to ravages of AIDS. The powerful, highly addictive drug is growing more popular among gays, and experts believe it's undermining efforts to promote safe sex, *Chicago Tribune*, 13 March 2005

590 Duesberg, Peter; Koehnlein, Claus; Rasnick, David, The Chemical Bases of the Various AIDS Epidemics: Recre-

ational Drugs, Anti-viral Chemotherapy and Malnutrition, *Journal of Biosciences*, June 2003, pp. 383-385

591 Cohen, Jon, Experts Question Danger of "AIDS Superbug", *Science*, 25 February 2005, p. 1185

592 Engelbrecht, Torsten, Sex and Drugs and Risk, interview with Jacques Normand, Director AIDS Research at the US National Institute on Drug Abuse, on New York's "Super AIDS Virus", and the link between highly toxic drugs like Poppers or Crystal Meth and AIDS, *Freitag*, 8 April 2005, p. 18

593 Lauritsen, John, The Poppers-Kaposi's Sarcoma Connection, *New York Native*, 13 June 1994

594 Jaffe, Harold, Kaposi's sarcoma among persons with AIDS: a sexually transmitted infection?, *Lancet*, 20 January 1990, pp. 123-128

595 Bittorf, Wilhelm, Die Lust ist da, aber ich verkneif's mir, *Der Spiegel*, 11/1987

596 Papadopulos-Eleopulos, Eleni; Turner, Valendar, A critique of the Montagnier evidence for the HIV/AIDS hypothesis, *Medical Hypotheses*, 4/2004, p. 598

597 Papadopulos-Eleopulos, Eleni; Turner, Valendar, Oxidative Stress, HIV and AIDS, *Research in Immunology*, February 1992, pp. 145-148

598 Beral, Valerie, Kaposi's sarcoma among persons with AIDS: a sexually transmitted infection? *Lancet*, 20 January 1990, pp. 123-128

599 Nancy Franklin, America, lost and found, *The New Yorker, 8 December 2003*

600 Engelbrecht, Torsten, Sex, Blut und Tod, „HIV verursacht AIDS." An der Verfestigung dieses Theorems lässt sich zeigen, wie der Wissenschafts-Journalismus folgenreiche Widersprüche ausblendet und Zweifel wegdrückt, *Message*, 1/2005, pp. 36-47

601 Duesberg, Peter, Inventing the AIDS Virus, Regnery Publishing, 1996, pp. 151-152

602 Fiala, Christian, Lieben wir gefährlich? Ein Arzt auf der Suche nach Fakten und Hintergründen von AIDS, Deuticke, 1997, p. 111

603 Die Bombe ist gelegt, *Der Spiegel* 45/1984

604 „Die Promiskuität ist der Motor der Seuche", *Der Spiegel*, 33/1985

605 Halter, Hans, Eine Epidemie, die erst beginnt, *Der Spiegel*, 23/1983

606 Noack, Hans-Joachim, „Plötzlich stirbst Du ein Stück weit", *Der Spiegel*, 5/1985

607 Bittorf, Wilhelm, Die Lust ist da, aber ich verkneif's mir, *Der Spiegel*, 11/1987

608 Schille, Peter, „Vergnügt euch, aber seht euch vor", Der Spiegel 44/1985

609 Bittorf, Wilhelm, Die Lust ist da, aber ich verkneif's mir, *Der Spiegel*, 11/1987

610 „Die Promiskuität ist der Motor der Seuche", *Der Spiegel*, 33/1985

611 Wiedemann, Erich, „In Afrika droht eine Apokalypse", *Der Spiegel*, 48/1986

612 Schille, Peter, „Vergnügt euch, aber seht euch vor", *Der Spiegel*, 44/1985

613 HIV and Its Transmission, Centers for Diseases Control and Prevention (CDC), Divisions of HIV/AIDS Prevention

614 Bittorf, Wilhelm, Die Lust ist da, aber ich verkneif's mir, *Der Spiegel*, 11/1987

615 *SPIEGEL*-Leser wissen mehr, *Spiegel*-Website, see media.spiegel.de/internet/media.nsf/0/6d9edf6dad-b75e51c1256ff1004584bc?OpenDocument

616 Mutter Natur verbessert, *Der Spiegel*, 26/1991

617 Grolle, Johann, Siege, aber kein Sieg, *Der Spiegel*, 29/1995

618 „AIDS hat ein neues Gesicht", *Der Spiegel*, 28/1996

619 Grolle, Johann, Sieg über die Seuche?, *Der Spiegel*, 2/1997

620 Hackenbroch, Veronika, „Der Optimismus ist verflogen." Der Virologe, AIDS-Forscher und Leiter des Berliner

Robert Koch Instituts, Reinhard Kurth, über die ersten HIV-Impfstoff-Tests in Deutschland, *Der Spiegel*, 9/2004, p. 153

[621] Tracey, Michael, Mere Smoke of Opinion; AIDS and the making of the public mind, *Continuum*, Summer/Fall 2001

[622] Bittorf, Wilhelm, Die Lust ist da, aber ich verkneif's mir, *Der Spiegel*, 11/1987

[623] Ibid.

[624] Gray, Kevin, Some Realities about HIV/AIDS, *Details*, 13 February 2004

[625] Duesberg, Peter; Koehnlein, Claus; Rasnick, David, The Chemical Bases of the Various AIDS Epidemics: Recreational Drugs, Anti-viral Chemotherapy and Malnutrition, *Journal of Biosciences*, June 2003, p. 391

[626] Facts zu HIV und AIDS, 2. Nationale Dimension, Welt AIDS Tag 2005, see www.welt-AIDS-tag.de/?p=33

[627] Duesberg, Peter; Koehnlein, Claus; Rasnick, David, The Chemical Bases of the Various AIDS Epidemics: Recreational Drugs, Anti-viral Chemotherapy and Malnutrition, *Journal of Biosciences*, June 2003, pp. 383-488

[628] Bartholomäus Grill, Die tödliche Ignoranz, *Die Zeit*, 15 July 2004, p. 1

[629] Gray, Kevin, Some Realities about HIV/AIDS, *Details*, 13 February 2004

[630] Papadopulos-Eleopulos, Eleni; Turner, Valendar, A critique of the Montagnier evidence for the HIV/AIDS hypothesis, *Medical Hypotheses*, 4/2004, p. 598

[631] Kamali, Anatoli, Syndromic management of sexually-transmitted infections and behaviour change interventions on transmission of HIV-1 in rural Uganda: a community randomised trial, *Lancet*, 22 February 2003, pp. 645-652

[632] Gray, Ronald, Probability of HIV-1 transmission per coital act in monogamous, heterosexual, HIV-1-discordant couples in Rakai, Uganda, *Lancet*, 14 April 2001, pp. 1149-53

[633] Padian, Nancy, Heterosexual transmission of human immunodeficiency virus (HIV) in northern California: results from a ten-year study, *American Journal of Epidemiology*, 15 August 1997, pp. 350-57

[634] Tracey, Michael, Mere Smoke of Opinion; AIDS and the making of the public mind, *Continuum*, Summer/Fall 2001

[635] Problems with HIV vaccine research, Wikipedia-Website, see en.wikipedia.org/wiki/HIV_vaccine

[636] Pahwa, Savita, Influence of the human T-lymphotropic virus/lymphadenopathy-associated virus on functions of human lymphocytes: evidence for immunosuppressive effects and polyclonal B-cell activation by Vol.ed viral preparations, in: *Proceedings of the National Academy of Sciences*, December 1985, pp. 8198-8202

[637] Epstein, Steven, Impure Science – AIDS, Activism and the Politics of Knowledge, University of California Press, 1996, p. 73

[638] Ibid., p. 83

[639] Ibid., p. 87

[640] Engelbrecht, Torsten, Spitze des Eisbergs: Warum Journalisten auch den angesehenen Wissenschaftszeitschriften nicht blindlings vertrauen sollten, *Message*, 3/2005, pp. 70-71

[641] Phillips, David, Importance of the lay press in the transmission of medical knowledge to the scientific community, *New England Journal of Medicine*, 17 October 1991, pp. 1180-1183

[642] Kinsella, James, Covering the Plague. AIDS and the American Media, Rutgers University Press, 1989, pp. 88-89

[643] Epstein, Steven, Impure Science – AIDS, Activism and the Politics of Knowledge, University of California Press, 1996, pp. 93-95

[644] Altman, Lawrence, Red Cross Evaluates Test To Detect AIDS In Donated Blood, *New York Times*, 15 May 1984

[645] Altman, Lawrence, The Doctor's World; How AIDS Researchers Strive For Virus Proof, *New York Times*, 24 October 1984

Literature

[646] Epstein, Steven, Impure Science—AIDS, Activism and the Politics of Knowledge, University of California Press, 1996, p. 93

[647] Duesberg, Peter, Inventing the AIDS Virus, Regnery Publishing, 1996, pp. 135-136

[648] Ibid., pp. 144-145

[649] About EIS, Website der Epidemic Intelligence Service, see www.cdc.gov/eis/about/about.htm

[650] Alumni, Website der Epidemic Intelligence Service, see www.cdc.gov/eis/alumni/alumni.htm

[651] Epstein, Steven, Impure Science—AIDS, Activism and the Politics of Knowledge, University of California Press, 1996, p. 72

[652] Koch, Klaus, Ist Europa jetzt vor Seuchen sicher?, Interview mit Hans Wigzell vom Karoliska-Institut in Stockholm, *Süddeutsche Zeitung*, 22 March 2005, p. 10

[653] Duesberg, Peter, Inventing the AIDS Virus, Regnery Publishing, 1996, pp. 135-136

[654] Cohen, Jon, Doing Science in the Spotlight's Glare, *Science*, 1992, Vol. 257, p. 1033

[655] Noelle-Neumann, Elisabeth, Die Schweigespirale: Öffentliche Meinung—unsere soziale Haut, Langen Müller, 2001, p. 322

[656] Epstein, Steven, Impure Science—AIDS, Activism and the Politics of Knowledge, University of California Press, 1996, pp. 105-106

[657] Celia Farber, AIDS: Words from the Front, *Spin*, January 1988, pp. 43-44, 73

[658] Penning, Randolph, Prävalenz der HIV-Infektion bei gerichtlich Obduzierten und speziell Drogentoten am Institut für Rechtsmedizin der Universität München von 1985 bis 1988, *AIDS-Forschung*, 4/1989, pp. 459–465

[659] Booth, William, A Rebel without a cause of AIDS, *Science*, 25 March 1988, p. 1485

[660] Epstein, Steven, Impure Science—AIDS, Activism and the Politics of Knowledge, University of California Press, 1996, p. 113

[661] see www.virusmyth.net/AIDS/index/cthomas.htm

[662] Hodgkinson, Neville, AIDS: Can We Be Positive?, *Sunday Times* (London), 26 April 1992

[663] Duesberg, Peter, Inventing the AIDS Virus, Regnery Publishing, 1996, p. 244

[664] Rapoport, Ron, AIDS: The Unanswered Questions, *Oakland Tribune*, 22 May 1989, pp. A1-A2

[665] Duesberg, Peter, Inventing the AIDS Virus, Regnery Publishing, 1996, p. 237

[666] Boffey, Phillip, A Solitary Dissenter Disputes Cause of AIDS, *New York Times*, 12 January 1988, p. C-3

[667] France, David, The HIV Disbelievers, *Newsweek*, 19 August 2000

[668] „Filtern und zensieren," Interview with John Maddox, *Der Spiegel*, 7 November 1994, p. 229

[669] Letter from John Maddox to Claus Köhnlein, 20 September 1995

[670] Ho, David, Rapid turnover of plasma virions and CD4 lymphocytes in HIV-1 infection, *Nature*, 12 January 1995, pp. 123-126

[671] Craddock, Mark, HIV: Science by press conference, in: AIDS: Virus- or Drug Induced? by Peter Duesberg (Ed.), Kluwer Academic Publishers, 1996, pp. 127-130

[672] Tahi, Djamel, AIDS—die großen Zweifel, Arte Television, 14 March 1996, see www.torstenengelbrecht.com/de/artikel_medien.html

[673] Langbein, Kurt; Ehgartner, Bert, Das Medizinkartell: Die sieben Todsünden der Gesundheitsindustrie, Piper, 2003, p. 347

[674] Wolthers, Katja, T Cell Telomere Length in HIV-1 Infection: No Evidence for increased CD4+ T Cell Turnover, *Science*, 29 November 1996, pp. 1543-1547

[675] Engelbrecht, Torsten, Sex, Blut und Tod, „HIV verursacht AIDS." An der Verfestigung dieses Theorems lässt sich zeigen, wie der Wissenschafts-Journalismus folgenreiche Widersprüche ausblendet und Zweifel wegdrückt, *Message*, 1/2005, pp. 41-42

[676] Cimons, Marlene, Bad Blood Two Groups of AIDS Researchers – One American, One French – Are Fighting More Than Just the Disease, *Los Angeles Times*, 25 May 1986, p. 16

[677] Remnick, David, Robert Gallo Goes To War, *Washington Post*, 9 August 1987, W 10

[678] Der lang erwartete Messias, *tageszeitung*, 24 December 1996, p. 11

[679] Hoffmann, Christian, ART 2004. Historie, see hiv.net/2010/haart.htm

[680] Chua-Eoan, Howard, 1996: David Ho, *TIME*, 30 December 1996

[681] Lawrence, Altman, US Panel seeks Changes in Treatment of AIDS Virus, *New York Times*, 4 February, 2001

[682] Berndt, Christina, Da-I, der Große, hat sich geirrt, *Süddeutsche Zeitung*, 27 January 2004

[683] Grolle, Johann, Sieg über die Seuche?, *Der Spiegel*, 2/1997

[684] Connolly, Ceci, States Offering Less Assistance For AIDS Drugs, *Washington Post*, 20 May 2004, p. A04

[685] Personal phone interview with Hans Halter

[686] Prange, Astrid, Hoffnung kostet 140 Dollar, *Rheinischer Merkur*, 48/2005, p. 14

[687] AIDS ist behandelbar, *Schleswig-Holsteinisches Ärzteblatt*, 2/2000, pp. 14-15

[688] AIDS Drugs extend Survival Times Fourfold, *Reuters NewMedia*, 14 March 2001

[689] Köhnlein, Claus, Die große Illusion. Das Dilemma der antiretroviralen Therapie/HAART aus einem kritischen Blickwinkel, see www.rethinkingaids.de/allg/koenl-2.htm

[690] Duesberg, Peter, Inventing the AIDS Virus, Regnery Publishing, 1996, p. 425

[691] Duesberg, Peter; Koehnlein, Claus; Rasnick, David, The Chemical Bases of the Various AIDS Epidemics: Recreational Drugs, Anti-viral Chemotherapy and Malnutrition, *Journal of Biosciences*, June 2003, p. 402

[692] Coghlan, Andy, Bid to solve riddle of 'natural resistance' to HIV, *New Scientist*, 15 August 2006

[693] Duesberg, Peter, Inventing the AIDS Virus, Regnery Publishing, 1996, p. 425

[694] Köhnlein, Claus, Die große Illusion. Das Dilemma der antiretroviralen Therapie/HAART aus einem kritischen Blickwinkel, see www.rethinkingaids.de/allg/koenl-2.htm

[695] HIV/AIDS-files, Robert Koch-Institute, June 2003

[696] Fleming, Thomas; DeMets, David, Surrogate end points in clinical trials: are we being misled?, *Annals of Internal Medicine*, 1 October 1996, pp. 605-613

[697] Revision Of The Surveillance Case Definition For AIDS In Canada, in: Canada Communicable Disease Report, Health and Welfare Canada, 15 December 1993, p. 196

[698] Koliadin, Vladimir, Some Facts behind de Expansion of the Definition of AIDS in 1993, March 1998; see www.virusmyth.net/aids/data/vknewdef.htm

[699] CASCADE (Concerted Action on SeroConversion to AIDS and Death in Europe) Collaboration, Determinants of survival following HIV-1 seroconversion after the introduction of HAART, *Lancet*, 18 October 2003, pp. 1267-1274

[700] Suspension of Disbelief??, Health Education AIDS Liaison (HEAL), Toronto, http://healtoronto.com/aidsdrop.html

[701] HIV treatment response and prognosis in Europe and North America in the first decade of highly active antiretroviral therapy: a collaborative analysis, Lancet, 5 August 2006, pp. 451-458

[702] New Studies Shake AIDS World ... and more interesting news from Alive & Well, news release from Christine Maggiore/Alive & Well, 30 November 2006

[703] Fischl, Margaret, The toxicity of azidothymidine (AZT) in the treatment of patients with AIDS and AIDS-related

complex. A double-blind, placebo-controlled trial, *New England Journal of Medicine*, 23 July 1987, pp. 192-197

[704] Law, Jacky, Big Pharma. How the world's biggest drug companies market illness, Constable & Robinson, 2006

[705] The fool's gold that heals, *Guardian*, 14 January 2006

[706] Temple, Robert, Placebo-Controlled Trials and Active-Control Trials in the Evaluation of New Treatments. Part 1: Ethical and Scientific Issues, *Annals of Internal Medicine*, 19 September 2000, pp. 455-463

[707] Ellenberg, Susan, Placebo-Controlled Trials and Active-Control Trials in the Evaluation of New Treatments. Part 2: Practical Issues and Specific Cases, *Annuals of Internal Medicine*, 19 September 2000, pp. 464-470

[708] Evans, David; Smith, Mike; Willen, Liz, Drug Industry Human Testing Masks Death, Injury, Compliant FDA, Bloomberg.com, 2 November 2005

[709] Sharav, Vera, New Evidence Uncovered About AIDS Drug/Vaccine Experiments on Foster Care Infants & Children, Alliance for Human Research Protection, 1 September 2005

[710] Scheff, Liam, The House that AIDS built, see www.altheal.org/toxicity/house.htm

[711] Montero, Douglas, AIDS Tots Used As 'Guinea Pigs', *New York Post*, 29 February 2004, p. 1

[712] Doran, Jamie, Guinea Pig Kids, 30 November 2004

[713] Solomon, John, Feds: Some AIDS Drug Tests Violated Rules, Associated Press, 16 June 2005

[714] Scott, Janny, Kaufman, Leslie, Belated Charge Ignites Furor Over AIDS Drug Trial, *New York Times*, 17 July 2005

[715] E-mail an Janny Scott und Leslie Kaufman, 17 July 2005

[716] Lewis, Linda, Lamivudine in children with human immunodeficiency virus infection: a phase I/II study, *Journal of Infectious Diseases*, July 1996, pp. 16-25

[717] Brown, Hannah, Marvellous microbicides, *Lancet*, 27 March 2003, pp. 1042-1043

[718] AIDS Chief says nonoxynol-9 not effective against HIV, July 2000, *AIDS Weekly*, pp. 2-3

[719] Brown, Hannah, Marvellous microbicides, *Lancet*, 27 March 2003, p. 1042

[720] Angell, Marcia, The Truth About the Drug Companies. How They Deceive Us And What To Do About It, Random House, 2004, p. 241

[721] Lauritsen, John, The AIDS War. Propaganda, Profeteering and Genocide from the Medical-Industrial Complex, Asklepios, 1993, pp. 381-397

[722] Müller, Roger, Skepsis gegenüber einem Medikament [AZT], das krank macht, *Weltwoche*, 25 June 1992, pp. 55-56

[723] John Lauritsen, The AIDS War. Propaganda, Profeteering and Genocide from the Medical-Industrial Complex, Asklepios, 1993, p. 73

[724] Personal e-mail communication with the *Neue Zürcher Zeitung*, 27 July 2004

[725] Köhnlein, Claus, Die große Illusion. Das Dilemma der antiretroviralen Therapie/HAART aus einem kritischen Blickwinkel, see www.rethinkingaids.de/allg/koenl-2.htm

[726] $95 billion a year spent on medical research, Associated Press, 20 September 2005

[727] Larisch, Katharina, Vioxx®-Rückzug, Netdoktor.de, 8 November 2004

[728] John Lauritsen, The AIDS War. Propaganda, Profeteering and Genocide from the Medical-Industrial Complex, Asklepios, 1993, pp. 140-141

[729] Ibid., p. 391

[730] Ibid., pp. 381-397

[731] Duesberg, Peter, HIV, AIDS, and zidovudine, *Lancet*, 28 March 1992, pp. 805-806

[732] John Lauritsen, The AIDS War. Propaganda, Profeteering and Genocide from the Medical-Industrial Complex, Asklepios, 1993, p. 74

[733] Ibid.

[734] Epstein, Steven, Impure Science – AIDS, Activism and the Politics of Knowledge, University of California Press, 1996, pp. 109, 119

[735] John Lauritsen, The AIDS War. Propaganda, Profeteering and Genocide from the Medical-Industrial Complex, Asklepios, 1993, pp. 59-69

[736] Personal interview, 25 January 2006

[737] E-mails to the NIAID on August 24 and 27, 2020

[738] Lauritsen, John, The AIDS War. Propaganda, Profeteering and Genocide from the Medical-Industrial Complex Asklepios, 1993, pp. 71-79

[739] Idrus, Amirah Al, Biotech: Gilead's remdesivir speeds COVID-19 recovery in first controlled trial readout, but it's no 'silver bullet'. www.fiercebiotech.com, 29 April 2020

[740] Epstein, Steven, Impure Science – AIDS, Activism and the Politics of Knowledge, University of California Press, 1996, p. 123

[741] Questionnaires sent out by e-mail in July 2004

[742] E-mail to Declan Butler, 19 December 2005

[743] Butler, Declan, Medical journal under attack as dissenters seize AIDS platform, Nature, 20 November 2003, p. 215

[744] Personal e-mail communication with John Moore, 16 February 2004

[745] Judson, Horace, The Great Betrayal. Fraud in Science, Harcourt, 2004, p. 6

[746] Cohen, Sheila, Antiretroviral therapy for AIDS, New England Journal of Medicine, 3 September 1987, pp. 629-630

[747] Bruce Nussbaum, Good Intentions: How Big Business and the Medical Establishment are Corrupting the Fight against AIDS, Alzheimer's, Cancer, and More, Penguin Books, 1990, pp. 177-178

[748] Duesberg, Peter, The toxicity of azidothymidine (AZT) on human and animal cells in culture at concentrations used for antiviral therapy, Genetica, 1-3/1995, pp. 103-109

[749] See website of Treatment Information Group: www.tig.org.za

[750] Kolata, Gina, Marrow suppression hampers AZT use in AIDS victims, Science, 20 March 1987, p. 1463

[751] Payne, Brendan A. I. et al., Mitochondrial aging is accelerated by anti-retroviral therapy through the clonal expansion of mtDNA mutations, Nature Genetics, 26 June 2011, pp. 806-810

[752] Buchholz, Bernd et al., HIV-Therapie in der Schwangerschaft Optimierung der Transmissionsverhinderung bei Minimierung unerwünschter Arzneimittelwirkungen, Deutsches Ärzteblatt, 14 June 2002, pp. A1674-A1683

[753] Prestes-Carneir, Luiz Euribel, Antiretroviral therapy, pregnancy, and birth defects: a discussion on the updated data, HIV AIDS (Auckland/New Zealand), 1 August 2013, pp. 181-189

[754] Goethe, Johann Wolfgang, Faust, 1. Teil, Insel, 1976, p. 51

[755] Freddie Mercury, Wikipedia-Website, see de.wikipedia.org/wiki/Freddie_Mercury

[756] John Lauritsen, The AIDS War. Propaganda, Profeteering and Genocide from the Medical-Industrial Complex, Asklepios, 1993, pp. 445-450

[757] Duesberg, Peter, Inventing the AIDS Virus, Regnery Publishing, 1996, pp. 356-358

[758] Ashe, Arthur, More Than Ever, Magical Things to Learn, Washington Post, 11 October 1992

[759] Duesberg, Peter, Inventing the AIDS Virus, Regnery Publishing, 1996, p. 357

[760] Iyer, Pico, "It Can Happen to Anybody. Even Magic Johnson." After testing positive for HIV, basketball's most beloved star retires and vows to become a spokesman in the battle against AIDS, TIME, 18 November 1991

[761] Elmer-Dewitt, Philip, How Safe Is Sex? When Magic Johnson announced he had the AIDS virus, he put the risk

of heterosexual transmission squarely in center court, *TIME*, 25 November 1991

762 Duesberg, Peter, Inventing the AIDS Virus, Regnery Publishing, 1996, p. 340

763 Nelson, J., Magic Reeling as Worst Nightmare Comes True—He's Getting Sicker, *National Enquirer*, 10 December 1991, p. 6

764 Iyer, Pico, "It Can Happen to Anybody. Even Magic Johnson." After testing positive for HIV, basketball's most beloved star retires and vows to become a spokesman in the battle against AIDS, *TIME*, 18 November 1991

765 Duesberg, Peter, Inventing the AIDS Virus, Regnery Publishing, 1996, p. 341

766 Duesberg, Peter, Inventing the AIDS Virus, Regnery Publishing, 1996, pp. 340-341

767 Polier, Alex, Ads are geared toward urban blacks, Associated Press, 21 January 2003

768 Darby, Sarah, Mortality before and after HIV infection in the complete UK population of haemophiliacs. UK Haemophilia Centre Directors' Organisation, *Nature*, 7 September 1995, pp. 79-82

769 Duesberg, Peter; Koehnlein, Claus; Rasnick, David, The Chemical Bases of the Various AIDS Epidemics: Recreational Drugs, Anti-viral Chemotherapy and Malnutrition, *Journal of Biosciences*, June 2003, pp. 396-398

770 Lang, Serge, Challenges, Springer, 1998, p. 687

771 Papdopulos-Eleopulos, Eleni; Turner, Valendar, HIV Seropositivity and Mortality in Persons with Heamophilia; Proof that HIV Causes AIDS?, see www.virusmyth.net/aids/data/epdarby.htm

772 Philpot, Paul. Darby Debunked: Pro-HIV hemophiliac study actually points towards non-contagious AIDS, re-thinkingaids.com, February 1996

773 Maddox, John, More Conviction on HIV and AIDS, *Nature*, 7 September 1995, Sep 7; p. 1

774 „Die Promiskuität ist der Motor der Seuche", *Der Spiegel*, 33/1985

775 Duesberg, Peter, Inventing the AIDS Virus, Regnery Publishing, 1996, pp. 445-451

776 HIV and Its Transmission, Centers for Diseases Control and Prevention (CDC), Divisions of HIV/AIDS Prevention, see www.cdc.gov/hiv/resources/factsheets/transmission.htm

777 Duesberg, Peter; Koehnlein, Claus; Rasnick, David, The Chemical Bases of the Various AIDS Epidemics: Recreational Drugs, Anti-viral Chemotherapy and Malnutrition, *Journal of Biosciences*, June 2003, p. 391

778 Rian Malan: Africa isn't dying of AIDS, The Spectator, 13 December 2003

779 Duesberg, Peter; Koehnlein, Claus; Rasnick, David, The Chemical Bases of the Various AIDS Epidemics: Recreational Drugs, Anti-viral Chemotherapy and Malnutrition, *Journal of Biosciences*, June 2003, p. 385

780 Thielke, Thilo, "Streicht diese Hilfe". Der kenianische Wirtschaftsexperte James Shikwati über die schädlichen Folgen der westlichen Entwicklungshilfe, korrupte Herrscher und aufgebauschte Horrormeldungen aus Afrika, *Der Spiegel*, 27/2005

781 Essex, Max; Kashala, Oscar, Infection with human immonodificiency virus type 1 (hiv-1) and human t-cell lymphotropic viruses among leprosy patients and contacts: correlation between hiv-1 cross-reactivity and antibodies to lipoarabinomanna; *Journal of Infectious Diseases*, February 1994, pp. 296-304

782 Tahi, Djamel, AIDS—The Doubt, Arte Television, 14 March 1996, see www.torstenengelbrecht.com/de/artikel_medien.html

783 Shenton, Joan, Positively False: Exposing the Myths Around HIV and AIDS, I.B. Tauris/St. Martin's Press, 1998

784 Lang, Serge, Challenges; Springer, New York, 1998, pp. 616-617

785 Geshekter, Charles; Mhlongo, Sam; Köhnlein, Claus, AIDS, Medicine and Public Health: The Scientific Value of Thabo Mbeki's Critique of AIDS Orthodoxy, Vortrag auf dem 47th Annual Meeting of the African Studies Association New Orleans, Louisiana, 11 November 2004

786 Duesberg, Peter; Koehnlein, Claus; Rasnick, David, The Chemical Bases of the Various AIDS Epidemics: Recreational Drugs, Anti-viral Chemotherapy and Malnutrition, *Journal of Biosciences*, June 2003, pp. 385-386

787 Katzenellenbogen, Jonathan, Third of Africans Undernourished, *Business Day* (Johannesburg), 20 August 2004

788 Fenton, Lynda, Preventing HIV/AIDS through poverty reduction: the only sustainable solution?, *Lancet*, 2004, 25 September 2004, pp. 1186-1187

Chapter 4
Hepatitis C: Toxins Such As Alcohol, Heroin, and Medical Drugs Suffice As Explanation

789 Köhnlein, Claus, Hepatitis C – the epidemic that never was?, *British Medical Journal* (online), 7 March 2002, see bmj.bmjjournals.com/cgi/eletters/324/7335/450

790 Larkin, Marylinn, Jay Hoofnagle: soldiering on against viral hepatitis, *Lancet*, 27 September 1997, p. 938

791 Intron-A, Rote Liste, 2005, p. 51025

792 Welche Nebenwirkungen haben Interferone?, Website of the Krebsinformationsdienst of the Deutsches Krebsforschungszentrum DKFZ (German Cancer Research Centre) in Heidelberg

793 Erstmals Vermehrung des Hepatitis C Virus im Labor möglich, press release of the Ruprechts-Karl-University in Heidelberg, 6 October 2004

794 Larkin, Marylinn, Jay Hoofnagle: soldiering on against viral hepatitis, *Lancet*, 27 September 1997, p. 938

795 Alter, Harvey, Transmissible agent in non-A, non-B hepatitis, *Lancet*, 4 March 1978, pp. 459-463

796 Houghton, Michael; Bradley, Daniel, Hepatitis C virus: the major causative agent of viral non-A, non-B hepatitis, *British Medical Bulletin*, April 1990, pp. 423-441

797 Chiron Advances Hepatitis C Vaccine Development Program, press release, Chiron Vaccines, 14 January 2004

798 Duesberg, Peter, Inventing the AIDS Virus, Regnery Publishing, 1996, p. 84

799 Köhnlein, Claus, Hepatitis C – the epidemic that never was?, *British Medical Journal* (online), 7 March 2002, see bmj.bmjjournals.com/cgi/eletters/324/7335/450

800 Chiron Reports First-Quarter 2005 Pro-Forma Earnings of 4 Cents Per Share, GAAP Loss of 5 Cents Per Share, press release of the Chiron Corporation, 27 April 2005

801 Duesberg, Peter, Inventing the AIDS Virus, Regnery Publishing, 1996, p. 84

802 Crowe, David, The ABCs of Hepatitis, *Alive Magazine*, May 2004

803 Chen, Zheng, Hepatitis C virus (HCV) specific sequences are demonstrable in the DNA fraction of peripheral blood mononuclear cells from healthy, anti-HCV antibody-negative individuals and cell lines of human origin, *European Journal of Clinical Chemistry and Clinical Biochemistry*, December 1997, pp. 899-905

804 Duesberg, Peter, Inventing the AIDS Virus, Regnery Publishing, 1996, pp. 84-85

805 Relman, David A.; Fredericks, David N., Sequence-Based Identification of Microbial Pathogens: a Reconsideration of Koch's Postulates, *Clinical Microbiology Reviews*, January 1996, p. 18-33

806 Syringe Exchange Programs, CDC's Website

807 Hagan, Holly, Syringe exchange and risk of infection with hepatitis B and C viruses, *American Journal of Epidemiology*, 1 February 1999, pp. 203-213

808 Crowe, David, The ABCs of Hepatitis, *Alive Magazine*, May 2004

809 Thomas, David, The natural history of hepatitis C virus infection: host, viral, and environmental factors, *Journal*

of the American Medical Association, 26 July 2000, p. 450

810 Hoofnagle, Jay, Hepatic Failure and Lactic Acidosis Due to Fialuridine (FIAU), an Investigational Nucleoside Analogue for Chronic Hepatitis B, New England Journal of Medicine, 26 October 1995, pp. 1099-105

811 Castillo, Inmaculada, Occult hepatitis C virus infection in patients in whom the etiology of persistently abnormal results of liver-function tests is unknown, Journal of Infectious Diseases, 1 January 2004, pp. 7-14

812 Thomas, David, The natural history of hepatitis C virus infection: host, viral, and environmental factors, Journal of the American Medical Association, 26 July 2000, p. 450

813 Köhnlein, Claus, Virale Seuchen, die es gar nicht gibt. BSE/AIDS/Hepatitis C, Raum & Zeit, 111/2001, p. 23

814 Laufs, Rainer, Was bedeutet der Befund „HCV-Antikörper positiv"?, Deutsches Ärzteblatt, 4 February 1994, p. A286

815 Siegmund-Schultze, Nicola, Die stille Seuche. 500.000 Deutsche sind mit Hepatitis C infiziert— nun werden die Aussichten auf einen Impfstoff besser, Süddeutsche Zeitung, 13 October 2004, p. 10

816 Laufs, Rainer, Was bedeutet der Befund „HCV-Antikörper positiv"?, Deutsches Ärzteblatt, 4 February 1994, p. A287

817 Hadziyannis, Stephanos, Interferon alpha therapy in HBeAg-negative chronic hepatitis B: new data in support of long-term efficacy, Journal of Hepatology, February 2002, pp. 280-282

818 Comment by the Deutsche Leberhilfe e.V. (German Liver Aid) to our book „Virus Mania", published on the Amazon.de website on 16 June 2006, see www.amazon.de/gp/product/customer-reviews/3891891474/ref=cm_cr_dp_2_1/303-3787228-9015431?ie=UTF8&customer-reviews.sort%5Fby=-SubmissionDate&n=299956

819 Comment from the authors of this book to the comment by the Deutsche Leberhilfe e.V. (German Liver Aid) to this book, published on the website of Torsten Engelbrecht on 4 July, 2006, see www.torstenengelbrecht.com/de/buch_viruswahn.html

820 Seeff, Leonard, 45-year follow-up of hepatitis C virus infection in healthy young adults, Annals of Internal Medicine, January 2000, pp. 105-11

821 Schentke, Klaus-Ulrich, Leberschäden durch Medikamente, Deutsche Medizinische Wochenschrift, 1995, Vol. 120, pp. 923-925

822 Personal e-mail communication, December 2005

823 See www.drruhland.com

824 V.I.P. Anderson Has Liver Disease, people.com, 21 March 2002

825 Pamela Anderson expects death in a decade, CNN.com, 22 October 2003

Chapter 5
BSE: The Epidemic that Never Was

826 Scholz, Roland, Phantom BSE-Gefahr. Irrwege von Wissenschaft und Politik im BSE-Skandal, Berenkamp, 2005

827 Riebsamen, Hans, BSE ist vergessen: Rare, medium oder well-done?, Frankfurter Allgemeine Sonntagszeitung, 17 November 2002, p. 6

828 Entwarnung: Creutzfeldt-Jakob-Krankheit fällt aus, Manager Magazin (online), 12 January 2005

829 Venters, George, New variant Creutzfeldt-Jakob disease: the epidemic that never was, British Medical Journal, 13 October 2001, pp. 858-861

830 Ghani, Azra, Projections of the future course of the primary vCJD epidemic in the UK: inclusion of subclinical infection and the possibility of wider genetic susceptibility, Journal of the Royal Society Interface, 22 March 2005, pp. 19-31

[831] Riebsamen, Hans, BSE ist vergessen: Rare, medium oder well-done?, *Frankfurter Allgemeine Sonntagszeitung*, 17 November 2002, p. 6

[832] New Generation BSE test approved by CFIA, press release, Prionics AG, 16 June 2005

[833] O'Brien, Jennifer, Prion finding offers insight into spontaneous protein diseases, News Release, University of California, San Francisco (UCSF), 29 July 2004, see pub.ucsf.edu/newsservices/releases/200407274?print

[834] Mayr, Anton, BSE und Creutzfeldt-Jakob-Krankheit (CJD): Falsche Begriffe und falsche Assoziationen, *Journal Med*, 57/2001, p. 6

[835] Scholz, Roland, Überlegungen zur Genese der bovinen spongiformen Encephalopathie (BSE), Biolab-Website, see www.biolab-muenchen.de/index.html?rightframe=http://www.biolab-muenchen.de/bse/scholz01.htm

[836] Parry, Herbert, Scrapie: a transmissible and hereditary disease of sheep, *Heredity*, February 1962, pp. 75-105

[837] Koch, Klaus, Nobelpreis für Prionenforschung: Eine gewagte These wird geadelt, *Deutsches Ärzteblatt*, 17 October 1997

[838] Scholz, Roland, Phantom BSE-Gefahr. Irrwege von Wissenschaft und Politik im BSE-Skandal, Berenkamp, 2005, pp. 11-12

[839] Deutschland im BSE-Schock. In Großbritannien hat man seit Jahren Erfahrung. Was weiß man definitiv, woher kommt BSE?, interview with *Zeit*-correspondent Jürgen Krönig, SWR 2, 27 November 2000

[840] Deutschland im BSE-Schock. In Großbritannien hat man seit Jahren Erfahrung. Was weiß man definitiv, woher kommt BSE?, interview with *Zeit*-correspondent Jürgen Krönig, SWR 2, 27 November 2000

[841] Prusiner, Stanley, Frühtests auf Rinderwahn, *Spektrum der Wissenschaft*, February 2005, pp. 62-69

[842] Ebringer, Alan, Bovine spongiform encephalopathy (BSE): Comparison between the "prion" hypothesis and the autoimmune theory, *Journal of Nutritional & Environmental Medicine*, 8/1998, pp. 265-276

[843] Ebringer, Alan, BSE as an autoimmune disease, *Immunology News*, 1997, Vol. 4, pp. 149-150

[844] Scholz, Roland, Phantom BSE-Gefahr. Irrwege von Wissenschaft und Politik im BSE-Skandal, Berenkamp, 2005, p. 153

[845] Legname, Giuseppe, Synthetic Mammalian Prions, *Science*, 30 July 2004, pp. 673-676

[846] Aguzzi, Adrioano, vCJD tissue distribution and transmission by transfusion – a worst-case scenario coming true?, *Lancet*, 7 February 2004, p. 411

[847] Scholz, Roland, Phantom BSE-Gefahr. Irrwege von Wissenschaft und Politik im BSE-Skandal, Berenkamp, 2005, pp. 12-13

[848] Scholz, Roland, 25 Thesen gegen die Behauptung, BSE und vCJK seien oral übertragbare Infektionskrankheiten und BSE gefährdet die menschliche Gesundheit, *Deutsche Medizinische Wochenschrift*, 15 February 2002, pp. 341-342

[849] Raine, Cedric, Chronic experimental allergic encephalomyelitis in inbred guinea pigs. An ultrastructural study, *Laboratory Investigation*, October 1974, pp. 369-380

[850] Scholz, Roland, 25 Thesen gegen die Behauptung, BSE und vCJK seien oral übertragbare Infektionskrankheiten und BSE gefährdet die menschliche Gesundheit, *Deutsche Medizinische Wochenschrift*, 15 February 2002, p. 341

[851] Scholz, Roland, Überlegungen zur Genese der bovinen spongiformen Encephalopathie (BSE), Biolab-Website, see www.biolab-muenchen.de/index.html?rightframe=http://www.biolab-muenchen.de/bse/scholz01.htm

[852] Prusiner, Stanley, Novel proteinaceous infectious particles cause scrapie, *Science*, 9 April 1982, pp. 136-144

[853] Scholz, Roland, Phantom BSE-Gefahr. Irrwege von Wissenschaft und Politik im BSE-Skandal, Berenkamp, 2005, pp. 27-28

[854] Poser, Sigrid, Die neue Variante der Creutzfeldt-Jakob-Krankheit, *Deutsche Medizinische Wochenschrift*, 15 Feb-

ruary 2002, p. 333

[855]   Anderson, Robert, Transmission dynamics and epidemiology of BSE in British cattle, *Nature*, 29 August 1996, p. 781

[856]   Köhnlein, Claus, BSE (Leserbrief zum Artikel von Sucharit Bhakdi: Prionen und der „BSE-Wahnsinn": Eine kritische Bestandsaufnahme), *Deutsches Ärzteblatt*, 13 September 2002, p. A2404

[857]   Köhnlein, Claus, Virale Seuchen, die es gar nicht gibt. BSE/AIDS/Hepatitis C, *Raum & Zeit*, 111/2001, pp. 23-24

[858]   Köhnlein, Claus, Virale Seuchen, die es gar nicht gibt. BSE/AIDS/Hepatitis C, *Raum & Zeit*, 111/2001, p. 24

[859]   Wucher, Petra; Ehlers, Hans-Joachim, BSE: Ein Pharma-Unfall?, *Raum & Zeit*, 84/1996, p. 90

[860]   Lüllmann, Heinz, Pharmakologie und Toxikologie, Thieme, 2003, p. 504

[861]   Jetzt wird das Pestizid als BSE-Auslöser diskutiert, *Ärzte Zeitung*, 15 April 1998

[862]   Whatley, Stephen, Phosmet induces up-regulation of surface levels of the cellular prion protein, *Neuroreport*, 11 May 1998, pp. 1391-1395

[863]   Personal interview, 8 February 2006

[864]   Köhnlein, Claus, Virale Seuchen, die es gar nicht gibt. BSE/AIDS/Hepatitis C, *Raum & Zeit*, 111/2001, pp. 24-25

[865]   Purdey, Mark, Ecosystems supporting clusters of sporadic TSEs demonstrate excesses of the radical-generating divalent cation manganese and deficiencies of antioxidant co-factors Cu, Se, Fe, Zn, *Medical Hypotheses*, 2/2002, pp. 278-306

[866]   Scholz, Roland, Phantom BSE-Gefahr. Irrwege von Wissenschaft und Politik im BSE-Skandal, Berenkamp, 2005, pp. 38-40

[867]   Bergmann, Werner; Beringer, Helmut, Kupfermangel. Ein möglicher BSE-auslösender Faktor?, *Journal of Plant Nutrition and Soil Science*, April 2001, pp. 233-235

[868]   Scholz, Roland, Phantom BSE-Gefahr. Irrwege von Wissenschaft und Politik im BSE-Skandal, Berenkamp, 2005

Chapter 6
SARS: Hysteria on the Heels of AIDS and BSE

[869]   Watzlawick, Paul, Wie wirklich ist die Wirklichkeit? Wahn, Täuschung, Verstehen, Piper, 2005, pp. 66-67

[870]   Schuh, Hans, Unheimliche Keime. Die Lungenkrankheit SARS infiziert Mensch und Börse, ist aber nur selten tödlich, *Die Zeit*, 15/2003

[871]   Nagy, Ursula, SARS in der Provinz—das Beispiel Ningbo, *China Fokus*, 28 May 2003

[872]   China 'laundering money' over SARS fears, *breakingnews.com*, 29 April 2003

[873]   Brost, Marc; Heuser, Uwe Jan, Die infizierte Weltwirtschaft, *Die Zeit*, 20/2003

[874]   Volksrepublik China, Wikipedia, see de.wikipedia.org/wiki/China

[875]   Summary of probable SARS cases with onset of illness from 1 November 2002 to 31 July 2003, World Health Organization, see www.who.int/csr/sars/country/table2003_09_23/en/

[876]   Zylka-Menhorn, Vera, SARS: Hysterie, *Deutsches Ärzteblatt*, 18 April.2003

[877]   Neue Erreger von Atemwegserkrankungen werden oft unterschätzt, *Ärzte Zeitung*, 10 July 2006

[878]   Schuh, Hans, Unheimliche Keime. Die Lungenkrankheit SARS infiziert Mensch und Börse, ist aber nur selten tödlich, *Die Zeit*, 15/2003

[879]   SARS-Hysterie: Uni Berkely sperrt Asiaten aus, *Spiegel Online*, 6 May 2003

[880]   Schuh, Hans, Unheimliche Keime. Die Lungenkrankheit SARS infiziert Mensch und Börse, ist aber nur selten tödlich, *Die Zeit*, 15/2003

[881] Foreman, William, Flutwelle schadet der Wirtschaft weniger als SARS, *Financial Times Deutschland* (online), 8 January 2005

[882] Watzlawick, Paul, Wie wirklich ist die Wirklichkeit? Wahn, Täuschung, Verstehen, Piper, 2005, pp. 84-85

[883] Köhnlein, Claus, Die SARS-Hysterie. SARS auf den Spuren von AIDS und BSE, *Eigentümlich Frei*, July 2003, p. 40

[884] Reilley, Brigg, SARS and Carlo Urbani, *New England Journal of Medicine*, 15 May 2003, p. 1951

[885] Wenzel, Richard, Managing SARS admist Uncertainty, *New England Journal of Medicine*, 15 May 2003, pp. 1947-1948

[886] Altman, Lawrence, Lessons of AIDS, Applied to SARS, *New York Times*, 6 May 2003

[887] Reilley, Brigg, SARS and Carlo Urbani, *New England Journal of Medicine*, 15 May 2003, p. 1951

[888] Wenzel, Richard, Managing SARS admist Uncertainty, *New England Journal of Medicine*, 15 May 2003, pp. 1947-1948

[889] Altman, Lawrence, Lessons of AIDS, Applied to SARS, *New York Times*, 6 May 2003

[890] Peiris, Malik, Coronavirus as a possible cause of severe acute respiratory syndrome, *Lancet*, 19 April, pp. 1319-1325

[891] *New England Journal of Medicine*, 15 May 2003

[892] Winn, Washington, Legionnaires' Disease: Historical Perspective, *Clinical Microbiology Review*, January 1988, p. 60

[893] Winn, Washington, Legionnaires' Disease: Historical Perspective, *Clinical Microbiology Review*, January 1988, p. 61

[894] Ibid., p. 72

[895] Ibid., p. 71

[896] Haley, Charles, Nosocomial Legionnaires' disease: a continuing common-source epidemic at Wadsworth Medical Center, *Annals of Internal Medicine*, April 1979, pp. 583-586

[897] England III, Albert, Sporadic and epidemic nosocomial legionellosis in the United States. Epidemiologic features, *American Journal of Medicine*, March 1981, pp. 707-711

[898] Zovirax, Rote Liste, 2005, p. 10487

[899] Tolzin, Hans, SARS: Wie ein Mythos entsteht, 25 May 2003, impfkritik.de, see www.impfkritik.de/sars/

[900] Zylka-Menhorn, Vera, Schweres akutes respiratorisches Syndrom: Erregernachweis durch weltweite Kooperation, *Ärzte Zeitung*, 4 April 2003, p. C701

[901] Wenzel, Richard, Managing SARS admist Uncertainty, *New England Journal of Medicine*, 15 May 2003, p. 1947

[902] Harrison, Pamela, Major International Conference a Landmark in Battle Against SARS: Presented at SARS-Toronto, *docguide.com*

[903] Zylka-Menhorn, Vera, Schweres akutes respiratorisches Syndrom: Erregernachweis durch weltweite Kooperation, *Ärzte Zeitung*, 4 April 2003, p. C701

[904] Fouchier, Ron, Aetiology: Koch's postulates fulfilled for SARS virus, *Nature*, 15 May 2003, p. 240

[905] Kuiken, Thijs, Newly discovered coronavirus as the primary cause of severe acute respiratory syndrome, *Lancet*, 26 July 2003, pp. 263-70

[906] Feldmeier, Hermann, Die Welt atmet auf, *Tagesspiegel*, 30 June 2003, p. 24

[907] WHO SARS Scientific Research Advisory Committee concludes its first meeting, WHO-Website, 22 October 2003

[908] Kuiken, Thijs, Newly discovered coronavirus as the primary cause of severe acute respiratory syndrome, *Lancet*, 26 July 2003, p. 263

[909] SARS: Angebliche Erfüllung der Koch-Postulate voller Fehler?, *Impf-Report*, 19 November 2003

[910] Kuiken, Thijs, Newly discovered coronavirus as the primary cause of severe acute respiratory syndrome, *Lancet*, 26 July 2003, p. 264

[911] Ibid., p. 266

[912] Ketamin, Rote Liste, 2005, p. 65011

[913] SARS: Angebliche Erfüllung der Koch-Postulate voller Fehler?, *Impf-Report*, 19 November 2003

[914] Personal communication with Francsico Guarner, 20 January 2005

[915] Guarner, Francisco, Gut flora in health and disease, *Lancet*, 8 February 2003, pp. 512-519

[916] Eckburg, Paul, Diversity of the human intestinal microbial flora, *Science*, 10 June 2005, pp. 1635-1638

[917] Tannock, Gerald, New Perspectives of the gut microbiota: implications for future research, *Gastroenterology Clinical North America*, September 2005, pp. 361-382

[918] Kuiken, Thijs, Newly discovered coronavirus as the primary cause of severe acute respiratory syndrome, *Lancet*, 26 July 2003, pp. 264

[919] Wenzel, Richard, Managing SARS admist Uncertainty, *New England Journal of Medicine*, 15 May 2003, pp. 1947-1947

[920] Schuh, Hans, Unheimliche Keime. Die Lungenkrankheit SARS infiziert Mensch und Börse, ist aber nur selten tödlich, *Die Zeit*, 15/2003

[921] Puckett, Jim, Exporting Harm. The High-Tech Trashing of Asia, Report der Basel Action Network und Silicon Valley Toxics Coalition, 25 February 2002

[922] Personal interview with Jim Puckett, 23 February 2006

[923] Chea, Terence, American Electronic Waste Contaminates China and India, Associated Press, 17 August 2005

Chapter 7
H5N1: Avian Flu and Not a Glimmer of Proof

[924] Wetlands International's Position Statement, November 2005

[925] Albrecht, Harro, Der Tod auf leisen Schwingen. Die Vogelgrippe ist im Anmarsch – höchste Zeit, dass Deutschland Impfstoffe und genügend Medikamente kauft, *Die Zeit*, 35/2005

[926] Grippe-Pandemie: Uno rechnet mit 150 Millionen Tote, *Spiegel Online*, 30 September 2005

[927] Schwägerl, Christian, „Die Gefahr wird unterschätzt", Interview mit Reinhard Kurth, *Frankfurter Allgemeine Zeitung*, 18 August 2005

[928] George, Lianne, Forget SARS, West Nile, Ebola and avian flu. The real epidemic is fear, *Macleans.ca*, 29 September 2005

[929] Siegel, Marc, Why we shouldn't fear bird flu, *Ottawa Citizen*, 19 September 2005, p. A15

[930] Siegel, Marc, An epidemic of overreaction, *Los Angeles Times*, 11 October 2005

[931] Siegel, Marc, Alive and well: The fear epidemic, *USA Today*, 19 October 2005

[932] Baureithel, Ulrike, Am Anfang steht die Angst. Aus dem Rollenbuch einer Seuche: Killervögel, Menschenzüge und vorsorglich Verdächtige, *Freitag*, 20 January 2006, p. 1

[933] Krönig, Jürgen, Die Panikindustrie, *Berliner Republik*, 6/2005

[934] Engelbrecht, Torsten; Crowe, David; West, Jim; Vormarsch der Killer-Enten. Schenkt man manchen Medien Glauben, so wird die Welt in naher Zukunft von einer Epidemie heimgesucht, ausgelöst durch Mutation eines Vogelgrippevirus mit dem faszinierend-schaurigen Namen H5N1. Auf welchen Fakten basieren die Horrormeldungen? Eine Recherche, *Journalist*, 11/2005, pp. 35-36

[935] Zimmermann, Kurt, Piep, piep, piiiiiiiep, *Weltwoche*, 27 October 2005, p. 29

[936] E-mails sent out to the managing science editors at *Spiegel*, *Spiegel Online*, *Frankfurter Allgemeine Zeitung*,

Frankfurter Allgemeine Sonntagszeitung, 6 October 2005; keine Antworten erhalten

[937] E-mail to the science desk of *Die Zeit*, 6 October 2005; answer received at the same day

[938] Lieberman, Trudy, Bitter Pill, *Columbia Journalism Review*, July 2005

[939] Siegel, Marc, Why we shouldn't fear bird flu, *Ottawa Citizen*, 19 September 2005, p. A15

[940] Avian Flu Pandemic Could Cost World 2 Trillion Dollars, *Medical News Today*, 18 September 2006

[941] Engelbrecht, Torsten; Crowe, David; West, Jim; Vormarsch der Killer-Enten. Schenkt man manchen Medien Glauben, so wird die Welt in naher Zukunft von einer Epidemie heimgesucht, ausgelöst durch Mutation eines Vogelgrippevirus mit dem faszinierend-schaurigen Namen H5N1. Auf welchen Fakten basieren die Horrormeldungen? Eine Recherche, *Journalist*, 11/2005, pp. 35-36

[942] German National Consumer Protection Ministry (Bundesministerium für Verbraucherschutz, Ernährung und Landwirtschaft, BMVEL), Vogelgrippe, press release for the press conference on 19 August 2005

[943] E-mail from the German National Consumer Protection Ministry (Bundesministerium für Verbraucherschutz, Ernährung und Landwirtschaft, BMVEL), 23 August 2005

[944] Bundesministerium für Verbraucherschutz, Ernährung und Landwirtschaft (BMVEL), Vogelgrippe. Presss release, 19 August 2005

[945] Hulse-Post, Diane; Webster, Robert, Role of domestic ducks in the propagation and biological evolution of highly pathogenic H5N1 influenza viruses in Asia, *Proceedings of the National Academy of Sciences USA*, 26 July 2006, pp. 10682-10687

[946] Hatta, Mochammad, Molecular basis for high virulence of Hong Kong H5N1 influenza A viruses, *Science*, 7 September 2001, pp. 1840-1842

[947] Hulse, Diane; Webster, Robert, Molecular determinants within the surface proteins involved in the pathogenicity of H5N1 influenza viruses in chickens, *Journal of Virology*, September 2004, pp. 9954-9964

[948] Uiprasertkul, Mongkol, Influenza A H5N1 replication sites in humans, *Emerging Infectious Diseases*, July 2005, pp. 1036-1041

[949] Subbarao, Kanta, Characterization of an avian influenza A (H5N1) virus isolated from a child with a fatal respiratory illness, *Science*, 16 January 1998, pp. 393-396

[950] Engelbrecht, Torsten; Crowe, David, Avian Flu Virus H5N1: No Proof for Existence, Pathogenicity, or Pandemic Potential; Non-'H5N1' Causation Omitted, *Medical Hypotheses*, 4/2006; pp. 855-857

[951] Ibid.

[952] Brandis, Henning; Pulverer, Gerhard, Lehrbuch der Medizinischen Mikrobiologie, Gustav Fischer, 1988, p. 633

[953] Engelbrecht, Torsten; Crowe, David, Avian Flu Virus H5N1: No Proof for Existence, Pathogenicity, or Pandemic Potential; Non-'H5N1' Causation Omitted, *Medical Hypotheses*, 4/2006; pp. 855-857

[954] Hulse-Post, Diane; Webster, Robert, Role of domestic ducks in the propagation and biological evolution of highly pathogenic H5N1 influenza viruses in Asia, *Proceedings of the National Academy of Sciences USA*, 26 July 2006, pp. 10682-10683

[955] Gen-Veränderung: H5N1-Virus passt sich dem Menschen an, *Spiegel Online*, 13 January 2006

[956] E-mails sent to the press department of the WHO and and its virologist Mike Perdue on 13, 19 und 27 January 2006

[957] Klassische Geflügelpest (Hochpathogene Form der Aviären Influenza), Friedrich-Loeffler-Institut, p. 2

[958] Ibid., p. 4

[959] Engelbrecht, Torsten; Crowe, David, Avian Flu Virus H5N1: No Proof for Existence, Pathogenicity, or Pandemic Potential; Non-'H5N1' Causation Omitted, *Medical Hypotheses*, 4/2006; pp. 855-857

960 Robbins, John, The Food Revolution, 2001 p. 196

961 Turner, Jacky; Garcés, Leah; Smith, Wendy, The Welfare Of Broiler Chickens In The European Union, Compassion in World Farming Trust, 2003, p. 2

962 Julian, Richard, Rapid Growth Problems: Ascites and Skeletal Deformities in Broilers, *Poultry Science*, December 1998, pp. 1773-1780

963 Turner, Jacky; Garcés, Leah; Smith, Wendy, The Welfare Of Broiler Chickens In The European Union, Compassion in World Farming Trust, 2003, p. 11

964 Scientific Committee on Animal health and Animal Welfare (SCAHAW), The Welfare of Chickens Kept for Meat Production (Broilers), European Commission, Health and Consumer Protection Directorate-General, March 2000

965 Turner, Jacky; Garcés, Leah; Smith, Wendy, The Welfare Of Broiler Chickens In The European Union, Compassion in World Farming Trust, 2003, p. 2

966 Ibid., p. 18

967 Scientific Committee on Animal health and Animal Welfare (SCAHAW), The Welfare of Chickens Kept for Meat Production (Broilers), European Commission, Health and Consumer Protection Directorate-General, March 2000

968 Julian, Richard, Rapid Growth Problems: Ascites and Skeletal Deformities in Broilers, *Poultry Science*, December 1998, pp. 1773-1780

969 Tolzin, Hans, Die Vogelgrippe und das Tabu der Massentierhaltung. Der merkwürdige Tunnelblick der Gesundheitsbehörden am Beispiel der holländischen Epidemie von 2003, *Impf-Report*, July/August 2005, p. 29

970 Klassische Geflügelpest (Hochpathogene Form der Aviären Influenza), Friedrich-Loeffler-Institut, p. 5

971 Tolzin, Hans, Die Vogelgrippe und das Tabu der Massentierhaltung. Der merkwürdige Tunnelblick der Gesundheitsbehörden am Beispiel der holländischen Epidemie von 2003, *Impf-Report*, July/August 2005, p. 29

972 Knierim, Ute, Studie zur Tiergerechtheit von Haltungssystemen für Legehennen im Auftrag des Bund für Umwelt und Naturschutz e.V. (BUND), 11/2003, p. 12

973 Ibid., p. 9

974 Hirt, Helen; Zeltner, Esther; Bapst, Bea, Arbeitsbericht: Fachgruppe Tierhaltung und Tierzucht. Forschungsarbeiten 2000-2004, Forschungsinstitut für Biologischen Landbau (FiBL)

975 Knierim, Ute, Studie zur Tiergerechtheit von Haltungssystemen für Legehennen im Auftrag des Bund für Umwelt und Naturschutz e.V. (BUND), 11/2003, p. 9

976 Hirt, Helen; Zeltner, Esther; Bapst, Bea, Arbeitsbericht: Fachgruppe Tierhaltung und Tierzucht. Forschungsarbeiten 2000-2004, Forschungsinstitut für biologischen Landbau (FiBL)

977 Legehennenauslauf: tiergerecht und nachhaltig, Forschungsinstitut für Biologischen Landbau (FiBL)

978 Rätselraten über Herkunft des Virus, *Spiegel Online*/AP/dpa, 15 February 2006

979 Bundesministerium für Verbraucherschutz, Ernährung und Landwirtschaft (BMVEL), Vogelgrippe. Press release, 19 August 2005

980 Tolzin, Hans, Die Vogelgrippe und das Tabu der Massentierhaltung. Der merkwürdige Tunnelblick der Gesundheitsbehörden am Beispiel der holländischen Epidemie von 2003, *Impf-Report*, July/August 2005, p. 27

981 Rathke, Martina, Vogelgrippe, ein uralter Begleiter, *Stern* (online), 16 September 2005

982 Albrecht, Harro, Der Tod auf leisen Schwingen. Die Vogelgrippe ist im Anmarsch – höchste Zeit, dass Deutschland Impfstoffe und genügend Medikamente kauft, *Die Zeit*, 35/2005

983 Tolzin, Hans, Die Vogelgrippe und das Tabu der Massentierhaltung. Der merkwürdige Tunnelblick der Gesundheitsbehörden am Beispiel der holländischen Epidemie von 2003, *Impf-Report*, July/August 2005, pp. 28-29

⁹⁸⁴ Virus In BC Duck Confirmed As Low Pathogenic North American Strain, press release, Canadian Food Inspection Agency, 20 November 2005

⁹⁸⁵ Wild Bird Survey Detects Avian Influenza In Ducks — No New Threat To Human Health, press release from the Canadian Food Inspection Agency, 31 October 2005

⁹⁸⁶ Branswell, Helen, Heightened climate of bird flu fear made B.C. slaughter inevitable: experts, Canada.com, 23 November 2005

⁹⁸⁷ Vogelgrippeverdacht: Tote Gänse bei Koblenz und Göttingen, N24.de, 25 October 2005

⁹⁸⁸ Gänse bei Neuwied an Gift verende, ZDFheute.de, 26 October 2005

⁹⁸⁹ Routes of infection of highly pathogenic avian influenza in Japan, Food Safety and Consumer Bureau, Ministry of Agriculture, Forestry & Fisheries, Japan, 30 June 2004, p. 16

⁹⁹⁰ Massonnet, Philippe, Chinas Wunderwirtschaft. Land der vergifteten Flüsse, Spiegel Online/AFP, 25 November 2005

⁹⁹¹ Wetlands International's Position Statement, November 2005

⁹⁹² Stop Ducking Hard Facts And Though Policy Options On Bird Flu, Says New Scientific Task Force, press release from the Convention on the Conservation of Migratory Species of Wild Animals und des United Nations Environment Programme, 24 October 2005

⁹⁹³ Khabir, Ahmad, Infectious diseases high on agenda under new WHO leadership, Lancet Infectious Diseases, September 2003, p. 524

⁹⁹⁴ Avian influenza frequently asked questions, World Health Organization (online), 5 December 2005

⁹⁹⁵ Cumulative Number of Confirmed Human Cases of Avian Influenza A/(H5N1) Reported to WHO, 13 November 2006

⁹⁹⁶ Methylprednisolone: Who should not take methylprednisolone?, Drugs.com

⁹⁹⁷ Subbarao, Kanta, Characterization of an avian influenza A (H5N1) virus isolated from a child with a fatal respiratory illness, Science, 16 January 1998, pp. 393-396

⁹⁹⁸ Töpfer, Carolina, Reye-Syndrom bei Baby & Kind, Netdoctor.de

⁹⁹⁹ Reye's Syndrome, National Reye's Syndrome Foundation, see www.reyessyndrome.org

¹⁰⁰⁰ Hurwitz, Eugene, Public Health Service study of Reye's syndrome and medications. Report of the Mayn study, Journal of the American Medical Association, 10 April 1987, pp. 1905-1911

¹⁰⁰¹ Pugliese, Agostino et al., Reye's and Reye's-like syndromes, Cell Biochemistry & Function, 18 August 2008, pp. 741-746

¹⁰⁰² Reye's Syndrome: Facts, National Reye's Syndrome Foundation; see www.reyessyndrome.org/facts.htm

¹⁰⁰³ Subbarao, Kanta, Characterization of an avian influenza A (H5N1) virus isolated from a child with a fatal respiratory illness, Science, 16 January 1998, p. 396

¹⁰⁰⁴ Herbermann, Jan, Der Doktor und das böse Vieh. Der Deutsche Klaus Stöhr letiet das Anti-Influenza-Programm der WHO. Er ist der oberste Kämpfer gegen die Vogelgrippe — ein Blick in seinen unterirdischen War-Room, Handelsblatt, 18 January 2006, p. 10

¹⁰⁰⁵ Engelbrecht, Torsten, Kollaps. Im Gespräch: Der Leipziger Infektionsmediziner Bernhard Ruf zum Influenza-Virus H5N1, Freitag, 21 January 2005, p. 18

¹⁰⁰⁶ E-mail from the Friedrich-Loeffler-Institut, 22 September 2005

¹⁰⁰⁷ Macfarlane, John, Bird flu and pandemic flu. What's the message for GPs and hospital doctors?, British Medical Journal, 29 Oktober 2005, pp. 975-976

¹⁰⁰⁸ Otto, Alexander, Bird flu threat not so grave, CDC chief says, The News Tribune (online), 17 April 2006

¹⁰⁰⁹ UNO-Erhebung. Vogelgrippe tötete bisher 100 Menschen, Spiegel-Online, 27 April 2006

[1010] Vogelgrippe-Schutz. Züchterselbstmorde – Bauern wettern gegen Stallpflicht, *Spiegel Online*, 27 April 2006

[1011] Albrecht, Harro, Der Tod auf leisen Schwingen. Die Vogelgrippe ist im Anmarsch – höchste Zeit, dass Deutschland Impfstoffe und genügend Medikamente kauft, *Die Zeit*, 35/2005

[1012] Franzen, Christof, Angst-Geschäft, Rundschau, 19 October 2005

[1013] Roche: Weltweite Grippe-Vorsorge beschert Gewinnsprung, *FTD.de*/Reuters, 20 July 2005

[1014] Vogelgrippe wird Milliarden-Geschäft, *Handelsblatt*, 2 February 2006, p. 14

[1015] Albrecht, Harro, Der Tod auf leisen Schwingen. Die Vogelgrippe ist im Anmarsch – höchste Zeit, dass Deutschland Impfstoffe und genügend Medikamente kauft, *Die Zeit*, 35/2005

[1016] Flu pill ads make some uneasy, *Boston Globe* (online), 1 November 2006

[1017] Mrusek, Konrad, Vom Ladenhüter zum Welterfolg, *Frankfurter Allgemeine Zeitung*, 16 January 2005, p. 3

[1018] Franzen, Christof, Angst-Geschäft, *Rundschau* (Swiss newscast), 19 October 2005

[1019] Outbreak! Tamiflu "useless" against avian flu. Doctor who has treated 41 victims of virus says "we place no importance on this drug", *Worldnetdaily.com*, 4 December 2005

[1020] Chugai says two deaths have possible Tamiflu link, *Chinadaily.com*/Reuters, 14 November 2005

[1021] Grippemittel Tamiflu unter Verdacht, *FAZ.net*/AFP/Reuters, 18 November 2005

[1022] Health Canada warns of hallucinations among Tamiflu users, *CBS News* (online), 30 November 2006

[1023] Bhattacharya, Shaoni, FDA considers Tamiflu safety in children, *Newscientist.com*, 18 November 2005

[1024] FDA Probes Tamiflu's Effect on Kids, Consumeraffairs.com, 18 November 2005

[1025] Bhattacharya, Shaoni, FDA considers Tamiflu safety in children, *Newscientist.com*, 18 November 2005

[1026] Patient Information: Tamiflu (oseltamivir phosphate), Roche

[1027] Hartmann, Gunther, Querschnittsbereich Klinische Pharmakologie/Allgemeinmedizin: Neue Arzneimittel, Tamiflu, Universitätsklinikum Bonn

[1028] Rokuro, Hama et al., Oseltamivir and early deterioration leading to death: a proportional mortality study for 2009A/H1N1 influenza, *International Journal of Risk & Safety in Medicine*, 2011, pp. 201-215

[1029] Tamiflu: Side effects, ratings, and patient comments, Askapatient.com

[1030] Engelbrecht, Torsten; Crowe, David; West, Jim; Vormarsch der Killer-Enten. Schenkt man manchen Medien Glauben, so wird die Welt in naher Zukunft von einer Epidemie heimgesucht, ausgelöst durch Mutation eines Vogelgrippevirus mit dem faszinierend-schaurigen Namen H5N1. Auf welchen Fakten basieren die Horrormeldungen? Eine Recherche, *Journalist*, 11/2005, p. 36

[1031] Nicholson, Karl, Effectiveness of neuraminidase inhibitors in treatment and prevention of influenza A and B: systematic review and meta-analyses of randomised controlled trials, *British Medical Journal*, 7 June 2003, p. 1239

[1032] House of Commons Health Committee, The Influence of the Pharmaceutical Industry, Forth Report of Session 2004-05, Volume 1, 22 March 2005, p. 53

[1033] Association between industry funding and statistically significant pro-industry findings in medical and surgical randomized trials, *Canadian Medical Association Journal*, 17 February 2004, pp. 477-480

[1034] Smith, Richard, Medical Journals Are an Extension of the Marketing Arm of Pharmaceutical Companies, *Plos Medicine*, May 2005, p. e138

[1035] Drazen, Jeffrey, Financial Associations of Authors, *New England Journal of Medicine*, 13 June 2002, pp. 1901-1902

[1036] Moynihan, Ray, Who pays for the pizza? Redefining the relationships between doctors and drug companies, *British Medical Journal*, 31 May 2003, p. 1190

[1037] Sharav, Vera, NIH Conflict of Interest Rules, "Option of Corruption," children victimized, press release from the

Allicance for Human Researach Protection (AHRP), 18 May 2004

[1038] Willman, David, Lawmakers Assail NIH Conflict Rules, *Los Angeles Times*, 13 May 2004

[1039] Vogelgrippe. Bush will Milliarden für Seuchenbekämpfung, *Spiegel Online*, 2 November 2005

[1040] Mercola, Joseph, Rumsfeld To Profit From Bird Flu Hoax, Mercola.com

[1041] Cole, Andrew, Experts question wisdom of stockpiling oseltamivir, *British Medical Journal*, 5 November 2005, p. 1041

[1042] Schwartz, Nelson, Rumsfeld's growing stake in Tamiflu, *CNN.com*, 31 October 2005

[1043] Tolzin, Hans, Tamiflu — Eine Erfolgsgeschichte aus Seilschaften und Korruption, *Impf-Report*, September/October 2005, p. 20

[1044] Schwartz, Nelson, Rumsfeld's growing stake in Tamiflu, *CNN.com*, 31 October 2005

[1045] Sucher, Jörn, Rumsfeld profitiert vom Tamiflu-Boom, *Spiegel Online*, 1 November 2005

[1046] Rumsfeld's growing stake in Tamiflu, Schwartz, Nelson, *CNN.com*, 31 October 2005

[1047] Krüger, Frank, Von Tamiflu zu "Rummy Flu": Vogelgrippe lässt Rumsfelds Kasse sprudeln, *Saar-Echo*, 31 October 2005

[1048] Tolzin, Hans, Tamiflu — Eine Erfolgsgeschichte aus Seilschaften und Korruption, *Impf-Report*, September/October 2005, pp. 21-22

[1049] Schmiester, Carsten, Versorgung der Truppen im Irak. Neuer Auftrag für Halliburton trotz Betrugsverdachts, *Tagesschau.de*, 11 February 2006

[1050] Pleming, Sue, Army gives $5 bln of work to Halliburton, 6 July 2005, Reuters

[1051] O'Harrow, Robert, Waxman Raises New Questions on Cheney, *Washington Post*, 14 June 2004; p. A04

[1052] Waxman, Henry, Fact Sheet. Halliburton's Iraq Contracts Now Worth Over $10 Billion, Committee on Government Reform, US House of Representatives, 9 December 2004

[1053] Jarecki, Eugene, Why we fight — Amerikas Kriege, documentary (USA 2003), aired on Arte television, 31 January 2006, 20.40 Uhr

[1054] Wetzel, Hubert, Bush legt Milliardenprogramm gegen Vogelgrippe auf, *Financial Times Deutschland*, 2 November 2005

[1055] Sharav, Vera, Biodefense Vaccine /Drug Development Act--S. 1873, press release, Alliance for Human Research Protection, 2 November 2005

[1056] Congressional Set To Pass Law Eliminating Liability For Vaccine Injuries, press release, National Vaccine Information Center, 19 October 2005

[1057] Wetzel, Hubert, Bush legt Milliardenprogramm gegen Vogelgrippe auf, *Financial Times Deutschland*, 2 November 2005

[1058] Becker; Markus, Kampf gegen Vogelgrippe. US-Forscher beleben altes Killervirus, *Spiegel Online*, 5 October 2005

[1059] Engelbrecht, Torsten; Crowe, David; West, Jim; Vormarsch der Killer-Enten. Schenkt man manchen Medien Glauben, so wird die Welt in naher Zukunft von einer Epidemie heimgesucht, ausgelöst durch Mutation eines Vogelgrippevirus mit dem faszinierend-schaurigen Namen H5N1. Auf welchen Fakten basieren die Horrormeldungen? Eine Recherche, *Journalist*, 11/2005, p. 36

[1060] Taubenberger, Jeffrey, Characterization of the 1918 influenza virus polymerase genes, *Nature*, 6 October 2005, pp. 889-293

[1061] Kelly, Thaddeus, Mucolipidosis I (acid neuraminidase deficiency). Three cases and delineation of the variability of the phenotype, *American Journal of Diseases of Children*, August 1981, pp. 703-708

[1062] Taubenberger, Jeffery, Characterization of the Reconstructed 1918 Spanish Influenza Pandemic Virus, *Science*, 7 October 2005, pp. 77-80

[1063] Becker, Markus, US-Forscher beleben altes Killervirus, *Spiegel Online*, 5 October 2005

[1064] Kolata, Gina, Influenza. Die Jagd nach dem Virus, Fischer, 2003, p. 18

[1065] Tolzin, Hans, Die Spanische Grippe, *Impf-Report*, July/August 2005, pp. 21-22

[1066] Ibid., p. 23

[1067] Kolata, Gina, Influenza. Die Jagd nach dem Virus, Fischer, 2003, pp. 75-77

[1068] Kratzer, Hans, Seuchen: „Niemand ist in Familien zur Pflege da, an die Kartoffelernte ist nicht zu denken," *sueddeutsche.de*, 16 April 2020

[1069] Ibid., p. 78

[1070] Kolata, Gina, Influenza. Die Jagd nach dem Virus, Fischer, 2003

[1071] Crosby, Alfred, Epidemic and Peace, 1918, Greenwood Press, 1976

[1072] Collier, Richard, Plague of the Spanish Lady: Influenza Pandemic, October 1918 to Januaryy 1919, Macmillan, 1974

[1073] Hoehling, Adolph, The Great Epidemic, Little, Brown & Company, 1961

[1074] Interview with David Crowe, 12 February 2006

[1075] Gemma, Simonetta, Metabolism of Chloroform in the Human Liver and Identification of the Competent P450s, *Drug Metabolism And Disposition*, March 2003, p. 266

[1076] Fernandez, Humberto, Heroin, Hazelden Information & Educational Services, 1998

[1077] Formaldehyd, Stoffbezogene Betriebsanweisungen, Ruhr-Universität Bochum

[1078] Herrlich, Andreas, Die Pocken. Erreger, Epidemiologie und klinisches Bild, Thieme, 1960, pp. 162-163

[1079] MacBean, Eleanora, The Spanish Influenza Epidemic of 1918 Was Caused By Vaccinations, chapter 2 of her work Swine Flu Expose, 1977, see www.whale.to/a/mcbean2.html#CHAPTER%202

[1080] Hale, Annie, The Medical Voodoo, Gotham House, 1935

[1081] Tolzin, Hans, Die Spanische Grippe, *Impf-Report*, July/August 2005, p.20

[1082] Kolata, Gina, Influenza. Die Jagd nach dem Virus, Fischer, 2003, pp. 65-66

[1083] Ibid., p. 70

Chapter 8
Cervical Cancer and Other Vaccines: Policy vs. Evidence

[1084] Burnet, Sir Frank Macfarlane, Genes, Dreams and Realities, Medical and Technical Publishing, 1971, p. 144

[1085] Sharav, Vera, Addendum: Theory suggests that a shortage of vitamin D triggers outbreaks of flu, press release from the Alliance for Human Research Protection (AHRP), 28 November 2006

[1086] Simonsen, Lone, Impact of influenza vaccination on seasonal mortality in the US elderly population. *Archives of Internal Medicine*, 14 February 2005, pp. 265-272

[1087] Thompson, William, Mortality Associated With Influenza and Respiratory Syncytial Virus in the United States, *Journal of the American Medical Association*, 8 January 2003, pp. 179-186

[1088] Demicheli, Vittorio et al., Vaccines for preventing influenza in the elderly, *Cochrane Database of Systematic Reviews*, 1 February 2018

[1089] Kennedy Townsend, Kathleen; Kennedy II, Joseph P.; McKean Kennedy, Maeve, RFK Jr. Is Our Brother and Uncle. He's Tragically Wrong About Vaccines, *politico.com*, May 08, 2019

[1090] Thompson, William, Mortality Associated With Influenza and Respiratory Syncytial Virus in the United States, *Journal of the American Medical Association*, 8 January 2003, pp. 179-186

[1091] Doshi, Peter, Are US flu death figures more PR than science?, *British Medical Journal*, 10 December 2005, pp. 1412-1413

[1092] Jefferson, Tom, Influenza vaccination: policy versus evidence, *British Medical Journal*, 28 October 2006, pp. 912-915

[1093] Yazback, Edward, Influenza Vaccination of Children: A Useless Risk, *Red Flags*, 28 November 2006

[1094] Sharav, Vera, Addendum: Theory suggests that a shortage of vitamin D triggers outbreaks of flu, press release from the Alliance for Human Research Protection (AHRP), 28 November 2006

[1095] Influenza data from the seasonal final report 2004/2005 from the AGI, Robert Koch-Institute (online)

[1096] Kögel-Schauz, Angelika, Influenza-Viropoly. Das globale Spiel um Milliarden-Gewinne, *Impf-Report*, September/October 2005, pp. 5-7

[1097] Haas, Walter, Why do official statistics of "influenza deaths" underestimate the real burden?, *British Medical Journal* (online), 2 January 2006

[1098] Engelbrecht, Torsten, Can we trust blindly the figures of CDC, RKI, etc.? Part 2, *British Medical Journal* (online), 4 January 2006, http://bmj.bmjjournals.com/cgi/eletters/331/7529/1412#125243

[1099] Inquiry sent to the Robert Koch-Institute, 13 Decmber 2005

[1100] Haas, Walter, Why do official statistics of "influenza deaths" underestimate the real burden?, *British Medical Journal* (online), 2 January 2006

[1101] E-mail from the Robert Koch-Institute, 13 December 2005

[1102] Influenza data from the seasonal final report 2004/2005 from the AGI, Robert Koch-Institute (online)

[1103] Influenza-Schutzimpfung jetzt!, press release from the Robert Koch-Institute, 4 October 2004

[1104] Engelbrecht, Torsten, Can we trust blindly the figures of CDC, RKI, etc.?, *British Medical Journal* (online), 11 December 2005, see http://bmj.bmjjournals.com/cgi/eletters/331/7529/1412#123609

[1105] Engelbrecht, Torsten, Can we trust blindly the figures of CDC, RKI, etc.? Part 2, *British Medical Journal* (online), 4 January 2006, see http://bmj.bmjjournals.com/cgi/eletters/331/7529/1412#125243

[1106] Website der Stiftung Präventive Pädiatrie, see www.stiftung-praeventive-paediatrie.de/ueberuns.html

[1107] Website der Stiftung Präventive Pädiatrie; see www.stiftung-praeventive-paediatrie.de/kooperation.html

[1108] Website of the organisation "Gesundes Kind," see www.gesundes-kind.de/gsk/home/impressum.htm

[1109] Ibid.

[1110] Desselberger, Axel; Krischer, Markus, Als Geldquelle genutzt. Ein Gesundheitsbeamter hat das ehrwürdige Robert-Koch-Institut offenbar zu seinem privaten Vorteil ausgebeutet, Focus, 14/2006, pp. 52-53

[1111] Müller, Thomas, Ein Pandemie-Impfstoff im nächsten Jahr? Davon kann Ulla Schmidt nur träumen, Äzte Zeitung, 27 March 2006

[1112] Sleegers, Anna, Impfstoff gegen Vogelgrippe. Große Pharmakonzerne arbeiten an schnelleren Produktionsverfahren für den Fall einer Pandemie, *Handelsblatt*, 31 March 2006, p. 19

[1113] Engelbrecht, Torsten; Crowe, David, Avian Flu Virus H5N1: No Proof for Existence, Pathogenicity, or Pandemic Potential; Non-'H5N1' Causation Omitted, *Medical Hypotheses*, 4/2006; pp. 855-857

[1114] Jahrbuch Korruption 2006: Schwerpunkt Korruption im Gesundheitswesen, Transparency International, Parthas Verlag, 2006

[1115] Müller-Jung, Joachim, Impfen gegen Krebs – in der Apotheke wird ein Traum wahr, *Frankfurter Allgemeine Zeitung*, 11 October 2006, p. N1

[1116] E-mails to the German Cancer Research Centre (Deutsches Krebsforschungszentrum, DKFZ), 11 and 12 October 2006

[1117] E-Mail from the DKFZ, 11 October 2006

[1118] Bosch, Xaver, The causal relation between human papillomavirus and cervical cancer, Journal of Clinical Pathology, 28 November 2006, pp. 245

[1119] Tolzin, Hans, Erster Krebsimpfstoff im Zulassungsverfahren, *Impf-Report*, January/February 2006, p. 32

[1120] Hein, Thomas, Impfungen bei Gebärmutterhalskrebs. Eine neue Attacke auf Patientinnen, *Raum&Zeit*, 144/2006, p. 11

[1121] zur Hausen, Harald, A papillomavirus DNA from a cervical carcinoma and its prevalence in cancer biopsy samples from different geographic regions, *Proceedings of the National Academy of Sciences USA*, June 1983, pp. 3812-3815

[1122] zur Hausen, Harald, A new type of papillomavirus DNA, its presence in genital cancer biopsies and in cell lines derived from cervical cancer, *EMBO Journal*, 3 May 1984, pp. 1151-1157

[1123] E-Mails to the DKFZ (Sibylle Kohlstädt) on 28 November and 1 December 2006

[1124] Hein, Thomas, Impfungen bei Gebärmutterhalskrebs. Eine neue Attacke auf Patientinnen, *Raum&Zeit*, 144/2006, p. 11

[1125] Ibid., p. 12

[1126] Raffle, Angela, Outcomes of screening to prevent cancer: analysis of cumulative incidence of cervical abnormality and modelling of cases and deaths prevented, *British Medical Journal*, 26 April 2003, pp. 901-904

[1127] Koch, Klaus, Mythos Krebsvorsorge, Eichborn 2003, p. 187

[1128] Burnet, Sir Frank Macfarlane, Genes, Dreams and Realities, Medical and Technical Publishing, 1971, pp. 139-140, 144

[1129] Sharav, Vera, National Vaccine Info Center Calls Merck & FDA "Not Completely Honest" about pre-adolescent HPV Vaccine Safety, press release from the Alliance for Human Research Protection (AHRP), 29 June 2006

[1130] HPV-Impfstoff Gardasil, *Arznei-Telegramm*, 12/2006, p. 118

[1131] Hein, Thomas, Impfungen bei Gebärmutterhalskrebs. Eine neue Attacke auf Patientinnen, *Raum&Zeit*, 144/2006, p. 15

[1132] www.cancer.gov/cancertopics/factsheet/Risk/DES

[1133] HPV-Impfstoff Gardasil, *Arznei-Telegramm*, 12/2006, p. 118

[1134] Impfen gegen Krebs: Impfstoff gegen Gebärmutterhalskrebs soll 2007 auch in Europa erhältlich sein, Deutsches Grünes Kreuz, see www.dgk.de

[1135] Merck's Gardasil Vaccine Not Proven Safe for Little Girls, press release from the National Vaccine Information Center (NVIC), 27 June 2006

[1136] Brower, Vicki, Cancer vaccine field gets shot of optimism from positive results, *Nature Medicine*, April 2005, p. 360

[1137] Engelbrecht, Torsten, Sailor-Shooting, interview with US molecular biologist Peter Duesberg on anti-smoking campaigns, gene-mutations, aneuploidy, and the failure of the established cancer research, *Freitag*, 27 May 2005, p. 18

[1138] Hein, Thomas, Impfungen bei Gebärmutterhalskrebs. Eine neue Attacke auf Patientinnen, *Raum&Zeit*, 144/2006, p. 16

[1139] Sharav, Vera, Addendum: Theory suggests that a shortage of vitamin D triggers outbreaks of flu, press release from the Alliance for Human Research Protection (AHRP), 28 November 2006

Chapter 9
The Big Swine Flu Hoax

[1140] Schweinegrippe: Streit um „Zwei-Klassen-Impfung", *fr-online.de*, October 18, 2009

[1141] Blaylock, Russell, Swine Flu – One of the Most Massive Cover-ups in American History, *Mercola.com*, November 3, 2009

[1142] Hoffmeister, Johannes (Hrsg.), Vorlesungen über die Philosophie der Weltgeschichte, Volume 1: Die Vernunft in der Geschichte, Hamburg, 1994, p. 19

[1143] Tolzin, Hans, Die Fakten zur „Schweinegrippe", impf-report, July/August 2009, p. 2

[1144] Photo exhibition of the Robert Koch-Institut for the Diagnosis of Influenza Viruses, Robert Koch-Institut, first published May 2006, updated June 2009

[1145] De Jone, Jørgen et al., Cellular gene transfer mediated by influenza virosomes with encapsulated plasmid DNA, Biochemical Journal, 1. July 2007, pp. 41-49

[1146] Tolzin, Hans, Die Ursprünge des Schweinegrippe-Mythos, impf-report, July/August 2009, p. 21

[1147] siehe http://www.cdc.gov/flu/

[1148] Attkisson, Sharyl, Swine Flu Cases Overestimated? CBS News Exclusive: Study Of State Results Finds H1N1 Not As Prevalent As Feared, CBSnewp.com, October 21, 2009

[1149] Spelsberg, Angela, Das Geschäft mit der Grippe, Blätter für deutsche und internationale Politik, 11/2009, p. 23

[1150] Finland downgrades swine influenza, Newsroom.finland.fi, 23. July 2009

[1151] Mercola, Joseph, Vaccine Doctor Given at Least $ 30 Million Dollars to Push Vaccines, Mercola.com, June 25, 2009

[1152] Dougherty, Jon, Feds' conflict of interest over vaccines? Committee eyes ,incestuous' ties between drug-makers, FDA, CDC, wnd.com, June 16, 2000

[1153] Spelsberg, Angela, Das Geschäft mit der Grippe, Blätter für deutsche und internationale Politik, 11/2009, p. 25

[1154] Nähe zur Pharmaindustrie: Pandemie-Beauftragter der Regierung hat umstrittenen Beraterjob, Spiegel Online, October 24, 2009

[1155] see Coordination gegen Bayer-Gefahren, www.cbgnetwork.org

[1156] Historiker-Bericht: Die dunkle Vergangenheit des Robert-Koch-Instituts, Spiegel Online, October 1, 2008

[1157] Engelbrecht, Torsten, Im Fake-News-Fieber: Spiegel & Co. haben die Schweinegrippe-Pandemie bis heute nicht aufgearbeitet – und verbreiten nun erneut Pharma-Propaganda, rubikon.news, 12 April 2020

[1158] Hackenbroch, Veronika; Traufetter, Gerald, Immun gegen die Impfung, Spiegel, 19 October 2009, p. 140

[1159] Spelsberg, Angela, Das Geschäft mit der Grippe, Blätter für deutsche und internationale Politik, 11/2009, p. 25

[1160] Pinzler, Jutta; Schwalfenberg, Steganie, Profiteure der Angst – das Geschäft mit der Schweinegrippe, Arte, October 21, 2009

[1161] Bartens, Werner, Schweinegrippe: Zu früh, zu unsicher, zu teuer?, Süddeutsche Zeitung, October 14, 2009

[1162] Thelen, Peter, Schweinegrippe: Vertrag mit Risiken und Nebenwirkungen. Bund und Länder haben Impfstoff gegen die Schweinegrippe bestellt – und haften nun für fast alles, tagesspiegel.de, November 23, 2009

[1163] Hackenbroch, Veronika; Traufetter, Gerald, Immun gegen die Impfung, Spiegel, October 19, 2009, p. 141

[1164] Engelbrecht, Torsten et al., Die Zukunft der Krebsmedizin: Klassische und alternative Therapien, Impfungen und Krebsgene: Was ist Fakt und was Fiktion?, naturaviva, 2009

[1165] Hackenbroch, Veronika; Traufetter, Gerald, Immun gegen die Impfung, Spiegel, October 19, 2009, p. 141

[1166] Spelsberg, Angela, Das Geschäft mit der Grippe, Blätter für deutsche und internationale Politik, 11/2009, p. 24

[1167] Wegen Schweinegrippe: In Frankreich wird das Küssen verboten, Bild.de, September 7, 2009

[1168] Schweinegrippe im Karneval: Närrisches Treiben: Küssen verboten!, Abendblatt.de, November 8, 2009

[1169] Interview von Brent Leung, maker oft he documentary „House of Numbers", with Luc Montagnier

[1170] Peric, Mark et al., Vitamin D Analogs Differentially Control Antimicrobial Peptide/„Alarmin" Expression in Psoriasis, PLoS One, July 2009, p. E634

[1171] Melamed, Michal et al., 25-Hydroxyvitamin D Levels and the Risk of Mortality in the General Population,

Archives of Internal Medicine, August 11, 2008; pp. 1629-1637

[1172] Rickmann, A., „Ich wäre fast an Schweinegrippe gestorben", *bild.de*, 16. October 2009

[1173] Blaylock, Russell, Swine Flu—One of the Most Massive Cover-ups in American History, *Mercola.com*, November 3, 2009

[1174] *Nature Insight*: Obesity and Diabetes, *Nature*, December 14, 2006, Supplement, pp. 839-888

[1175] Thun, Michael et al., Overweight, Obesity, and Mortality from Cancer in a Prospectively Studied Cohort of U.P. Adults, *New England Journal of Medicine*, 24. April 2003, pp. 1625-1638

[1176] The ANZIC Influenza Investigators, Critical Care Services and 2009 H1N1 Influenza in Australia and New Zealand, *New England Journal of Medicine*, November 12, 2009, pp. 1925-1934

[1177] Le Ker, Heike, Schweinegrippe: Gesundheitliche Probleme nicht immer Folge der Impfung, *Spiegel Online*, November 2, 2009

[1178] Tolzin, Hans, Editorial, *impf-report*, July/August 2009, p. 2

[1179] Ema, Makoto et al., Evaluation of developmental neurotoxicity of polysorbate 80 in rats, R*eproductive Toxicology*, January 2008, p. 89-99

[1180] Gajdová, M. et al., Delayed effects of neonatal exposure to Tween 80 on female reproductive organs in rats, *Food and Chemical Toxicology*, March 1993, pp. 183-190

[1181] Shoenfeld, Yehuda; Rose, Noel (Hrsg.), Infection and Autoimmunity, Elsevier Science & Technology, 2004, pp. 87-104

[1182] Carlson, Barbro et al., The endogenous adjuvant squalene can induce a chronic T-cell-mediated arthritis in rats, *American Journal of Pathology*, June 2000, pp. 2057-2065

[1183] A study overview of squalene can be found at http://www.whale.to/vaccine/squalene_c.html

[1184] Engelbrecht, Torsten et al., Die Zukunft der Krebsmedizin: Klassische und alternative Therapien, Impfungen und Krebsgene: Was ist Fakt und was Fiktion?, naturaviva, 2009

[1185] Spiess, Heinz; Heiniger, Ulrich (Hrsg.), Impfkompendium, Thieme Verlag, 2005

[1186] Tolzin, Hans, Illegal & gefährlich für Schwangere?, *impf-report*, July/August 2009, p. 6

[1187] Tonne, Dominic, Death link to swine flu vaccine, *Sunday Times*, August 16, 2009

[1188] Leitner, Michael, Verstärkerimpfstoffe in Impfungen—Terror gegen unser Immunsystem, *impf-report*, July/August 2009, pp. 8-10

[1189] Hackenbroch, Veronika; Traufetter, Gerald, Immun gegen die Impfung, *Spiegel*, October 19, 2009, p. 142

[1190] Kinder oft stärker mit Chemikalien belastet als ihre Mütter: WWF-Test findet 73 bedenkliche Schadstoffe im Blut europäischer Familien, World Wide Fund for Nature, October 16, 2005

[1191] Mutter, Joachim, Is dental amalgam safe for humans? The opinion of the scientific committee of the European Commission, *Journal of Occupational Medicine and Toxicology*, January 13, 2011

[1192] Engelbrecht, Torsten, Die Amalgam-Kontroverse: Was steckt wirklich dahinter?, *Natur&Heilen*, 9/2008

[1193] Drasch, Gustav, et al.: Mercury burden of human fetal and infant tissues, *European Journal of Pediatrics*, August 1994, pp. 607-610

[1194] Hartmann, Klaus, Stuttgarter Impfsymposium 2009, DVD

[1195] „Solchen Wissenschaftlern würde ich gerne Kamera oder Mikrofon entziehen", Interview mit dem Gesundheitsstatistiker Gerd Bosbach zur Corona-Debatte, *nachdenkseiten.de*, March 26, 2020

[1196] Engelbrecht, Torsten, Im Fake-News-Fieber: *Spiegel* & Co. haben die Schweinegrippe-Pandemie bis heute nicht aufgearbeitet—und verbreiten nun erneut Pharma-Propaganda, *Rubikon*, April 12, 2020

Chapter 10
Postscript to Chapter 3 about AIDS

[1197] Interview by Brent Leung, Director oft he 2009 documentary „House of Numbers", mit Luc Montagnier, see https://www.youtube.com/watch?v=tKyIBYKoT20

[1198] Research on AIDS virus and cancer wins Nobel Medicine Prize, AFP, October 6, 2008

[1199] Papadopulos-Eleopulos, Eleni; Turner, Valendar, A critique of the Montagnier evidence fort he HIV/AIDS hypothesis, *Medical Hypotheses*, Volume 63, Issue 4, 2004, p. 597-601

[1200] Montagnier, Luc et al., Molecular cloning of lymphadenopathy-associated virus, *Nature*, 20. December 1984, pp. 757-760

[1201] Tahi, Djamel, Did Luc Montagnier discover HIV? „I repeat, we did not pur ify!", *Continuum*, Winter 1997/1998, pp. 31-35

[1202] Sharav, Vera, Another Nobel Foundation member is being investigated, press release of the Alliance for Human Research Protection (AHRP), December 22, 2008

[1203] Moniz develops lobotomy for mental illness 1935, see www.pbp.org/wgbh/aso/databank/entries/dh35lo.html

[1204] Diefenbach, Gretchen, Portrayal of Lobotomy in the Popular Press: 1935 - 1960, Journal of the History of Neurosciences, April 1999, pp. 60-69

[1205] Laurence, William, Lobotomy banned in Soviet Union as Cruel; Brain Operation in the Insane is Inhumane, Russian Tells Vienna Health Session, *New York Times*, August 22, 1953

[1206] Breggin, Peter, Elektroschock ist keine Therapie, 1989, Urban & Schwarzenberg, p. 175

[1207] Frequently Asked Questions About Lobotomies, *www.npr.org*, November 16, 2005

[1208] Surgery of the Soul, *zoecormier.com*, November 30, 2010

[1209] Sharav, Vera, Another Nobel Foundation member is being investigated, press release of the Alliance for Human Research Protection (AHRP), December 22, 2008

[1210] see http://de.wikipedia.org/wiki/Lobotomie

[1211] Valenstein, Elliot, The psychosurgery debate, W. H. Freeman, San Francisco 1980

[1212] Jonathan Ned Katz: Gay American History, Avon Books, 1978, pp. 129-207

[1213] Mark, Vernon et al., Role of Brain Disease in Riots and Urban Violence, *Journal of the American Medical Association*, September 11, 1967, p. 895

[1214] see http://de.wikipedia.org/wiki/Lobotomie

[1215] Sharav, Vera, Another Nobel Foundation member is being investigated, press release of the Alliance for Human Research Protection (AHRP), December 22, 2008

[1216] see http://www.houseofnumberp.com/

[1217] see http://www.youtube.com/watch?v=tKyIBYKoT20

[1218] see http://nymag.com/health/features/61740/

[1219] Aids: Mitochondrien könnten Erkrankungszeitpunkt beeinflussen, *Spiegel Online*, December 15, 2008

[1220] Kruis, Wolfgang. Informationen über eine Therapiestudie: Rezidivprophylaxe bei Patienten mit Colitis ulcerosa durch Mutaflor im Vergleich zu Mesalazin, *Der Bauchredner*, 3/1996, pp. 64-68

[1221] Mai, Volker; Draganov, Peter, Recent advances and remaining gaps in our knowledge of associations between gut microbiota and human health, *World Journal of Gastroenterology*, Januar 7, 2009, pp. 81-85

[1222] Bjorksten, Bengt, Effects of intestinal microflora and the environment on the development of asthma and allergy, *Springer Seminars in Immunopathology*, February 25, 2004, pp. 257-270

[1223] Knight, David, Gut flora in health and disease, *Lancet*, May 24, 2003, p. 1831

[1224] Tannock, Gerald. Medical Importance of the Normal Microflora, Kluwer Academic Publishers, 1999

[1225] Langosch, Angelika, Einfluss der Ernährung insbesondere der Rohkost auf die Darmflora und Infektabwehr, Institut für Medizinische Balneologie und Klimatologie der Universität München, 1984 (dissertation)

[1226] Lance, Tony, GRID = Gay Related Intestinal Dysbiosis? Explaining HIV/AIDS Paradoxes in Terms of Intestinal Dysbiosis, http://www.heallondon.org, December 14, 2008

[1227] Koliadin, Vladimir, Destruction of normal resident microflora as the main cause of AIDS, see http://www.virusmyth.com/aids/hiv/vkmicro.htm

[1228] Koliadin, Vladimir, What causes a positive test for HIV-antibodies?, see http://www.virusmyth.com/aids/hiv/vktest.htm431

[1229] Anukam, Kingsley et al., Yogurt containing probiotic Lactobacillus rhamnosus GR-1 and L. reuteri RC-14 helps resolve moderate diarrhea and increases CD4 count in HIV/AIDS patients, *Journal of Clinical Gastroenterology*. March 2008, pp. 239-243

[1230] Mutter, Joachim, Gesund statt chronisch krank! Der ganzheitliche Weg: Vorbeugung und Heilung sind möglich, fit fürs Leben Verlag, 2009, p. 388

[1231] Reduced glutathione-L-cysteine-anthocyanins gel, NCI Drug Dictionary, Website of the U. P. National Cancer Institute

[1232] Ohlenschläger, Gerhard, Glutathionsystem, Ordnungs- und informationserhaltende Grundregulation lebender Systeme, Verlag für Medizin Dr. Ewald Fischer, Heidelberg 1991

[1233] Zachara, Bronislaw et al., Decreased selenium concentration and glutathione peroxidase activity in blood and increase of these parameters in malignant tissue of lung cancer patients, *Lung*, September 1, 1997, pp. 321-332

[1234] Qiu, Fa-Bo et al., Predominant expression of Th1-type cytokines in primary hepatic cancer and adjacent liver tissues, *Hepatobiliary & Pancreatic Diseases International*, February 2007, pp. 63-66

[1235] Locigno, Roberto; Castronovo, Vincent, Reduced glutathione system: role in cancer development, prevention and treatment (review), *International Journal of Oncology*, August 2001, pp. 221-236

[1236] Bianchini, Franba; Vainio, Harri, Allium vegetables and organosulfur compounds: do they help prevent cancer?, *Environmental Health Perspectives*, September 2001, pp. 893-902

[1237] Pinto, John et al., Effects of garlic thioallyl derivatives on growth, glutathione concentration, and polyamine formation of human prostate carcinoma cells in culture, *American Journal of Clinical Nutrition*, August 1997, pp. 398-405

[1238] Olivieri, Gianfranco et al., The effects of beta-estradiol on SHSY5Y neuroblastoma cells during heavy metal induced oxidative stress, neurotoxicity and beta-amyloid secretion, *Neuroscience*, September 10, 2002, pp. 849-855

[1239] Mutter, Joachim, Gesund statt chronisch krank! Der ganzheitliche Weg: Vorbeugung und Heilung sind möglich, fit fürs Leben Verlag, 2009, p. 394

[1240] ibid., pp. 253-255

[1241] Galon, Jérôme et al., Coordination of intratumoral immune reaction and human colorectal cancer recurrence, *Cancer Research*, March 15, 2009, pp. 2685-2693

[1242] Deer, Brian, Death by denial: The campaigners who continue to deny HIV causes Aids, *The Guardian*, Februar 21, 2012

[1243] Schweinsburg, Brian et al., Brain mitochondrial injury in human immunodeficiency virusseropositive (HIV+) individuals taking nucleoside reverse transcriptase inhibitors, *Journal of NeuroVirology*, August 2005, pp. 356-364

[1244] Payne, Brendan A. I. et al., Mitochondrial aging is accelerated by anti-retroviral therapy through the clonal expansion of mtDNA mutations, *Nature Genetics*, June 26, 2011, pp. 806-810

[1245] Barnes, Martik K.; Engelbrecht, Torsten, Stricken Heroine Rethinkers Died from Toxic Drugs, Not AIDS: Christine Maggiore, Karri Stokely, Maria Papagiannidou, *rethinkingaids.com*

[1246] de Fries, Felix, Therapieempfehlungen für HIV-Test-Positive und AIDS-Patienten, *ummafrapp.de*

[1247] see the Facebook site of Eneko Llandaburu

Chapter 11
10 Reasons against Measles Vaccination

[1248] Mawson, Anthony R., Special Issue „Vaccination and Health Outcomes," *International Journal of Environmental Research and Public Health*, July 15, 2018

[1249] Dubos, René, Mirage of Health: Utopias, Progress, and Biological Change, Rutgers University Press, 1987, p. 102

[1250] Alm, Johan et al., Atopy in children of families with an anthroposophic lifestyle; *Lancet*, May 1999, pp. 1485-1488

[1251] Kass, Edward H., Infectious Diseases and Social Change, *The Journal of Infectious Diseases*, January 1971, pp. 110-114

[1252] Mawson, Anthony R., Special Issue „Vaccination and Health Outcomes," *International Journal of Environmental Research and Public Health*, July 15, 2018

[1253] Berndt, Christina, Urteil gegen Impfgegner: 100 000 Euro für ein "Hirngespinst", *www.sueddeutsche.de*, March 12, 2015

[1254] E-mail from *Süddeutsche Zeitung* editor Christina Berndt from April 7, 2015

[1255] Gerß, Wolfgang, Das Ende der DDR als konsequente mathematische Katastrophe, *Duisburger Beiträge zur Soziologischen Forschung*, No. 1/2008 (University of Duisburg-Essen)

[1256] We answered to the e-mail from *Süddeutsche Zeitung* editor Christina Berndt from April 7, 2018 (see endnote 8) on April 15 an 29 and on May 5, 2015 and asked for comments

[1257] Miller, Neil Z., Vaccines: Are They Really Safe & Effective? New Atlantean Press, 2005, p. 26

[1258] Buchwald, Gerhard, Impfen: Das Geschäft mit der Angst, emu-Verlag, 1994

[1259] De Serres, Gaston et al., Largest Measles Epidemic in North America in a Decade – Quebec, Canada, 2011: Contribution of Susceptibility, Serendipity, and Superspreading Events, *The Journal of Infectious Diseases*, March 15, 2013, pp. 990-998

[1260] Prikazsky, Vladimir et al., An increase in the number of mumps cases in the czech republic, 2005-2006, *Eurosurveillance*, April 17, 2008

[1261] Schönberger, Katharina et al., Epidemiology of Subacute Sclerosing Panencephalitis (SSPE) in Germany from 2003 to 2009: A Risk Estimation, *PLOS One*, July 9, 2013

[1262] Angelika Müller, Tod nach Masern? Der Fall Aliana, *impf-report*, issue 106/1st quarter 2015, pp. 43-45

[1263] Weber, Nina, „Unspezifische Effekte": Wie eine provokante These die Sicht aufs Impfen ändern könnte, *www.spiegel.de*, September 11, 2018

[1264] E-mail from August 27, 2018

[1265] Kennedy Jr., Robert F., Americans Can Handle an Open Discussion on Vaccines – RFK, Jr. Responds to Criticism from His Family, childrenshealthdefese.org, August 15, 2019

[1266] Trial of BCG vaccines in south India for tuberculosis prevention, *Indian Journal of Medical Research*, September 1979

[1267] Cowling, Benjamin J. et al., Increased risk of non-influenza respiratory virus infections associated with receipt of inactivated influenza vaccine, *Clinical Infectious Diseases*, June 2012, pp. 1778-83

[1268] Turner, Louise, Flu Vaccine Causes 5.5 Times More Respiratory Infections: Study, *Yournewswire.com*, January 10, 2015

[1269] Hooker, Brian S.; Miller, Neil Z., Analysis of health outcomes in vaccinated and unvaccinated children: Developmental delays, asthma, ear infections and gastrointestinal disorders, *SAGE Open Medicine*, May 27, 2020

[1270] Vaxxed Unvaxxed: The Science, Full-Presentation-Parts-I-VII, childrenshealthdefense.org,

[1271] Miller, Neil Z.; Goldman, Gary S., Relative trends in hospitaliza-tions and mortality among infants by the number of vaccine doses and age, based on the VAERS, 1990-2010, *Human & Experimental Toxicology*, October 2012, pp. 1012-1021

[1272] Miller, Neil Z.; Goldman, Gary S., Infant mortality rates regressed against number of vaccine doses routinely given: Is there a biochemical or synergistic toxicity?; *Human & Experimental Toxicology*, September 2011, pp. 1420-1428

[1273] ibid.

[1274] Martin Hirte et al., Impfzeitpunkt von Bedeutung, *Deutsches Ärzteblatt*, October 14, 2011, pp. 696-697

[1275] McDonald, Karla L. et al., Delay in Diphtheria, pertussis, tetanus vaccination is associated with a reduced risk of childhood asthma; *Journal of Allergy and Clinical Immunology*, March 2008, pp. 626-631

[1276] E-Mail from August 27, 2018

[1277] Fisher, Barbara Loe, The Vaccine Culture War in America: Are You Ready?, *www.mercola.com*, March 17, 201

[1278] Bryant, Alison, 20 Top-selling Vaccines--H1 2012, *www.fiercevaccines.com*, September 25, 2012

[1279] Global vaccine market revenues from 2014 to 2020 (in billion U.S. Dollars), *www.statista.co*

[1280] Demicheli, Vittorio et al., Vaccines for measles, mumps and rubella in children, *The Cochrane Database Systematic Reviews*, February 15, 2012

[1281] Mawson, Anthony R., Special Issue „Vaccination and Health Outcomes," *International Journal of Environmental Research and Public Health*, July 15, 2018

[1282] *impf-report*, 1st quarter 2015, p. 36

[1283] see www.impfkritik.de/antikoerpertiter

[1284] Tolzin, Hans U. P., Das Ansteckungs-Experiment von 1911: Wirklich ein Meilenstein der Forschung?, *impf-report*, 1st quarter 2016, pp. 28-31

[1285] Pressemitteilung: Anderthalbjähriges Kind an Masern verstorben, www.berlin.de, Februar 23, 2015

[1286] Bergmann, Jörg et al., Masern-Angst: Wie viele Sorgen muss ich mir um mein Kind machen?, *www.bild.de*, Februar 25, 2015

[1287] Bartens, Werner, Masern-Impfung: Gefährliche Ignoranz, *www.sueddeutsche.de*, March 1, 2015

[1288] Rabe, Steffen. Masern in Berlin: zwei Arten Schweigepflicht?, *www.individuelle-impfentscheidung.de*, February 26, 2015

[1289] Lanka, Stefan, Der Bundesgerichtshof hat entschieden: Wir haben den Masern-Virus-Prozess endgültig gewonnen!, *www.wissenschaftplus.de*

Chapter 12
Total Corona Mania: Worthless PCR Tests, Lethal Medication and Mortality Data that Makes a Viral Cause Impossible

[1290] James, David, PCR Inventor: "It doesn't tell you that you are sick", *OffGuardian,* October 5, 2020

[1291] Lauritsen, John, Has Provincetown become protease town?, *New York Native*, December 9, 1996

[1292] Grabar, Eddar, Coronavirus: „Diskussionen sind unerwünscht", Interview mit Jürgen Windeler, *Die Zeit*, December 3, 2020

[1293] Prof. Matthias Schrappe in an interview with the German *heute* newscast of the ZDF, November 23, 2020

[1294] Schrappe, Matthias et al., Thesenpapier 6, Teil 6.1: Epidemiologie. Die Pandemie durch SARS-CoV-2/CoViD-19, Zur Notwendigkeit eines Strategiewechsels. Köln, Berlin, Bremen; Hamburg, November 22, 2020

[1295] „Solchen Wissenschaftlern würde ich gerne Kamera oder Mikrofon entziehen", Interview mit dem Gesundheitsstatistiker Gerd Bosbach zur Corona-Debatte, *www.nachdenkseiten.de*, March 26, 2020

[1296] Cevik, Muge et al., SARS-CoV-2, SARS-CoV, and MERS-CoV viral load dynamics, duration of viral shedding, and infectiousness: a systematic review and meta-analysis, *The Lancet*, November 19, 2020

[1297] File number (in Germany) 19 B 1780/20 NE

[1298] Judson, Horace, The Great Betrayal. Fraud in Science, Harcourt, 2004, p.6

[1299] Red Cross Knew of AIDS Blood Threat, *San Francisco Chronicle*, May 16, 1994

[1300] Engelbrecht, Torsten; Köhnlein, Claus. Das trügerische AIDS-Erbe von Rock Hudson, *www.rubikon.news*, December 1, 2017

[1301] Pascal, Mathilde et al., The mortality impacts of fine particles in France, *The Science of the Total Environment*, November 15, 2016, pp.416-425

[1302] Neue Ergebnisse: Studie: Feinstaub verursacht deutlich mehr Todesfälle als angenommen, *www.stern.de*, January 18, 2019

[1303] Air pollution costs France € 100 billion per year, www.euractiv.com, July 16, 2015

[1304] Schmid, Fred, Der Rüstungs-Rekord: Die weltweiten Rüstungausgaben haben ein neues Rekordhoch erreicht, *www.rubikon.news*, June 8, 2019

[1305] Jean Ziegler über Hunger in Afrika: „Es gibt genügend Nahrungsmittel", *www.taz.de*, April 19, 2017

[1306] Quick facts: What you need to know about global hunger, *www.mercycorps.org*, October 1, 2018

[1307] see www.worldometers.info/coronavirus/

[1308] Viner, Russell et al.. School closure and management practices during coronavirus outbreaks including COVID-19: a rapid systematic review, *Lancet Child & Adolescent Health*, Mai 2020, pp. 397-404

[1309] Thomma, Norbert, Aktivist Jean Ziegler: „Ich bin so radikal, weil ich die Opfer kenne", *www.tagesspiegel.de*, January 7, 2013

[1310] USA mit Abstand Spitzenreiter: Globale Rüstungsausgaben auf höchstem Stand seit 30 Jahren, *www.tagesspiegel.de*, April 29, 2019

[1311] Besser Spitze bei Hungerbekämpfung statt bei Aufrüstung, *www.newsroom.de*, April 29, 2020

[1312] Wolff, Reinhard, Kommentar Rüstungsausgaben: Ein halbes Prozent für den Hunger, *www.taz.de*, December 4, 2012

[1313] Brandt, Willy. Der organisierte Wahnsinn: Wettrüsten und Welthunger, Kiepenheuer & Witsch, 1985

[1314] D'Souza, Frances, Democracy as a Cure for Famine, *Journal of Peace Research*, November 1994, pp.369-373

[1315] Engelbrecht, Torsten; Demeter, Konstantin, Die Corona-Korruption: Die Lockdown-Entscheidungen vieler Länder wurden auf Empfehlung eines Wissenschaftlers forciert, der von massiven Interessenkonflikten betroffen ist, *www.rubikon.news*, May 10, 2020

[1316] Wodarg, Wolfgang, Lösung des Corona-Problems: Panikmacher isolieren, *Flensburger Tageblatt*, Februar 29, 2020, p.29

[1317] Engelbrecht, Torsten, Journalismus am Ende: Statt journalistisch zu arbeiten, verbreitet der *Spiegel* recherchelos die Propaganda der Reichen und Mächtigen unserer Welt, *www.rubikon.news*, April 17, 2020

1318   Schmidt, Tobias, 280 000 Tote in Deutschland denkbar. Charité-Virologe Drosten über das Coronavirus: „Wir stehen erst am Anfang", *www.noz.de*, March 6, 2020

1319   Gøtzsche, Peter C., Corona: an epidemic of mass panic, *Deadly Medicine & Organized Crime—a blog about drugs*, March 21, 2020

1320   Ioannidis, John P.A., A fiasco in the making? As the coronavirus pandemic takes hold, we are making decisions without reliable data, *www.statnews.com*, March 17, 2020

1321   Statistikwissenschaftler John Ioannidis, Daten-Fiasko bei Corona-Krise: Stanford-Professor warnt vor Blindflug bei Maßnahmen, *www.focus.de*, March 21, 2020

1322   Millionen Tote: WHO hält globale Seuche für unvermeidbar, *Spiegel Online*, November 26, 2004

1323   Hager, Angelika, Interview mit Gerd Gigerenzer „Angst ist ein Markt", *Profil*, 8. März 2020

1324   „Solchen Wissenschaftlern würde ich gerne Kamera oder Mikrofon entziehen", Interview mit dem Gesundheitsstatistiker Gerd Bosbach zur Corona-Debatte, *www.nachdenkseiten*.de, March 26, 2020

1325   Gøtzsche, Peter C., Our prescription drugs kill us in large numbers, *Polskie Archiwum Medycyny Wewnetrznej*, Epub October 30, 2014

1326   Drosten warnt nach Studie: Viele Infizierte stecken andere an, bevor sie sich selbst krank fühlen, *www.focus.de*, March 24, 2020

1327   Xuhua Guan et al., Pneumonia Incidence and Mortality in Mainland China: Systematic Review of Chinese and English Literature, 1985-2008, *PLoS ONE*, July 23, 2010, e11721

1328   Qun Li et al., Early Transmission Dynamics in Wuhan, China, of Novel Coronavirus—Infected Pneumonia, *New England Journal Medicine*, January 29, 2020

1329   Huang, Chaolin et al., Clinical features of patients infected with 2019 novel coronavirus in Wuhan, China, *Lancet*, January 24, 2020, pp. 497-506

1330   Chen, Nanshan et al., Epidemiological and clinical characteristics of 99 cases of 2019 novel coronavirus pneumonia in Wuhan, China: a descriptive study, *Lancet*, February 15, 2020, pp. 507-513

1331   Crowe, David, Is the 2019 Coronavirus Really a Pandemic?, *www.theinfectiousmyth.com*

1332   Kolata, Gina, Faith in Quick Test Leads to Epidemic That Wasn't, *New York Times*, January 22, 2007

1333   Schmitt, Peter-Philipp, Virologe Hendrik Streeck: „Wir haben neue Symptome entdeckt, *www.faz.net*, March 16, 2020

1334   Prof. Dr. med. Thomas Löscher geht in den Ruhestand … aber nicht ganz!, www.klinikum.uni-muenchen.de

1335   Kotlar, Kerstin, Er behandelte erste deutsche Patienten. Mehr als 52 000 Geheilte: Professor sagt, wie das Immunsystem den Erreger bekämpft, *www.focus.de*, March 6, 2020

1336   E-mail von Prof. Thomas Löscher from March 6, 2020

1337   Nickbakhsh, Sema et al., Virus-virus interactions impact the population dynamics of influenza and the common cold, *Proceedings of the National Academy of Sciences*, December 26, 2019, pp. 27142-27150

1338   Wodarg, Wolfgang, Lösung des Corona-Problems: Panikmacher isolieren, *Flensburger Tageblatt*, February 29, 2020, p. 29

1339   Phone call on March 8, 2020

1340   Corman, Victor M. et al., Detection of 2019 novel coronavirus (2019-nCoV) by real-time RT-PCR, *Eurosurveillance*, January 23, 2020

1341   Hohmann-Jeddi, Christina, Coronavirus-Diagnostik: Roche erhält Notfall-Zulassung der FDA für Hochdurchsatztest, *www.pharmazeutische-zeitung.de*, March 14, 2020

1342   Wildermuth, Volkart, Neues Coronavirus Diagnostischer Test aus Berlin weltweit gefragt, *www.deutschlandfunk*.

de, January 23, 2020

[1343] Hohmann-Jeddi, Christina, Coronavirus-Diagnostik: Roche erhält Notfall-Zulassung der FDA für Hochdurch-satztest, *www.pharmazeutische-zeitung.de*, March 14, 2020

[1344] Phone Call on March 8, 2020

[1345] Berndt, Christina, Coronavirus: Zu schön, um wahr zu sein, *www.sueddeutsche.de*, March 24, 2020

[1346] SARS-CoV-2 Coronavirus Multiplex RT-qPCR Kit, CD Creative Diagnostics

[1347] Berndt, Christina, Coronavirus: Zu schön, um wahr zu sein, *www.sueddeutsche.de*, March 24, 2020

[1348] Gorguner, Metin; Akgun, Metin, Acute Inhalation Injury, *The Eurasian Journal of Medicine*, April 2010, pp. 28-35

[1349] Laporte, Joan-Ramon, In the midst of the SARS-CoV-2 pandemia, caution is needed with commonly used drugs that increase the risk of pneumonia, *www.rxisk.org*, April 2, 2020

[1350] Susan Payne, Viruses: From Understanding to Investigation, Academic Press, 2017

[1351] White/Fenner, Medical Virology, San Diego Academic Press, 1986, p.9

[1352] Engelbrecht, Torsten; Demeter, Konstantin, COVID-19 PCR-Tests Are Scientifically Meaninless, *OffGuardian*, 27. Juni 2020

[1353] Na Zhu et al., A Novel Coronavirus from Patients with Pneumonia in China, 2019, *New England Journal of Medicine*, March 5, 2020, pp. 727-733

[1354] Oh, Myoung-don et al., Virus Isolation from the First Patient with SARS-CoV-2 in Korea, *Journal of Korean Medical Science*, February 24, 2020

[1355] Ensering, Martin. Virology, Old guard urges virologists to go back to basics, *Science*, July 6, 2001, p. 24

[1356] Engelbrecht, Torsten; Demeter, Konstantin, COVID-19 PCR Tests Are Scientifically Meaningless, *OffGuardian*, June 27, 2020

[1357] Centers for Disease Control and Prevention, CDC 2019-Novel Coronavirus (2019-nCoV) Real-Time RT-PCR Diagnostic Panel, For Emergency Use Only, Instructions for Use, Jul 13, 2020

[1358] Scoglio, Stefano, THE INVENTED PANDEMIC, the lack of VIRUS ISOLATION and the INVALID COVID-19 test, www.facebook.com/stefano.scoglio/, September 23, 2020

[1359] Cowan, Thomas, Only Poisoned Monkey Kidney Cells ‚Grew' the „Virus", *drtomcowan.com*, October 15, 2020

[1360] Engelbrecht, Torsten; Demeter, Konstantin, COVID-19 PCR Tests Are Scientifically Meaningless, *OffGuardian*, June 27, 2020

[1361] Corona-Ausschuss, session 26, from 3:13:50, corona-ausschuss.de/sitzungen, November 6, 2020

[1362] Mandavilli, Apoorva, Your Coronavirus Test Is Positive. Maybe It Shouldn't Be, *www.nyt.com*, August 29, 2020

[1363] Engelbrecht, Torsten; Demeter, Konstantin, COVID-19 PCR Tests Are Scientifically Meaningless, *OffGuardian*, June 27, 2020

[1364] Emails of the Robert Koch-Institute from November 9 and December 3, 2020

[1365] Engelbrecht, Torsten; Demeter, Konstantin, COVID-19 PCR Tests Are Scientifically Meaningless, *OffGuardian*, June 27, 2020

[1366] Crowe, David, Is the 2019 Coronavirus Really a Pandemic?, *www.theinfectiousmyth.com*

[1367] Feng, Coco; Hu, Minghe, Race to diagnose coronavirus patients constrained by shortage of reliable detection kits, *scmp.com*, February 11, 2020

[1368] Koop, Fermin, A startling number of coronavirus patients get reinfected Patients in the Guangdong province were tested positive again with the virus, *www.zmescience.com*, February 26, 2020

[1369] Crowe, David, Is the 2019 Coronavirus Really a Pandemic?, *www.theinfectiousmyth.com*

[1370] Emails of the Robert Koch-Institute from November 9 and December 3, 2020

[1371] Kämmerer, Ulrike et al., Review report Corman-Drosten et al. Eurosurveillance 2020: External peer review of the RTPCR test to detect SARS-CoV-2 reveals 10 major scientific flaws at the molecular and methodological level: consequences for false positive results, cormandrostenreview.com/report, November 27, 2020

[1372] Jeschke, Wolfgang, Wissenschaftler demontieren Drosten-Test, *laufpass.com*, November 30, 2020

[1373] Ioannidis, John P.A., A fiasco in the making? As the coronavirus pandemic takes hold, we are making decisions without reliable data, *www.statnews.com*, March 17, 2020

[1374] Müller-Jung, Joachim, Forscher für härtere Maßnahmen: Kurve abflachen? Das reicht nicht mehr, *www.faz.net*, March 20, 2020

[1375] Aust, Stefan, Denn sie wissen nicht, was sie tun, *Welt am Sonntag*, September 6, 2020

[1376] Schmitt, Peter-Philipp, Rock Hudson: Er gab Aids ein Gesicht, *www.faz.net*, September 30, 2010

[1377] Italien: Priester spendet sein Beatmungsgerät und verstirbt, *www.vaticannews.va*, March 24, 2020

[1378] Berndt, Christina, Coronavirus: Zu schön, um wahr zu sein, *www.sueddeutsche.de*, March 24, 2020

[1379] "Solchen Wissenschaftlern würde ich gerne Kamera oder Mikrofon entziehen", Interview mit dem Gesundheitsstatistiker Gerd Bosbach zur Corona-Debatte, *www.nachdenkseiten.de*, March 26, 2020

[1380] Ravizza, Simona, l'emergenza: Milano, terapie intensive al collasso per l'influenza: già 48 malati gravi molte operazioni rinviate, *www.milano.corriere.it*, January 10, 2018

[1381] Newey, Sarah, Why have so many coronavirus patients died in Italy?, *www.telegraph.co.uk*, March 23, 2020

[1382] Ebhardt, Tommaso et al., World 99 % of Those Who Died From Virus Had Other Illness, Italy Says, *www.bloomberg.com,* March 18, 2020

[1383] Sawicki, Peter, Palliativmediziner zu COVID-19-Behandlungen: „Sehr falsche Prioritäten gesetzt und alle ethischen Prinzipien verletzt", *www.deutschlandfunk.de*, April 11, 2020

[1384] „Solchen Wissenschaftlern würde ich gerne Kamera oder Mikrofon entziehen", Interview mit dem Gesundheitsstatistiker Gerd Bosbach zur Corona-Debatte, *www.nachdenkseiten.de*, March 26, 2020

[1385] Schmitt, Peter-Philipp, Virologe Hendrik Streeck: „Wir haben neue Symptome entdeckt", *www.faz.net*, March 16, 2020

[1386] Sen. Dr. Jensen's Shocking Admission About Coronavirus, *www.valleynewslive.com*, April 7, 2020

[1387] Gøtzsche, Peter C., Our prescription drugs kill us in large numbers, *Polskie Archiwum Medycyny Wewnetrznej*, Epub October 30, 2014

[1388] Engelbrecht, Torsten; Köhnlein, Claus, COVID-19 (excess) mortalities: viral cause impossible — drugs with key role in about 200,000 extra deaths in Europe and the US alone, *www.realnewsaustralia.com*, October 1, 2020

[1389] Hüttemann, Daniela, Lungeninfektionen: Wie wird eine Coronavirus-Infektion behandelt?, *www.pharmazeutische-zeitung.de*, January 28, 2020

[1390] Lopinavir / Ritonavir, www.aidsinfo.niv.gov

[1391] Engelbrecht, Torsten; Köhnlein, Claus, COVID-19 (excess) mortalities: viral cause impossible — drugs with key role in about 200,000 extra deaths in Europe and the US alone, *www.realnewsaustralia.com*, October 1, 2020

[1392] Email of Andrew Kaufman from November 14, 2020

[1393] Engelbrecht, Torsten; Köhnlein, Claus, COVID-19 (excess) mortalities: viral cause impossible — drugs with key role in about 200,000 extra deaths in Europe and the US alone, *www.realnewsaustralia.com*, October 1, 2020

[1394] Hüttemann, Daniela, Lungeninfektionen: Wie wird eine Coronavirus-Infektion behandelt?, *www.pharmazeutische-zeitung.de*, January 28, 2020

[1395] Stockman, Lauren J. et al., SARS: Systematic Review of Treatment Effects, *PLoS Medicine*, September 12, 2006, e343

[1396] Gebauer, Thomas, Die Macht des Geldes, *Dr. med. Mabuse*, September/October 2011

[1397] Engelbrecht, Torsten, Pandemie ohne Pandemie, www.rubikon.news, 1. September 2020

[1398] Engelbrecht, Torsten; Demeter, Konstantin, Die Corona-Korruption, *www.rubikon.news*, May 10, 2020

[1399] Hofmann, Siegfried, HIV- und Tuberkulose-Impfstoffe Bill und Melinda Gates investieren in deutsche Biotech-firma Biontech, *www.handelsblatt.com*, September 4, 2019

[1400] Hartmann, Kathrin, Interview mit Medizinexperten McCoy: "Die Gates-Stiftung ist ein Mittel, um Macht auszuü-ben", *www.spiegel.de*, July 27, 2014

[1401] Demeter, Konstantin; Engelbrecht, Torsten, Die Corona-Korruption: Die Lockdown-Entscheidungen vieler Länder wurden auf Empfehlung eines Wissenschaftlers forciert, der von massiven Interessenkonflikten be-troffen ist, *rubikon.news*, May 10, 2020

van Dongen, Johan, Why The World Health Organization Treats Bill Gates Like A President, *www.modernghana.com*, February 14, 2019

[3] Gates Foundation calls for global cooperation on vaccine for 7 billion people, www.euractiv.com, April 16, 2020

[4] Schlak, Martin, Impfstoff gegen Coronavirus: Das riskante Wettrennen der Pharmakonzerne, *spiegel.de*, March 14, 2020

[1405] Stüwe, Christian, Virologe Drosten: Wir müssen schauen, wo wir einen Impfstoff herzaubern, *gmx.net*, March 19, 2020

[1406] Coronavirus: Das ist der Stand der Impfstoff-Entwicklung, www.bundesregierung.de, Stand: December 3, 2020

[1407] Die Jagd nach dem Impfstoff: Impfstoff erhält Notfall-Zulassung, *www.ndr.de*, Stand: Dezember 2, 2020, 10:22

[1408] Dr. Wodarg und Dr. Yeadon beantragen den Stopp sämtlicher Corona-Impfstudien und rufen zum Mitzeichnen der Petition auf, *2020news.de*, December 1, 2020

[1409] Vorsitzender der Arzneimittelkommission der deutschen Ärzteschaft kritisiert Corona- Impfungen, *www.jour-nalistenwatch.com*, December 2, 2020

[1410] Mercola, Joseph, Emergency COVID-19 Vaccines May Cause Massive Sidde Effects, *mercola.com*, December 8, 2020

[1411] Cardozo, Timothy; Veazey, Ronald, Informed consent disclosure to vaccine trial subjects of risk of COVID-19 vaccines worsening clinical disease, International Journal of Clinical Practice, 28. Oktober 2020

[1412] Lyons-Weiler, James; Thomas, Paul, Relative Incidence of Office Visits and CumulativeRates of Billed Diagnoses Along the Axisof Vaccination, *International Journal of Environmental Research and Public Health*, November 22, 2020

[1413] Atkeson, Andrew, NBER Working Paper Series: Four Stylized Facts About COVID-19, nber.org, August 2020

[1414] Cowling, Benjamin J. et al., Nonpharmaceutical Measures for Pandemic Influenza in Nonhealthcare Settings – Personal Protective and Environmental Measures, *Emerging Infectious Diseases*, May 2020, pp. 967-975

[1415] www.aerzteklaerenauf.de/masken

[1416] Bundgaard, Henning et al. Effectiveness of Adding a Mask Recommendation to Other Public Health Measures to Prevent SARS-CoV-2 Infection in Danish Mask Wearers, A Randomized Controlled Trial, *Annals of Internal Medicine*, November 18, 2020

[1417] https://twitter.com/yinonw/status/1321177359601393664

[1418] Erfassung der SARS-CoV-2-Testzahlen in Deutschland: Tabellen zu Testzahlen, Testkapazitäten und Proben-rückstau pro Woche (23.12.2020), rki.de, December 23, 2020

[1419] https://coronavirus.data.gov.uk/details/testing

[1420] Robert Koch-Institute, *Epidemiologisches Bulletin*, 45/2020 vom November 5, 2020, p. 20

Literature

[1421] Nationale Teststrategie – wer wird in Deutschland auf das Vorliegen einer SARS-CoV-2 Infektion getestet?, rki. de (as of December 18, 2020)

[1422] Sterbefälle und Lebenserwartung: Sonderauswertung zu Sterbefallzahlen des Jahres 2020, www.destatis.de, December 30, 2020

[1423] Statistisches Bundesamt: Übersterblichkeit in Deutschland steigt auf 14 Prozent, *www.faz.net*, December 30, 2020

[1424] Breyer, Friedrich, Die ökonomische Frage: Mehr Tote in Deutschland durch Corona?, *Südkurier*, June 6, 2020

[1425] Erfassung der SARS-CoV-2-Testzahlen in Deutschland: Tabellen zu Testzahlen, Testkapazitäten und Proben-rückstau pro Woche (23.12.2020), rki.de, Dezember 23, 2020

[1426] Lewis, Dyani, Is the coronavirus airborne? Experts can't agree, *Nature*, April 9, 2020

[1427] *Markus Lanz*, December 9, 2020, minutes 48:40-50:27

[1428] Engelbrecht, Torsten; Demeter, Konstantin, Fatale Therapie:Die Behandlung von positiv auf SARS-CoV-2 testeten Patienten mit hochtoxischen Medikamenten und riskanten Intubationen kann tödlich sein, *ww rubikon.news*, May 28, 2020

[1429] Engelbrecht, Torsten; Demeter, Konstantin, Anthony Fauci: 40 Years of Lies From AZT to Remdesivi, *OffGuardiar* October 27, 2020

[1430] "Solchen Wissenschaftlern würde ich gerne Kamera oder Mikrofon entziehen", Interview mit dem Gesund-heitsstatistiker Gerd Bosbach zur Corona-Debatte, *nachdenkseiten*.de, March 26, 2020

Epilog
Rock Hudson Gave „AIDS" a Face – and His Fallacious Story the Virus Hunters Godlike Status

[1431] How One Test Changed HIV: March 2nd marks 30 years since an Abbott breakthrough: the first licensed test for HIV, Abbott press release, March 2, 2015

[1432] Cowley Geoffrey, The day they discovered the AIDS virus, *www.msnbc.com*, April 23, 2014

[1433] Ely, Elizabeth; Crilly, Cal, How „We All" Came to „Have AIDS": Rock Hudson's False „Legacy", *www.omsj.org*, March 5, 2014

[1434] Schock, Axel, „Möge Gott verhüten, dass Rock vergebens gestorben ist", *Deutsche AIDS-Hilfemagazin.hiv*, 2. Okt. 2015

[1435] see https://en.wikipedia.org/wiki/Rock_Hudson#Illness_and_death

[1436] „Die Promiskuität ist der Motor der Seuche", *Spiegel*, 33/1985

[1437] Yarbrough, Jeff, Rock Hudson: On Camera and Off, *www.people.com*, August 12, 1985 (revised on February 12, 2011)

[1438] Armistead Maupin tells Patrick Gale how he took the rap for outing Rock Hudson. „A friend rang me and said how could I do that to such a beautiful, beautiful man?", *www.guardian.com*, June 24, 1999

[1439] Gavilanes, Grace, 10 Secrets of Rock Hudson's Heartbreaking Final Days, *www.people.com*, October 2, 2015

[1440] „Tense" Rock Hudson continues smokig despite heart surgery, *Lakeland Ledger*, October 1, 1982

[1441] One Year After Heart Surgery, Rock Hudson Is Rolling Again, but His „Devlin Connection" Is Ailing, *www.people.com*, November 15, 1982

[1442] Doris Day & Rock Hudson – forever friends, www.youtube.com/watch?v=z21shqPRTP8

[1443] Rock Hudson is Ill With Liver Cancer in Paris Hospital, *Associated Press/New York Times*, April 23, 1985

[1444] Ely, Elizabeth; Crilly, Cal, How „We All" Came to „Have AIDS": Rock Hudson's False „Legacy", *omsj.org*, March 5, 2014

[1445] Bittorf, Wilhelm, Die Lust ist da, aber ich verkneif's mir, *Spiegel*, 11/1987

[1446] Schock, Axel, „Möge Gott verhüten, dass Rock vergebens gestorben ist", *Deutsche AIDS-Hilfe magazin.hiv*, October 2, 2015

[1447] Ely, Elizabeth; Crilly, Cal, How „We All" Came to „Have AIDS": Rock Hudson's False „Legacy", *www.omsj.org*, March 5, 2014

[1448] Altman, Lawrence. The Doctor's World; Search for an AIDS Drug is Case History in Frustration, *New York Times*, July 30, 1985

[1449] Jon, Van, Hudson Aids Case Turns Spotlight On Drug Approval Process, *Chicago Tribune*, August 4, 1985

[1450] Schille, Peter, „Vergnügt euch, aber seht euch vor", *Spiegel*, 44/1985

[1451] Ely, Elizabeth; Crilly, Cal, How „We All" Came to „Have AIDS": Rock Hudson's False „Legacy", *www.omsj.org*, March 5, 2014

Moskovitz, Bruce L., Clinical Trial of Tolerance of HPA-23 in Patients with Acquired Immune Deficiency Syndrome, *Animicrobial Agents and Chemotherapy*, September 1988, pp. 1300-1313

Woo, Elaine, Marc Christian MacGinnis dies at 56; Rock Hudson's ex-lover, *Los Angeles Times*, December 5, 2009

Schock, Axel, „Möge Gott verhüten, dass Rock vergebens gestorben ist", *Deutsche AIDS-Hilfe magazin.hiv*, October 2, 2015

Rock Hudson, victim of Aids, dies aged 59, *Guardian*, October 3, 1985

Ely, Elizabeth; Crilly, Cal, How „We All" Came to „Have AIDS": Rock Hudson's False „Legacy", *www.omsj.org*, March 5, 2014

Lightning Source UK Ltd.
Milton Keynes UK
UKHW011047240221
379311UK00005B/339